Hyperlipidaemia and Atherosclerosis

Hyperlipidaemia and Atherosclerosis

Edited by

KEITH E. SUCKLING

Smith Kline & French Research Limited
Welwyn, Hertfordshire, UK

PIETER H. E. GROOT

Smith Kline & French Research Limited
Welwyn, Hertfordshire, UK

1988

ACADEMIC PRESS

Harcourt Brace Jovanovich, Publishers

London San Diego New York
Boston Sydney Tokyo Toronto

ACADEMIC PRESS LIMITED
24/28 Oval Road
London NW1 7DX

United States Edition published by
ACADEMIC PRESS INC.
San Diego, CA 92101

British Library Cataloguing in Publication Data

Hyperlipidaemia and atherosclerosis.
1. Man. Arteries. Atherosclerosis related to hyperlipidaemia 2. Man. Blood. Hyperlipidaemia related to atherosclerosis
I. Suckling, Keith E., *1947–* II. Groot, P. H. E.
616.1′36
ISBN 0–12–675645–7

Typeset by Paston Press, Loddon, Norfolk
Printed in Great Britain at The Alden Press, Oxford

Contributors

R. Y. Ball Department of Pathology, University of Cambridge, Tennis Court Road, Cambridge CB2 1QP, UK

M. Been Department of Cardiology, Freeman Hospital, Newcastle upon Tyne, UK

G. Bondjers Arterial Biology Group, Wallenberg Laboratory for Cardiovascular Research, University of Göteborg, Sahlgren's Hospital, 413 45 Göteborg, Sweden

D. P. de Bono Department of Medicine, Royal Infirmary, Edinburgh University, Edinburgh EH3 9YW, UK

H. B. Brewer Molecular Disease Branch, National Heart, Lung and Blood Institute, National Institute of Health, Bethesda, Maryland 20205, USA

G. Camejo Arterial Biology Group, Wallenberg Laboratory for Cardiovascular Research, University of Göteborg, Sahlgren's Hospital, 413 45 Göteborg, Sweden

K. L. H. Carpenter Department of Pathology, University of Cambridge, Tennis Court Road, Cambridge CB2 1QP, UK

D. Collen Center for Thrombosis and Vascular Research, University of Leuven, Leuven, Belgium

J. M. Dietschy Department of Internal Medicine, University of Texas, Southwestern Medical Center at Dallas, Dallas, Texas 75235–9030, USA

S. Eisenberg Department of Medicine B, Hadassah University Hospital, Jerusalem, Israel

G. Fager Arterial Biology Group, Wallenberg Laboratory for Cardiovascular Research, University of Göteborg, Sahlgren's Hospital, 413 45 Göteborg, Sweden

J. Fingerle Department of Pathology, University of Washington, Seattle WA 98195, USA

R. E. Gregg Molecular Disease Branch, National Heart, Lung and Blood Institute, National Institute of Health, Bethesda, Maryland 20205, USA

P. H. E. Groot Smith Kline & French Research Ltd, The Frythe, Welwyn, Hertfordshire AL6 9AR, UK

K. Higuchi Molecular Disease Branch, National Heart, Lung and Blood Institute, National Institute of Health, Bethesda, Maryland 20205, USA

J. Hoeg Molecular Disease Branch, National Heart, Lung and Blood Institute, National Institute of Health, Bethesda, Maryland 20205, USA

A. Hospattankar Molecular Disease Branch, National Heart, Lung and Blood Institute, National Institute of Health, Bethesda, Maryland 20205, USA

E. Hurt Arterial Biology Group, Wallenberg Laboratory for Cardiovascular Research, University of Göteborg, Sahlgren's Hospital, 413 45 Göteborg, Sweden

M. Kano MRC Liopoprotein Team, Hammersmith Hospital, Ducane Road, London W12 OHS, UK

Y. A. Kesäniemi Department of Medicine, University of Oulu, Finland

T. J. Knott Division of Molecular Medicine, MRC Clinical Research Centre, Watford Road, Harrow, Middlesex HA1 3UJ, UK

J. Koizumi MRC Lipoprotein Team, Hammersmith Hospital, Ducane Road, London W12 OHS, UK

M. W. Majesky Department of Pathology, University of Washington, Seattle WA 98195, USA

D. McAreavey Department of Medicine, The Royal Infirmary, Edinburgh University, Edinburgh EH3 9WY, UK

T. W. Meade MRC Epidemiology and Medical Care Unit, Northwick Park Hospital, Harrow HA1 3UJ, UK

J. D. Meddings Department of Internal Medicine, University of Texas, Southwestern Medical Center at Dallas, Dallas, Texas 75235–9030, USA

T. A. Miettinen Second Department of Medicine, University of Helsinki, Finland

M. J. Mitchinson Department of Pathology, University of Cambridge, Tennis Court Road, Cambridge CB2 1QP, UK

S.-O. Olofsson Arterial Biology Group, Wallenberg Laboratory for Cardiovascular Research, University of Göteborg, Sahlgren's Hospital, 413 45 Göteborg, Sweden

D. V. Parums Department of Pathology, University of Cambridge, Tennis Court Road, Cambridge CB2 1QP, UK

J. Pease Division of Molecular Medicine, MRC Clinical Research Centre, Watford Road, Harrow, Middlesex HA1 3UJ, UK

H. Peterson Department of Medicine, The Royal Infirmary, Edinburgh University, Edinburgh EH3 9YW, UK

L. Powell Division of Molecular Medicine, MRC Research Centre, Watford Road, Harrow, Middlesex HA1 3UJ, UK

M. A. Reidy Department of Pathology, University of Washington, Seattle, Washington 98195, USA

J. Scott Division of Molecular Research, Watford Road, Harrow, Middlesex HA1 3UJ, UK

D. K. Spady Department of Internal Medicine, University of Texas, Medical Center at Dallas, Dallas, Texas 75235–9030, USA

K. E. Suckling Smith Kline & French Research Ltd, The Frythe, Welwyn, Hertfordshire AL6 9AR, UK

G. R. Thompson MRC Lipoprotein Team, Hammersmith Hospital, Ducane Road, London W12 OHS, UK

S. C. Wallis Division of Molecular Medicine, Watford Road, Harrow, Middlesex HA1 3UJ, UK

O. Wiklund Arterial Biology Group, Wallenberg Laboratory for Cardiovascular Research, University of Göteborg, Sahlgren's Hospital, 413 45 Göteborg, Sweden

Foreword

Atherosclerosis is the greatest single cause of mortality in the "developed" world, accounting for up to 45% of all deaths; in some countries coronary heart disease alone, resulting from coronary artery atherosclerosis, causes one in four deaths. The disease is clearly multifactorial, and the development of the lesions involves a bewildering array of complex biological processes. Nonetheless, a multidisciplinary approach, including molecular genetics, cell biology, biochemistry, experimental pathology, epidemiology and clinical science, is providing substantial clues as to the aetiology of atherosclerosis. We can now identify critical risk factors and lifestyle changes that can reduce risk; novel therapies are coming on-stream, both to prevent or slow the progress of the atherosclerotic plaque, and to deal with one of the most devastating consequences, coronary thrombosis.

This book contains the proceedings of the Smith Kline & French Research Symposium on Hyperlipidaemia and Atherosclerosis, held in Cambridge, UK from 8 to 10 December 1987; in addition abstracts of posters presented by participants at the symposium are appended. During this meeting a group of leading experts presented current views and recent progress in lipoprotein synthesis, metabolism and transport, plaque formation, epidemiology of atherosclerosis and coronary heart disease, and therapeutic fibrinolysis. We believe that their contributions convey the excitement felt in this enormously important field, and provide an excellent overview of many of the approaches that are needed to increase our understanding of atherosclerosis and to identify new ways of preventing and treating this modern scourge.

George Poste, *Symposium Co-Chairman*
Timothy Rink, *Symposium Co-Chairman*

Contents

1

Hyperlipidaemia and Atherosclerosis: Introduction

PIETER H. E. GROOT and KEITH E. SUCKLING

Smith Kline & French Research Limited, The Frythe, Welwyn, Hertfordshire, UK

In this introduction we aim to guide readers through the different aspects of atherosclerosis research covered in detail by the various contributors. As reflected by the title, much emphasis has been given in this book to the role of plasma lipoproteins in atherosclerosis. Contributions are included on the structure and synthesis of plasma lipoproteins and apolipoproteins, the role of the different cellular plasma membrane receptors in lipoprotein metabolism, receptor-independent removal of plasma lipoprotein, familial dyslipoproteinaemias and clinical management of hyperlipoproteinaemias. Several contributions deal with the cell biology of the formation of the atherosclerotic lesion. Furthermore, this book includes contributions on the role of platelets and coagulation factors in the progression of the atherosclerotic lesion. Finally two chapters are included on the current therapeutic interventions in acute myocardial infarction with fibrinolytic agents.

1 The role of plasma lipoproteins in coronary artery disease

Since the results of the Lipid Research Clinic Coronary Primary Prevention Trial (LRCCPPT) became available in 1984, a widespread acceptance has been established among regulatory bodies and clinicians about the desirability of treatment of hypercholesterolaemia. In this study it was demonstrated using hard end-points (fatal and non-fatal myocardial infarction) that long-term treatment of hypercholesterolaemia using the bile acid sequestrant choles-

HYPERLIPIDAEMIA AND ATHEROSCLEROSIS
ISBN 0.12.675645-7

tyramine resulted in a decreased risk of coronary artery disease. In a subsequent secondary prevention study of Blankenhorn *et al.* (1987), in patients with manifest coronary artery disease (as documented by coronary angiography), it was demonstrated that vigorous hypocholesterolaemic therapy results in a pronounced inhibition of lesion development. In several cases even a regression of the coronary atherosclerotic lesion could be demonstrated. The combined results of these studies (and a vast amount of previously obtained evidence) indicate and explain that treatment of hypercholesterolaemia results in a lowering of risk for coronary artery disease.

The data from the LRCCPPT study showed that in the group tested a decrease in plasma LDL-cholesterol of 1% is associated with a decrease in risk for symptomatic coronary artery disease of 2%. Such a result was anticipated from data of several large prospective epidemiological studies. The data of the second large long-term primary prevention trial (The Helsinki Heart Study) have shown more pronounced results (Frick *et al.*, 1987). In a rather mixed group of patients with hyperlipoproteinaemia an average drop in plasma cholesterol of 8% was associated with a decrease in the incidence rate of fatal and non-fatal myocardial infarctions of 34%. In addition, HDL-cholesterol was increased in the treated group by an average of 10% while plasma triglycerides dropped by 34%. These data re-emphasize the possible roles of other plasma lipoproteins like HDL and triglyceride-rich lipoproteins or their remnants in the aetiology of coronary artery disease.

As a consequence of the abovementioned experimental evidence, consensus conferences have been organized by regulatory bodies and specialists in the field on management of hyperlipoproteinaemias both in the USA and in Europe. Their reports and recommendations have been published in the scientific literature (National Institute of Health Consensus Development Statement, 1985; Study Group European Atherosclerosis Society, 1987; The British Cardiac Society Working on Coronary Prevention, 1987; Shepherd *et al.* 1987) and widely discussed in both scientific and non-scientific journals. In general, it was considered that desirable levels of plasma cholesterol should be below 5.2 mM (200 mg/dl) for individuals above 40 years of age and below 4.7 mM (180 mg/dl) for individuals below the age of 40. For most persons with levels of 5.2–6.5 mM (200–250 mg/dl) dietary advice and correction of other risk factors are appropriate. Individuals with plasma cholesterol levels above 6.5 mM demand clinical care and need treatment, first by dietary measures, but if changes in diet fail to reduce plasma cholesterol concentrations to acceptable levels, drug treatment has to be considered. At the Cambridge conference the recommendations of the European Study Group for Atherosclerosis were discussed by Drs Assmann and Lewis. For details of these recommendations the reader is referred to the Recommendations for Management of Hyperlipoproteinaemia as published in the *European Heart Journal* (Study Group European Atherosclerosis Society, 1987).

In the first lecture in Cambridge, Dr D. M. Small discussed his work on the structure of plasma lipoproteins. Dr Small has investigated the role of lipid composition and fatty acid saturation on the stability of lipoproteins and their affinity for apolipoproteins using artificial triglyceride-rich lipid emulsions and natural triglyceride-rich plasma lipoproteins. It is evident from this work that both the composition of the core as well as the surface film of lipoproteins strongly affects their metabolic properties. This is partially due to differences in the affinity of the particle for apolipoproteins. It was found that high concentrations of unesterified cholesterol in the surface film of triglyceride-rich model lipoproteins is associated with a decrease in affinity for apolipoproteins A-IV and C and an increase in affinity for apolipoprotein E. As a consequence, such lipoproteins with a high content of cholesterol in the surface film are only sluggishly hydrolysed by lipoprotein lipase. They are channelled to the liver in an early phase of their metabolism owing to the high apoE content. These findings may be of physiological relevance in the metabolic fate of chylomicrons in animals on high cholesterol diets, as early uptake of chylomicrons by the liver may induce hepatic VLDL synthesis.

In the first contribution in this book Dr J. M. Dietschy discusses his approach to the quantification of plasma LDL metabolism in man and experimental animals. Steady-state plasma LDL concentrations are determined according to Dietschy and his colleagues by four factors: (1) the rate of LDL production; (2) the rate of LDL receptor-independent degradation of LDL; (3) the maximum receptor-dependent transport velocity of LDL from plasma; and (4) the Michaelis constant for the latter process. In experimental animals these parameters were measured directly in series of elegant experiments in which receptor-dependent and receptor-independent LDL catabolism in individual tissues was determined at different concentrations of plasma LDL raised artificially during the study by infusion of solutions of isolated LDL. According to Dr Dietschy, the major determinant of the steady-state concentration in plasma of LDL is the rate of LDL synthesis. LDL receptor number is also important, but changes in his parameter result under most conditions in a less dramatic change in steady-state plasma LDL concentrations. Of major interest are the data of Dr Dietschy on the effect of the fat composition and the cholesterol content of the diet on LDL metabolism. Addition of only small amounts of cholesterol to fat-free diets in hamsters results in a progressive decrease in receptor-dependent LDL transport from plasma. When saturated fat is added to such a diet this suppressive effect of cholesterol is augmented while the synthetic rate of LDL increases markedly at the same time. This results in a dramatic increase in steady-state plasma LDL concentration. Replacement of saturated fat by polyunsaturated fat suppresses LDL synthesis and enhances receptor-dependent LDL transport, resulting in a normalization of the plasma LDL concentrations. Ageing is in most animal species associated with an increase in plasma LDL concentration. According to Dr Dietschy, this effect is mainly due to an increase in LDL production rate. It was stressed by Dr Dietschy that his methods for studying LDL metabolism in experimental animals (hamsters) are very suitable for evaluating the effect of new hypolipidaemic drugs.

2 The role of oxidized LDL in atherosclerosis

LDL receptor-independent LDL transport from plasma is of major interest for our understanding of the role of LDL in the aetiology of atherosclerosis. Present evidence suggests that plasma LDL has to undergo a change in charge and/or structure of apoB, the sole protein of LDL, to be actively taken up by macrophages and to induce cholesterol accumulation in these cells. Changes in the properties of LDL resulting in a rapid and massive uptake by macrophages can be induced *in vitro* by chemical acetylation or by incubation of LDL under conditions that facilitate lipid peroxidation (either with cells that generate reactive oxygen species or in the test tube with enzymes that generate these oxygen species, both in the presence of transition metal ions). At the Cambridge meeting the state of the art was discussed by Dr D. Steinberg. His group is leading this field, and data were presented of experiments in Watanabe Hereditable Hyperlipidaemic (WHHL) rabbits treated with the hypolipidaemic drug probucol. In these studies *in vivo* evidence was obtained indicating that protection of LDL against reactive oxygen species diminished both uptake of LDL by the arterial wall and also plaque formation. Probucol is associated in plasma with LDL and has radical scavenger properties, thereby preventing LDL from oxidative modification. According to Dr Steinberg, generation of reactive oxygen species by tissue macrophages and endothelial cells in the arterial wall could create an environment that facilitates lipid peroxidation of the ultrafiltered plasma LDL in the arterial wall. Oxidized LDL is recognized by the acetyl-LDL receptor present on macrophages (and possibly endothelial cells) and rapidly internalized. Since the acetyl-LDL receptor is not down-regulated by cellular sterols (as is the LDL receptor), this process can result in a massive uptake of oxidatively modified LDL and lipid deposition in these macrophages. Furthermore, during the modification of LDL, products are formed that have a chemotactic effect on monocyte macrophages. This results in the infiltration of more of these plasma cells into the affected arterial tissue and more modification of LDL. Once inside the affected tissue, macrophages are prevented from exiting into plasma by the presence of factors in oxidized LDL (Quinn *et al.*, 1985), and all these processes together will stimulate the conversion of these trapped macrophages into foam cells. Dr Steinberg has found now that the arterial uptake and degradation of LDL is diminished in probucol-treated WHHL rabbits as compared with animals with identical plasma cholesterol concentrations, titrated to the level in probucol-treated animals by feeding low concentrations of the HMG-CoA inhibitor mevinolin. Aortic preparations of probucol-treated animals showed less fulminant atherosclerosis than seen in the naive control and mevinolin-treated animals. Dr Steinberg concluded from these experiments that a combination therapy of a hypocholesterolaemic agent with an antioxidant could be beneficial in combatting atherogenesis. It should be stated that the contribution of arterial tissue to the overall LDL receptor-independent LDL removal from plasma is very low. At present it is unknown whether high LDL receptor-independent removal from plasma of LDL implies that this process is also very active in arterial tissue.

3 The molecular mechanism of synthesis of apolipoprotein B48

For more than a decade it has been known that the species of apolipoprotein B produced by the gut (apoB48) is smaller than the counterparts produced by the liver (apoB100). Studies with monoclonal antibodies against different epitopes in apoB100 have further indicated that apoB48 is immunologically identical with the amino terminal half of apoB100. In his contribution, Dr J. Scott presented data showing that the mRNA for intestinal apoB48 in man and in rabbit is colinear with the message for the amino terminal half of hepatic apoB100. Termination of synthesis of apoB in the gut at amino acid 2152 was shown to be due to a single C to T conversion in triplet 2153 of the corresponding cDNA, which generates a stop codon. It was shown by Dr Scott that this is not due to a difference in genomic DNA but is caused by a co- or post-translational C to U change in the message for apoB in the gut. The concentration of unmodified mRNA in the gut preparation investigated by Dr Scott was below the detection limit, although full size (14.5 kb) mRNA species (containing the stop codon at triplet 2153) were present, as were smaller mRNA species of 7.0 kb. Whether this unprecedented finding represents an example of a more universal principle, is an intriguing question that awaits future studies. Dr Scott's data as published in *Cell* (Powell *et al.*, 1987) are in close agreement with data from the group of Dr L. Chan (Chan *et al.*, 1987) and Dr H. B. Brewer (see Chapter 3).

Dr Brewer also presented data on apoB synthesis and the apoB mRNA species in gut. His data indicate that the adult human gut synthesizes apoB48 as well as apoB100. In contrast with Dr Scott's observations, he also found full size (14.5 kb) mRNA in gut biopsies that did not contain the stop codon in addition to mRNA species in which the stop codon was present. As synthesis of apoB100 by foetal gut had been demonstrated earlier, the differences between Scott's and Brewer's findings are more of a quantitative nature than fundamentally different.

Of major interest were the data of Dr Brewer on the defects in apoB synthesis in abetalipoproteinaemia and hypobetalipoproteinaemia. In abetalipoproteinaemia increased mRNA levels were found for apoB in liver, while in hypobetalipoproteinaemia these levels were lower than in normal subjects. This suggests that in abetalipoproteinaemia the defect in apoB secretion is due to a post-transcriptional event, while in hypobetalipoproteinemia the defect would be expected to be found in the regulation of the transcription or the mRNA stability.

4 The role of apolipoproteins A and B in VLDL catabolism

Dr S. Eisenberg investigated the role of apoB and apoE in the interaction of VLDL, IDL and LDL with cellular receptors using the human hepatoma cell line HepG2 and human fibroblasts. His *in vitro* studies indicated that catabolism of VLDL and IDL by these cells is much lower than found with LDL, although affinities of these lipoproteins for the LDL (apoB,E) receptors are comparable. Addition of apoE3 does increase catabolism of VLDL and IDL, but the rates never exceeded the rate of LDL catabolism. Dr Eisenberg therefore challenges the concept that in normal man about half the number of the secreted VLDL particles are removed from the circulation as IDL (Kesäniemi *et al.*, 1985).

5 Studies of cholesterol transport

Dr G. R. Thompson presented data on his attempts in man and experimental animals to mobilize tissue cholesterol. Homozygous familial hypercholesterolaemic patients are not very responsive to lipid-lowering drug therapy. In order to decrease their plasma LDL concentration, Dr Thompson treats these patients by plasma exchange and more recently by LDL apheresis (extracorporal removal of LDL from patients' plasma by affinity chromatography). This treatment induced a regression of xanthomas in these patients. The results of the treatment on patients' life expectation are encouraging, but await more data before final conclusions can be drawn. Plasma exchange removes

LDL as well as HDL, while plasma apheresis selectively removes LDL. As HDL is supposed to play a role in the mobilization of cholesterol from peripheral tissues, LDL apheresis may be preferable. This question was addressed by Dr Thompson using WHHL rabbits that were pre-labelled in their body cholesterol pools with radioactive cholesterol. His experimental data do not indicate that in LDL apheresis a better mobilization of peripheral cholesterol is achieved than in animals treated by plasma exchange. In other studies Dr Thompson investigated whether a treatment with i.v. HDL analogues could induce a mobilization of tissue cholesterol and be of interest as future therapy for the fulminant atherosclerosis in familial hypercholesterolaemic patients. So far his data do not seem to be very encouraging for such a therapy.

Dr T. Miettinen has studied cholesterol balance in normal individuals in order to investigate the factors regulating the within-population variation in serum cholesterol concentration. The proportion of cholesterol absorbed did not correlate with the dietary intake of cholesterol, according to Dr Miettinen, at least not in the normal range of cholesterol intake seen in our western society. Therefore there does not seem to be a physiological threshold, a maximum cholesterol absorption, that would limit entrance of dietary cholesterol into our body. Individual variations in the proportion of cholesterol absorbed are large, and this is likely to be the major determinant of the inter-individual variation in plasma cholesterol concentration. As liver LDL receptors are down-regulated by a large inflow of absorbed cholesterol via the chylomicron remnant pathway, such a link seems feasible. The proportion of cholesterol absorbed was found to be related to the apoE phenotype of a subject, being low in E2/E2, intermediate in E2/E3 and E3/E3 and high in E3/E4 and E4/E4. Such an effect could explain the rise in plasma cholesterol concentration seen in this array, although others have explained this phenomenon on the basis of an increase in affinity and availability of apoE for the chylomicron remnant receptor (Ehnholm *et al.*, 1986). A low affinity (apoE2) would result in an inefficient chylomicron remnant uptake by the liver, up-regulation of hepatic LDL receptors and a decrease in plasma LDL.

6 The haemostatic system and risk for coronary artery disease

The role of the haemostatic system in coronary artery disease was discussed by Dr T. Meade. His work has revealed a strong association between the coagulating activity in plasma of factor VII (VII_c) as well as plasma levels of fibrinogen and mortality from coronary artery disease. High levels of plasma fibrinogen are also associated with the incidence of stroke. In many epidemiological studies, including Dr Meade's Northwick Park Heart Study, associations are seen between factor VII_c activity and plasma cholesterol concentrations. Such associations are not seen for fibrinogen. Factor VII_c activity is affected by dietary manipulation, and data of Dr Meade and others do suggest that conditions leading to increased concentrations of VLDL and LDL (high fat diet) are associated with increased factor VII_c activity. It is suggested that large (negatively charged) lipoproteins such as chylomicrons and VLDL could play a role in the intrinsic (contact) activation of factor XII and subsequent activation of factor VII. Along these lines, it would be of considerable interest to know if atherogenic lipoproteins such as betaVLDL or modified LDL (see above) are particularly potent in such an activation process. The relationship between fibrinogen and coronary artery disease is complex, and available data indicate that fibrinogen levels are only positively associated with the incidence of coronary artery disease in populations with high plasma cholesterol concentrations. Hypercoagulability could play a direct role in the progression of the lesion since fibrin is a component of more advanced atherosclerotic plaques. Obviously, hypercoagulability will promote thrombus formation and increase the risk of coronary infarction. The interactions between the haemostatic system, blood lipoproteins and atherosclerosis are a fascinating but still largely unexplored area.

7 The cell biology of the atherosclerotic lesion

The events and cellular responses involved in the formation and progression of the atherosclerotic lesion are discussed in contributions of Drs M. J. Mitchinson, G. Bondjers and M. A. Reidy. Foam cells in human atherosclerotic lesions are, according to Dr Mitchinson, nearly all derived from monocyte macrophages. Although smooth muscle cells do contain lipid droplets in human atherosclerotic artery material, they never become so engorged with lipids as macrophages. Lesions consisting mainly of smooth muscle cells are healing phases and not primary forms of future complicated lesions, according to Dr Mitchinson.

Foam cells contain ceroid. Ceroid is an autofluorescent substance that is insoluble in lipid solvents but that reacts positively with histological stains for lipid. It is thought to be composed of oxidized lipid and protein. According to Dr Mitchinson, ceroid represents an end-product of LDL oxidation that accumulates in the monocyte-derived macrophage. Ceroid is antigenic, and in many patients with coronary artery disease antibodies against this material have been observed in plasma. These antibodies may play a role in the progression of the lesion. Dr Mitchinson has found now that these antibodies cross-react with oxidized LDL and that the immuno-reactivity in plasma against ceroid can be removed in most cases by immuno-absorption with oxidized LDL. Therefore Dr Mitchinson believes that oxidized lipids and lipoproteins play a key role in atherogenesis, an opinion shared by Dr Steinberg, as discussed earlier.

Other processes in the arterial wall may also change the properties of LDL and initiate uptake of LDL by cells and arterial lipid accumulation. When LDL interacts with arterial proteoglycans, the conformation of apolipoprotein B on LDL changes, according to Dr Bondjers, and this process affects the metabolic fate of this lipoprotein. Proteoglycans are elements of the extracellular matrix of arterial tissue, only accessible to LDL particles that have penetrated through the endothelial cell lining. High concentrations of LDL in plasma and endothelial damage are factors that will favour such an infiltration process. As a consequence of the interaction of a specific site (amino acids 3359–3377) with arterial proteoglycans, an irreversible change in the composition of apoB on LDL is induced, resulting in accelerated uptake by smooth muscle cells and tissue macrophages, an uptake that is not efficiently down-regulated. The molecular mechanism of this process is not yet understood, but involvement of the acetyl-LDL receptor (the receptor on macrophages and other cells involved in the uptake of oxidized LDL) was excluded. A massive uptake of proteoglycan-modified LDL by macrophages (and smooth muscle cells) would lead to lipid accumulation and foam-cell formation.

Advanced atherosclerotic lesions are characterized by extracellular deposits of lipids, supposedly due to necrosis of foam cells. Necrosis could be the result of anoxia in those macrophages actively involved in the removal of proteoglycan-modified LDL. Dr Bondjers speculates that the uptake of massive quantities of cholesterol will simultaneously stimulate these macrophages to esterify cholesterol for storage and to hydrolyse these cholesteryl esters again in order to export the surplus cholesterol by HDL or phospholipid vesicle-mediated pathways. A futile metabolic cycle of esterification and hydrolysis would create net hydrolysis of ATP and may, if significant, result in hypoxia or anoxia in affected areas in the artery. Hypoxia, according to Dr Bondjers, would stimulate acidic proteoglycan synthesis (these proteoglycans are most active in LDL modification), and this process may play a catalytic role in disturbing the normal physiology of the vessel wall. Measurements of the turnover of the cholesteryl ester pool in macrophages are awaited to substantiate this theory.

It has been recognized for more than a decade that damage to the vascular endothelium results in proliferation of vascular smooth muscle cells. Adhesion of platelets to exposed vascular elements is thought to result in the release of platelet-derived growth factor(s), which have been shown to be mitogenic for smooth muscle cells. This process could explain the migration of smooth muscle cells into the intima and the intimal thickening seen after experimental endothelial denudation. Dr Reidy has challenged the physiological significance of this process for "normal" endothelial damage and atherosclerosis.

The experimental procedures for denuding the vessel wall of endothelium used in the past (balloon denudation) are so rough that intima as well as media are damaged. Under these conditions, repair mechanisms may be much more extensive and different from those taking place after superficial endothelial damage. Using a much more subtle technique of endothelial scratching, it was found that the endothelium could be repaired without smooth muscle cell migration into the intima. Regrowth of the endothelium is possibly associated with the production of a factor that inhibits smooth muscle cell migration and prevents intimal thickening.

Smooth muscle cell proliferation can also take place under an undamaged endothelium in cholesterol-fed animals. Under these conditions, platelets are unlikely to play a role, and other cells like macrophages and/or endothelial cells, able to synthesize platelet-derived growth factor (PDGF) *in vitro*, may be implicated. Dr Reidy discusses experiments showing that a subpopulation of arterial smooth muscle cells can synthesize PDGF and could "self-stimulate" a proliferation under certain conditions.

Although knowledge of the cell biology of the arterial wall has increased enormously in the last decade, many questions still remain about which of the large number of possible atherogenic factors and cellular responses are really implicated in atherogenesis. Current evidence indicates that the monocyte-derived macrophage plays a central role in early lesion formation. After penetration into the arterial wall in response to yet undefined initial signals, the macrophage modifies LDL, generates signals to attract more monocytes and becomes immobilized, unable to escape out of the arterial wall. As a result of these processes, it engorges itself on the product of its own action (oxidized LDL). It is not difficult to envisage that high concentrations of LDL in plasma would favour this. Monocyte penetration into the arterial wall could well be a normal process (possibly in response to physiologically occurring tissue damage). However, these cells are expected to leave the arterial wall again after being involved in those normal repair processes. A high concentration of LDL in the arterial wall would then be enough to explain the abovementioned sequence of events. Alternatively, high concentrations of LDL in the arterial wall could cause an extensive modification by proteoglycans leading to a stimulated uptake by smooth muscle cells, and this process could trigger smooth muscle cells to proliferate into the intima and attract monocytes. Smooth muscle cells themselves are probably not precursors of foam cells (although this is still debated), but they may synthesize a surplus of extracellular elements (proteoglycans, collagen and elastic fibres) that initiate the process of vascular sclerosis. As a result of a disturbed metabolism (a futile cycle of cholesterol esterification and hydrolysis or alternatively as a consequence of accumulation of lipid and debris), lipid-laden macrophages in the arterial wall die off and extracellular lipids start to accumulate in the lesion. In the presence of high concentrations of fibrinogen, activated factor VII and other factors fibrous clots could be formed, contributing to the further development of the atherosclerotic lesion. Involvement of these haemostatic elements in the conversion to the acute phase of coronary artery disease can easily be envisioned. All these processes and their relationships as discussed by the different contributors to this book, are summarized in Fig. 1.

8 Thrombolytic therapy in acute myocardial infarction

Progress in combatting the devastating effects of coronary artery disease has not only been made in the field of preventive action but also in the treatment of acute myocardial infarction. One of the most exciting new developments in this area is the use of thrombolytic agents in the acute myocardial infarction to induce fast re-perfusion of the anoxic tissue and to limit tissue necrosis. This area is discussed in the contributions of Drs D. Collen and D. de Bono. The fibrinolytic system is formed by a set of proteolytic zymogens converted into active proteases in a cascade of activation reactions, ending in the breakdown of fibrin clots by the protease plasmin. To be effective in fibrinolysis, plasminogen should be activated to plasmin on the fibrin clot. Plasmin generated in blood will not discriminate between fibrinogen and fibrin and in addition, will be rapidly inactivated by α_2-antiplasmin. Physiological activators of plasminogen, tissue-type plasminogen activator (t-PA) and single-chain urokinase plasminogen activator (scu-PA) exert activating activity at the fibrin clot. Thrombolytic therapy may also find application in treatment of cerebrovascular thrombosis and other thrombotic complications.

Several thrombolytic agents have been used during the last decade in the treatment of acute myocardial infarction. These include streptokinase (a bacterial inducer of plasminogen self-activation), urokinase, tissue-type plasminogen activator (t-PA), single-chain urokinase plasminogen activator (scu-PA) and acylated plasminogen streptokinase activator. Streptokinase, a short-acting first-generation thrombolytic, has been used in tens of thousands of patients, and early intravenous infusion (within a few hours after the infarction) has been shown to reduce mortality significantly (−18%) in the period of three weeks following the event. As plasminogen is activated in blood and not at the fibrin clot, this therapy is associated with extensive breakdown of the haemostatic system. Clot-directed plasminogen activators (t-PA and scu-PA) would not suffer from these drawbacks, and clinical experience with these second-generation thrombolytics is currently being collected and evaluated. Further improvements in thrombolytics are expected to come from work on site-directed mutagenesis and genetic engineering of t-PA, resulting in agents with longer *in vivo* half-life and higher affinity for fibrin.

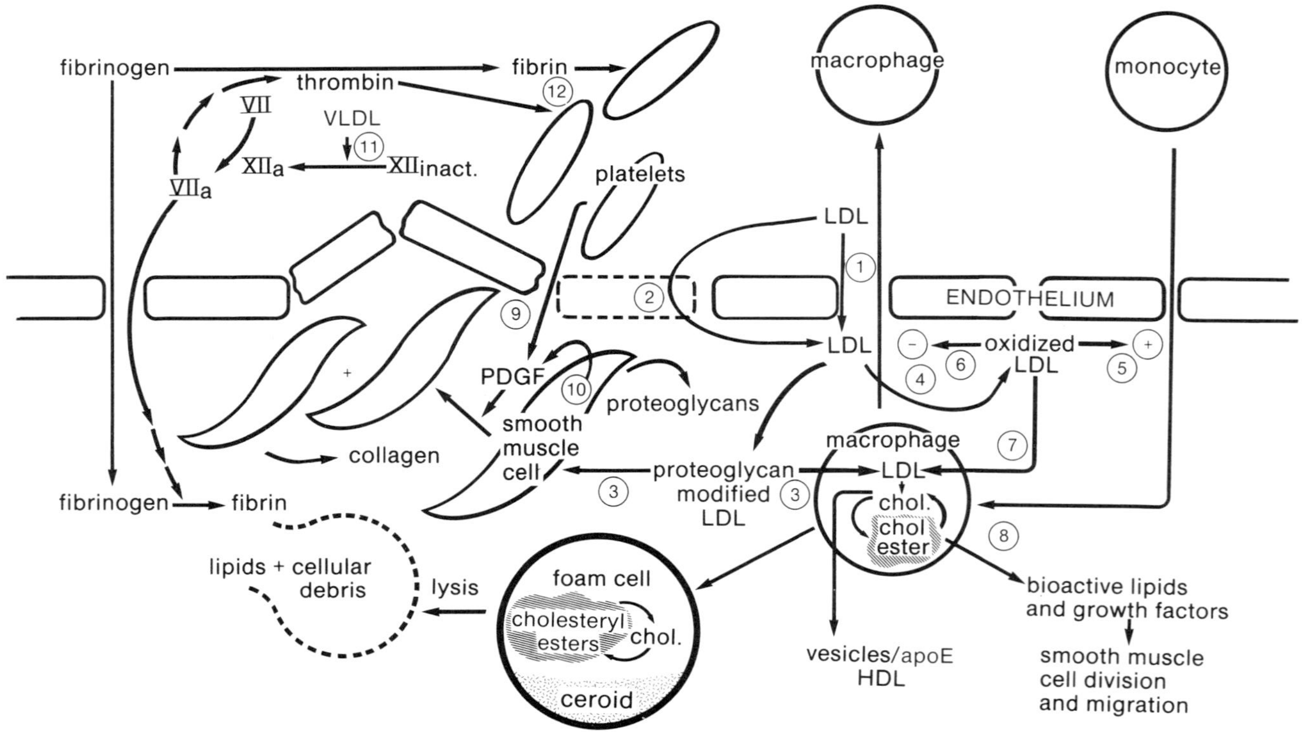

fibrinogen
fibrin
thrombin
VII
VLDL
XIIa
XIIinact.
VIIa
platelets
macrophage
monocyte
LDL
ENDOTHELIUM
oxidized LDL
PDGF
proteoglycans
smooth muscle cell
collagen
proteoglycan modified LDL
macrophage
chol.
chol ester
fibrinogen
fibrin
lipids + cellular debris
lysis
foam cell
cholesteryl esters
chol.
ceroid
vesicles/apoE HDL
bioactive lipids and growth factors
smooth muscle cell division and migration

Fig. 1 Biological processes involved in atherogenesis. The figure shows a schematic representation of the arterial wall (lower half of the figure) and the adjacent lumen (upper half of the figure). Plasma LDL penetrates into the subendothelial space by transendocytosis or through gaps between cells in the endothelial cell lining (1), or after endothelial damage (2). In the subendothelial space LDL is exposed to proteoglycans of the extracellular matrix and to monocyte-derived macrophages penetrated into the vessel wall. Interaction with proteoglycans modifies LDL in such a way that it is quickly taken up by smooth muscle cells and macrophages via non-LDL receptor pathways (3). LDL can also be modified by reactive oxygen species, generated by macrophages (4) and endothelial cells. Oxidation of LDL generates products with chemotatic properties for monocytes (5) and factors that inhibit macrophage mobility (6). Once monocytes have been attracted, the differentiated monocyte-derived macrophages are prevented from exiting, thereby creating conditions for further stimulation of LDL modification. Oxidized LDL is cytotoxic and is swiftly taken up by macrophages via their acetyl-LDL receptor (7). High rates of uptake result in a deposition of cholesteryl esters and accumulation of oxidized debris (ceroid) and conversion into foam cells. As a result of a disturbed metabolism (anoxia or due to engorgement with lipids and debris), foam cells may lyse and dump their cellular debris in the extracellular space. Activated tissue macrophages also secrete bioactive lipids and growth factors, which could stimulate smooth muscle cell proliferation and migration (8). Smooth muscle cell proliferation and migration could also be induced by platelet-derived growth factor (PDGF) from activated platelets (9) or by PDGF produced by smooth muscle cells itself in response to uptake of proteoglycan modified LDL (10). Fibrin deposition may further contribute to the growth of the lesion. High plasma concentrations of fibrinogen and activated factor VII will stimulate this process. Since factor VII can be activated by factor XII via the intrinsic (contact with negatively charged surfaces) pathway, large, negatively charged lipoproteins like VLDL may facilitate this process (11). An activated haemostatic system (12) and local endothelial damage also facilitate thrombus formation in the arterial lumen at the site of the lesion and induce stenosis.

Patients treated with thrombolytics during the acute phase of myocardial infarction run a higher risk for re-occlusion afterwards. Therefore supplementary therapy with anticoagulants, anti-platelet drugs or thromboxane antagonists has been proposed, as well as treatment by percutaneous coronary angioplasty (PTCA). In severe cases coronary bypass surgery would still be the follow-up treatment. Studies on the efficacy of different thrombolytic therapies and follow-up treatment are under way, and mortality and morbidity data are needed in large groups of patients to draw conclusions about what therapy has to be preferred. It is unlikely that control groups without thrombolytic therapy will be included in future studies, since its efficacy in general has been established.

It can be concluded that during the last decade enormous progress has been made in our understanding of the pathophysiology of atheroma formation. The role of plasma lipoproteins in atherogenesis is generally accepted and pharmacological intervention to treat hypercholesterolaemia is now possible. This should be seen as a starting point for therapeutic approaches. As knowledge about critical steps at the level of the atherosclerotic lesion increases, second-generation anti-atherosclerotic drugs will be developed and will reach the market. The stage is set for an effective battle against this devastating disease. In view of the chronic nature of atherosclerosis, long-term preventive and curative therapy is needed, demanding extremely high safety standards. This will be a challenge for the pharmaceutical industry, with high rewards for the well being of present and future generations.

References

The Lipid Research Clinics Coronary Primary Prevention Trial Results. (1984). (I) The reduction in incidence for coronary heart disease. (II) The relationship of reduction in incidence of coronary heart disease to cholesterol lowering. *J. Am. Med. Assoc.* **251**, 351–374.

Blankenhorn, D. H., Nessim, S. S., Johnson, R. L., Sanmarco, M. E., Azen, S. P. and Cashin-Hemphill, L. (1987). Beneficial effects of combined colestipol–niacin therapy on coronary atherosclerosis and coronary venous bypass grafts. *J. Am. Med. Assoc.* **257**, 3223–3240.

Frick, M. H. *et al.* (1987). Helsinki Heart Study: Primary-prevention trial with gemfibrozil in middle-aged men with dyslipidemia. *N. Engl. J. Med.* **317**, 1237–1245.

National Institute of Health Consensus Development Statement. (1985). Lowering blood cholesterol to prevent heart disease. *J. Am. Med. Assoc.* **253**, 2080–2086.

Study Group European Atherosclerosis Society. (1987). Strategies for the prevention of coronary heart disease: A policy statement of the European Atherosclerosis Society. *Eur. Heart J.* **8**, 77–88.

The British Cardiac Society Working Group on Coronary Prevention. (1987). Conclusions and recommendations. *Br. Heart J.* **57**, 188–189.

Shepherd, J. *et al.* (1987). Strategies for reducing coronary heart disease and desirable limits for blood lipid concentrations: guidelines of the British Hyperlipidaemia Association. *Br. Med. J.* **295**, 1245–1246.

Quinn, M. T., Parthasarathy, S. and Steinberg, D. (1985). Endothelial cell-derived chemotactic activity for mouse peritoneal macrophages and the effects of modified forms of low density lipoprotein. *Proc. Natl Acad. Sci. USA.* **82**, 5949–5953.

Powell, L. M., Wallis, S. C., Pease, R. J., Edwards, Y. H., Knott, T. J. and Scott, J. (1987). A novel form of tissue-specific RNA processing produces apolipoprotein B-48 in intestine. *Cell* **50**, 831–840.

Chen, S.-H. *et al.* (1987) Apolipoprotein B-48 is the product of a messenger RNA with an organ specific in frame stop codon. *Science* **238**, 363–366.

Kesäniemi, Y. A., Belz, W. F. and Grundy, S. M. (1985). Comparison of metabolism of apolipoprotein B in normal subjects and patients with coronary heart disease. *J. Clin. Invest.* **76**, 586–595.

Ehnholm, C., Lukka, M., Kuusi, T., Nikkila, E. and Uterman, G. (1986). Apolipoprotein E polymorphism in the Finnish population: gene frequencies and relation to lipoprotein concentration. *J. Lipid Res.* **27**, 227–235.

2

A Quantitative Approach to Low Density Lipoprotein Metabolism in Man and in Various Experimental Animals

JOHN M. DIETSCHY, DAVID K. SPADY and JONATHAN B. MEDDINGS

Department of Internal Medicine, University of Texas Southwestern Medical Center at Dallas, Texas, USA

1 Introduction

One of the major risk factors in the development of atherosclerotic vascular disease is the level of circulating low density lipoproteins (LDL). The steady-state level of LDL in man or in experimental animals is determined by four separate factors. These include the rate of LDL production, the rate of receptor-independent LDL degradation and the values for the maximum transport velocity and the Michaelis constant for the receptor-dependent LDL transport process. The values of these four factors have now been determined in man, hamster, rat and rabbit. Using the respective values for these different species, it is possible to predict the final plasma LDL-cholesterol concentration given any physiological change in the rate of LDL production or LDL degradation by the receptor-dependent and receptor-independent pathways. From an analysis of these kinetic relationships several important conclusions have emerged. First, the rate of LDL production is the most significant determinant of the plasma LDL-cholesterol concentration. Secondly, in man or in the experimental animal on a low-cholesterol, low-triacylglycerol diet, the total rate of LDL degradation is determined primarily by the rate of receptor-dependent LDL transport out of the plasma. Thirdly, in quantitative terms, receptor-dependent LDL degradation is limited to the liver and, to a lesser extent, the small intestine. Fourthly, with either an increase in the LDL

HYPERLIPIDAEMIA AND ATHEROSCLEROSIS
ISBN 0.12.675645-7

production rate or loss in receptor-dependent LDL transport, the peripheral extrahepatic organs become quantitatively more important in the degradation of LDL-cholesterol. Finally, this model also suggests that changes in the affinity of the LDL particle for the LDL receptor would have relatively less of an effect on plasma LDL-cholesterol concentrations.

2 Lipoprotein metabolism in the plasma

Cholesterol is an essential component of every cell membrane. As a consequence, nearly every tissue in the body of the growing or adult animal or man must have constant access to a source of sterol. Cholesterol can be added to the body pools from only two sources. Either preformed sterol is absorbed from dietary sources or, alternatively, the cholesterol molecule is synthesized *de novo* from acetyl-CoA in a variety of different tissues within the body. The sum of these two processes equals the total input of cholesterol into the body each day. Since in the adult there is no net accumulation of cholesterol within the tissues, each day an amount of cholesterol must be excreted that just equals this input of cholesterol. This takes place through the loss of the cholesterol molecule itself from the skin and through gastrointestinal secretions or after modification of the cholesterol molecule to bile acids and various steroid hormones. Thus in the growing animal approximately 1.4 g of cholesterol accumulates for each kilogram of body weight that is gained. Once adulthood is reached, however, the rate of cholesterol excretion through these two pathways must equal the rate of cholesterol accumulation through absorption and synthesis (Turley and Dietschy, 1988).

Recent data have confirmed that nearly all tissues in the body of every species have a significant rate of cholesterol synthesis (Dietschy, 1987). In general, however, the larger the animal, the lower the rate of cholesterol turnover and, hence, the lower the rate of cholesterol synthesis. Thus, for example, a small rodent such as the rat will synthesize approximately 120 mg/day per kg of body weight while man synthesizes only about 9 mg/day per kg (Turley and Dietschy, 1988). However, within any species the profile of synthetic activity in the various tissues is similar. Organs such as liver, intestine and various other intra-abdominal viscera have relatively high rates of sterol synthesis (Dietschy and Spady, 1986). There are important differences, however, in the absolute rates at which the liver can synthesize cholesterol. These are illustrated in Fig. 1. As is apparent in this figure, animals such as the rat and squirrel monkey have very high rates of hepatic cholesterol synthesis, while species such as man and the hamster can synthesize sterol at only much lower rates. This quantitative difference has very

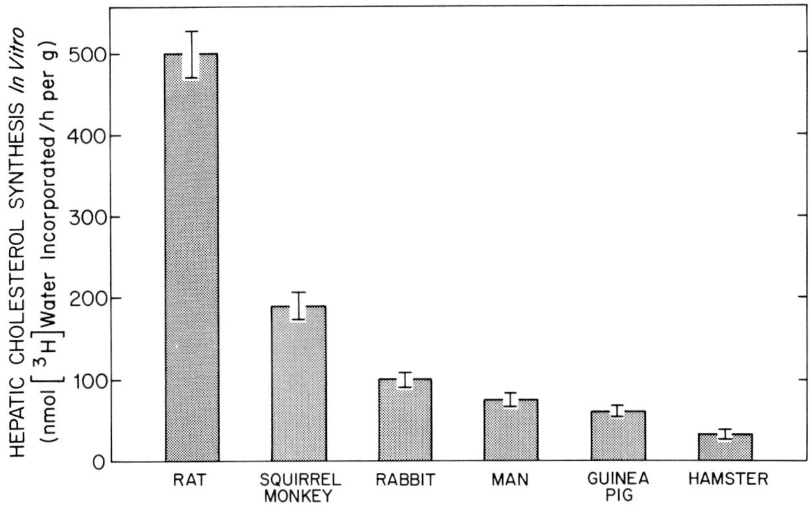

Fig. 1 Relative rates of hepatic cholesterol synthesis measured *in vitro*. In this diagram the rate of [^{3}H]water incorporation into cholesterol by liver tissue obtained from six different species is shown. In all situations the animals had been maintained on a low-cholesterol, low-triacylglycerol diet prior to the time these measurements were made. (From Turley and Dietschy, 1988.)

important implications with respect to regulation of plasma LDL-cholesterol levels. Most species respond to increased dietary intake of cholesterol by suppressing hepatic cholesterol synthesis. Animals such as the hamster and man have such low rates of hepatic synthesis that they have only very limited capacities to adapt to increasing loads of dietary cholesterol through this mechanism (Turley and Dietschy, 1988).

While the liver may not synthesize as much cholesterol as formerly believed, this organ is nevertheless key to the regulation of cholesterol balance within the intact animal and man. Furthermore, it is the liver that is largely responsible for regulating the level of circulating low density lipoproteins (LDL). The central role of the liver in these key processes is emphasized diagrammatically in Fig. 2. Dietary cholesterol, along with cholesterol that has been secreted into the intestinal lumen in bile, is absorbed by intestinal cells and incorporated into the chylomicron. Much of the triacylglycerol in this particle is removed in the peripheral organs, but the chylomicron remnant is quantitatively removed from the plasma by the liver. A second triacylglycerol-rich particle is synthesized and secreted by the liver. Much of the triacylglycerol carried in this very low density lipoprotein (VLDL) particle is also removed by peripheral tissues.

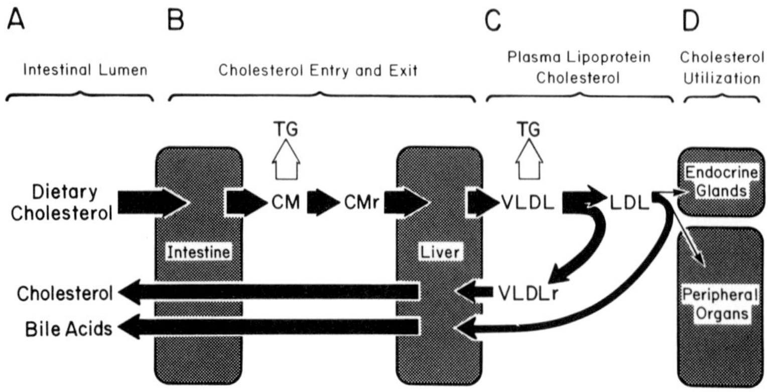

Fig. 2 Schematic representation of the metabolism of the major lipoprotein particles in the plasma. It should be noted that the rate of entry of LDL into the plasma space, i.e. the LDL production rate, can be changed by altering either the rate of VLDL secretion from the liver or the percentage of VLDL that is metabolized to LDL.

A portion of the VLDL is converted to a VLDL remnant and taken up by the liver, while the remaining VLDL is converted to LDL. It should be noted that the rate of LDL entry into the plasma space, i.e. the LDL production rate, can be altered by changing either the rate at which VLDL is secreted by the liver or by changing the fraction of the VLDL that is metabolized to LDL. The LDL particles are subsequently removed from the plasma space by several different organs, but predominantly by the liver. Thus the liver contains a pool of cholesterol that is complex and that is derived from dietary cholesterol: cholesterol that is newly synthesized in the intestine and liver, cholesterol that is taken up from the plasma space in VLDL remnants and LDL, and sterol that ultimately was synthesized in the extrahepatic organs and is delivered back to the liver, presumably in high density lipoproteins. Each day a portion of this pool is converted to bile acids, and these acidic sterols, along with cholesterol itself, are secreted into the gastrointestinal tract through the bile. In this manner sterol balance is maintained, and as much cholesterol is excreted in the faeces as enters the body through the diet or is acquired through *de novo* synthesis. It should be noted that the concentration of LDL-cholesterol in the plasma does not necessarily reflect directly either the entry of dietary cholesterol into the system or the rate of cholesterol synthesis in any of the organs. Rather it is a complex function of the rate at which LDL is produced relative to the rate at which it is removed from the plasma space (Meddings and Dietschy, 1987a).

3 Kinetics of low density lipoprotein metabolism

From the considerations outlined in Fig. 2, it is apparent that in order to understand the processes that regulate plasma LDL concentrations, one must begin to understand the regulation of LDL production and the transport mechanisms that are responsible for the removal of LDL particles from the plasma. It is now recognized that there are two discrete membrane transport processes that result in LDL uptake from the plasma space. One of these processes involves the interaction of the LDL particle with specific binding sites on the cell membrane, followed by the concentration of these LDL-receptor complexes into coated pits and their subsequent internalization through an endocytotic process (Brown and Goldstein, 1979). This is the process of receptor-dependent LDL transport. A second process also exists in which LDL is taken up from the plasma by a mechanism that apparently does not involve specific interactions with membrane receptors, and where the rate of uptake is a linear function of the plasma LDL concentration (Spady *et al.*, 1985b; Dietschy and Spady, 1986; Spady *et al.*, 1987). This process is referred to as receptor-independent LDL transport.

3.1 LDL clearance in the normal animal

The rates of both receptor-dependent and receptor-independent LDL transport have now been measured in the major organs of five animal species and, to a very limited degree, of man. The data obtained in three of these species are summarized in Fig. 3 (Spady *et al.*, 1983, 1985b, 1987). This figure shows the rate of LDL uptake by these two mechanisms in the whole animal, as well as in the individual organs of the animal, under *in vivo* conditions. It should be emphasized that the sum of the rates of uptake in the individual organs accounts for the rate of LDL turnover seen in the whole animal. As is apparent, there is little LDL uptake in any of the organs of these three species other than the liver and, to a much lesser extent, small bowel. In all species that have been examined so far, including man, approximately two-thirds to three-quarters of whole-body LDL turnover can be accounted for by the uptake of LDL into the liver. There is also now available detailed information on the extent to which both receptor-dependent and receptor-independent LDL transport take place in all of these organs. In tissues such as spleen, for example, the receptor-independent process is of greatest importance (Spady *et al.*, 1985b). In other organs such as the liver and endocrine glands, however, receptor-dependent LDL transport accounts for more than 90% of the observed tissue uptake (Spady *et al.*, 1983). Furthermore, since the liver (and small bowel) are such large

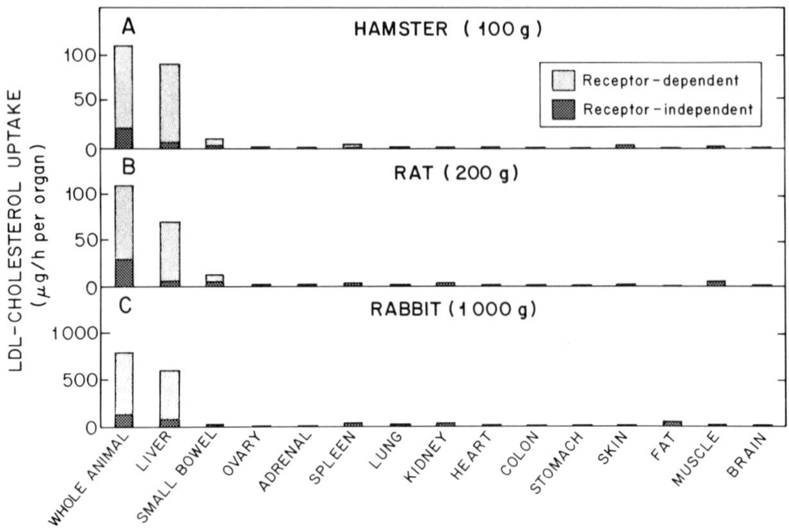

Fig. 3 Rates of receptor-dependent and receptor-independent LDL transport in the whole hamster, rat and rabbit, and in the individual organs of these animals. These rates are expressed as the mass (in μg) of LDL-cholesterol that is taken up per hour per whole animal or per whole organ. Both the receptor-dependent and receptor-independent components are shown. (From Meddings and Dietschy, 1987b.)

organs, essentially all of the receptor-dependent LDL transport that can be quantitated in the whole animal can be accounted for by receptor-dependent uptake in these two organs. Similar quantitative data have also been obtained in the mouse and dog and, to a more limited extent, man. The same general conclusions concerning LDL transport appear to apply to all of these species.

3.2 *Kinetic considerations*

Unfortunately these general conclusions are valid only in the control animal fed a low-fat diet and having a plasma LDL-cholesterol concentration that is normal for that species. Since the receptor-dependent LDL transport process involves interaction of the lipoprotein with a finite number of receptor sites, this transport process is saturable (Spady *et al.*, 1986a). The receptor-independent transport process, on the other hand, is not saturable (Spady *et al.*, 1986a). From these considerations it follows that in any situation in which the plasma LDL-cholesterol concentration increases, the quantitative significance of the receptor-dependent transport process in the whole animal, in general, and in the liver in particular will become less important. In order to understand these somewhat complex interrelationships, it is necessary to obtain detailed kinetic constants for each of these transport processes in each of the major organs of the body.

In the steady state where the plasma LDL-cholesterol concentration is constant, the rate of LDL-cholesterol production must equal the rate at which LDL is removed from the plasma space by the various transport mechanisms in all organs in the body. Thus the rate of LDL production must equal the rate of total LDL uptake and degradation J_t. This rate of LDL degradation, in turn, must equal the rate of receptor-dependent (J_d) and receptor-independent (J_i) uptake and degradation by the various tissues of the body. Thus the following relationship must hold:

$$J_t = J_d + J_i. \tag{1}$$

Both J_d and J_i are critically dependent upon the concentration C_2 of LDL-cholesterol at the surface of each cell. This value, however, is difficult to measure experimentally. Since plasma LDL is separated from the surface of the cells by a series of diffusion barriers, it is clear that the concentration C_1 of LDL-cholesterol in the plasma may be greater than the concentration C_2 that exists at the cell surface. The difference between these two values is proportional to two parameters. First, the diffusion barrier that separates the plasma space from the cell surface offers a finite resistance R to the diffusion of LDL particles. Secondly, if the rate of LDL-cholesterol uptake by parenchymal cells is rapid compared with the ability of the plasma LDL to diffuse across the resistance barrier then C_2 may be much lower than C_1. Thus C_2 can be calculated in any tissue from the following relationship (Thomas and Dietschy, 1984; Westergaard *et al.*, 1986), where J_t now represents the rate of total LDL transport into that organ:

$$C_2 = C_1 - J_t R. \tag{2}$$

It should be noted that in tissues like the liver, C_2 essentially equals C_1 since the resistance term is essentially zero.

The magnitude of receptor-dependent LDL-cholesterol uptake in a given organ can be described by classical Michaelis–Menton kinetics:

$$J_d = \frac{J^m C_2}{K_m + C_2}. \tag{3}$$

Thus J_d approaches the maximum transport rate J^m when either C_2 becomes very large or K_m approaches zero (infinite receptor affinity). In this formulation J^m is a manifestation of functional number in any given tissue. However, this parameter has the units of a transport term and defines the maximum mass of LDL-cholesterol that is taken up by a given organ per hour per gram of tissue when the plasma concentration of LDL-cholesterol is sufficiently high to saturate fully all functional receptors. The values of J^m have been measured in a variety of organs, and in the hamster, for example, these vary from 5.5 to 126 μg of LDL-cholesterol transported per hour per gram of tissue in the kidney and liver respectively (Spady *et al.*, 1986a).

Unlike the variability seen in J^m values, the affinity of the LDL receptor, expressed as the functional K_m value for the receptor-dependent transport process, is remarkably constant among the various organs. For example, in all tissues of both the rat and hamster, K_m values for the receptor-dependent LDL transport process are very close to 90 mg/dl of LDL-cholesterol. Since this functional K_m value represents the concentration of plasma LDL-cholesterol that is necessary to achieve half the value of J^m, it follows that this receptor-dependent transport process is almost never saturated, even at the very high concentrations of LDL-cholesterol seen in pathological states in man.

In contrast with the curvilinear, saturable relationship that exists between the plasma LDL-cholesterol concentration and receptor-dependent uptake, receptor-independent LDL transport has been shown to be a linear function of the concentration of plasma LDL-cholesterol (Spady *et al.*, 1985b, 1986a). The slope P of this relationship represents the mass of LDL-cholesterol taken up and degraded per hour per gram of tissue for each 1.0 mg/dl increase in the LDL-cholesterol concentration. The value of P represents a type of membrane permeability coefficient for the LDL particle. Thus the rate of receptor-independent LDL-cholesterol degradation J_i in a given organ can be calculated from the following relationship:

$$J_i = PC_2. \tag{4}$$

The value of P can be determined in each organ of the experimental animal (or in intact man) using modified forms of LDL that do not interact with the LDL receptor (Koelz *et al.*, 1982; Spady *et al.*, 1983).

Since the rate of total LDL-cholesterol uptake J_t in a given tissue must equal the sum of the receptor-dependent and receptor-independent uptakes, the following relationship must apply:

$$J_t = \frac{J^m C_2 + C_2}{K_m + C_2} + PC_2. \tag{5}$$

Equation (5) is written in terms of C_2. However, in at least two animal species the values of R in several organs have been found to be so low that the value of C_2 approaches C_1. Thus equation (5) can be rearranged to give a new expression that allows calculation of the rate of total LDL uptake and degradation by a particular organ J_t in terms of the four variables J^m, K_m, P and C_1 that are appropriate for that organ:

$$J_t = \frac{J^m C_1 + PC_1K_m + PC_1^2}{K_m + C_1}. \tag{6}$$

Thus this expression defines the relationship between LDL transport in any organ and the concentration of LDL-cholesterol in the plasma. This expression takes into account both the receptor-dependent and the receptor-independent components of this uptake process.

3.3 Whole-animal kinetic parameters in different species

Equation (6) defines the total rate of LDL transport taking place in a given whole organ. When the individual values for J^m, K_m and P are experimentally determined in different tissues, the value of J_t as a function of C_1 can be calculated, and when plotted yields curves such as those shown in Fig. 4. When such curves are available for all organs in the body, it follows that the sum of these curves must give a single curve that represents the kinetic characteristics of LDL-cholesterol uptake in the whole animal as a function of the plasma LDL-cholesterol concentration. Such a curve is also shown in Fig. 4 (labelled "Total").

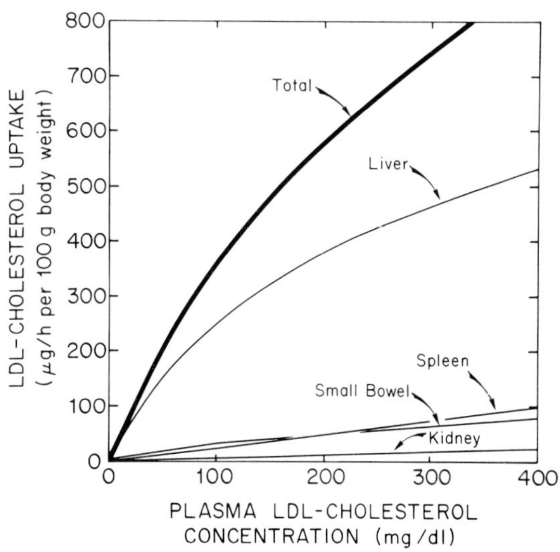

Fig. 4 Kinetic curves showing the rate of total LDL-cholesterol uptake J_t in different organs and in the whole animal as a function of the plasma LDL-cholesterol concentration C_1. These curves illustrate the typical relationships seen in individual organs and in the whole animal when appropriate values for the various kinetic constants are entered into equation (6). (From Meddings and Dietschy, 1987b.)

Table 1 Values for the various kinetic parameters of low density lipoprotein metabolism in four different species.

Species	Receptor-dependent		Receptor-independent	Transport rates		Receptor-dependent transport
	J^m	K_m	P	J_t	J_i	
	(mg/h per kg)	(mg/dl)	(mg/h per kg per mg/dl)	(mg/h per kg)	(mg/h per kg)	(%)
Hamster	4.85	91	0.012	3.11	0.92	70
Rat	4.06	97	0.006	2.18	0.41	81
Rabbit	2.13	90	0.009	1.67	0.71	58
Man	0.78	90	0.003	0.58	0.23	61

This table gives approximate values for the three parameters J^m, K_m and P that determine plasma LDL-cholesterol concentrations in the normal animal or man. The last three columns show the absolute rates of total LDL-cholesterol removal from the plasma (J_t) and the receptor-independent component (J_i) as well as the percentage of J_t that is receptor-dependent. These last three values are concentration-dependent and were calculated assuming that the plasma LDL-cholesterol concentration was 75 mg/dl in all four species. It should also be noted that these values of J_t are equal to the metabolic production rates of LDL-cholesterol at this value of C_1. All rate constants are given in terms of the mass (in mg) of LDL-cholesterol that is taken up from the plasma by the various transport processes.

In this formulation where the rate of whole-animal uptake and degradation of LDL-cholesterol J_t is plotted as a function of C_1, J^m represents the maximum rate of receptor-dependent LDL transport in all organs of the body, K_m equals the mean Michaelis constant for all of these organs and P represents the proportionality constant for receptor-independent LDL uptake by all tissues in the body. Such whole-body rate constants for LDL turnover have now been determined directly in three animal species including the rat, hamster and rabbit (Spady *et al.*, 1986a, 1987) and indirectly in man (Meddings and Dietschy, 1986).

Table 1 summarizes these whole-animal kinetic parameters in four species. Column 1 shows the values for J^m expressed as the mass (in milligrams) of LDL-cholesterol that can be transported per hour per kilogram of body weight provided that the plasma LDL-cholesterol concentration is sufficiently high to saturate fully the receptor-dependent transport process in all organs. In general, it is apparent that such receptor-dependent transport decreases in magnitude with an increase in animal size. J^m, for example, in the hamster and rat is five-fold higher than in man. In contrast with these variations, however, the data in the second column show that the functional K_m values for the receptor-dependent transport process are essentially the same in all of the species in which they have been determined. Thus, in all of these species, the maximum receptor-dependent transport rates shown in column 1 will not be achieved until the plasma LDL-cholesterol concentration is well in excess of 400 mg/dl. The values of P for the receptor-independent transport process are shown in column 3. Again, these tend to decrease with increasing animal size.

In columns 4 and 5 these parameters of LDL uptake have been used to calculate the absolute rate of total LDL transport J_t and the receptor-independent component J_i under circumstances where the plasma LDL-cholesterol concentration was set equal to 75 mg/dl in all species. As can be seen, the absolute rate of total transport, and the receptor-independent component, both decrease with increasing animal size so that the relative importance of the receptor-dependent component (column 6) remains relatively constant and about 60–80%.

4 Regulation of LDL metabolism

Utilizing these various relationships and the experimentally determined values for the various transport parameters, it is now possible to make a series of predictions concerning the manner in which the steady-state plasma LDL-cholesterol concentration will vary under circumstances where there has been a change in the amount of receptor-dependent transport, the affinity of the LDL receptor for the LDL particle or the LDL production rate.

4.1 Effect of varying different transport parameters

In order to illustrate the manner in which a change in one or more transport parameters alters the steady-state concentrations of LDL-cholesterol, it is useful to rearrange equation (6) and solve for the quantity C_1. When this is done the following expression is obtained:

$$C_1 = \frac{J_t - J^m - PK_m + [(J_t - J^m - PK_m)^2 + 4K_mJ_t]^{1/2}}{2P}. \qquad (7)$$

Thus, utilizing this expression, it is possible to calculate the value of C_1, the concentration of LDL-cholesterol in the plasma, under circumstances where there has been a change in the whole-animal LDL production rate J_t, a change in the amount of receptor-dependent LDL transport J^m, a change in the affinity of the LDL particle for the LDL receptor K_m, or an alteration in the magnitude of receptor-independent LDL transport P. In most situations in which there has been an alteration in the plasma LDL-cholesterol concentration, it has been found that this alteration is due to either a change in production rate or the amount of receptor-dependent LDL transport. Hence the other two variables will not be further discussed in this paper.

Figure 5 illustrates graphically how changes in either the amount of receptor-dependent transport or the production rate alter the steady-state plasma LDL-cholesterol concentrations in man. In this presentation the absolute magnitude of J^m and J_t have been set equal to 1.0 in the control population. Thus changes in these two parameters are expressed in terms of multiples of the normal value. The point labelled (a) represents the young, healthy individual with a normal production rate and normal receptor number and a mean plasma LDL-cholesterol concentration of approximately 70 mg/dl. If the LDL production rate is kept constant then loss of 50% of the receptor activity will increase the plasma LDL-cholesterol concentration to about 110 mg/dl (point (b)). Alternatively, doubling receptor activity will lower the plasma LDL-cholesterol concentration to about 40 mg/dl (point (e)). If there is a 50% loss in receptor activity and, at the same time, a 1.7-fold increase in production rate (point (c)) then the plasma LDL-cholesterol concentration will increase more dramatically to approximately 220 mg/dl. It should be noted that the plasma LDL-cholesterol concentration would increase to about the same level even if receptor number were twice normal but the production rate were increased just over three-fold (point (d)). Thus this graphical formulation of equation (7) illustrates the very important interplay of total receptor activity and production rate in determining the plasma LDL-cholesterol concentration. It should again be emphasized that in this particular presentation the values for K_m and P were assumed to be constant. Using this

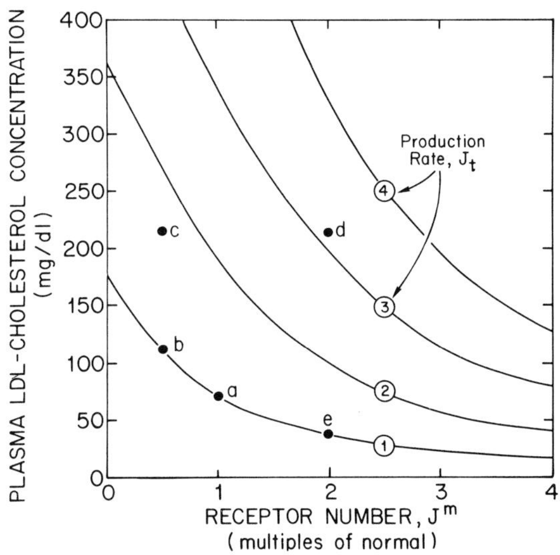

Fig. 5 Relationship between LDL production rates, LDL receptor number and plasma LDL-cholesterol concentrations. These curves illustrate how the plasma LDL-cholesterol concentration in man changes when there has been a systematic alteration in either the amount of receptor-dependent LDL transport J^m or an alteration in the LDL production rate J_t. The specific points labelled (a)–(e) are discussed in the text.

formulation, it is now possible to determine much more precisely what event or events resulted in a change in the plasma LDL-cholesterol concentration given any physiological, dietary or pharmacological manipulation of an experimental animal or man.

A variety of situations have now been described in which there are significant alterations in these parameters. For example, during malignant transformation, receptor-dependent LDL uptake appears to be deleted in several types of malignancies (Clayman *et al.*, 1986a,b). Furthermore, any change in the size or composition of the bile acid pool circulating within the enterohepatic circulation can alter receptor-dependent LDL uptake in the liver (Spady *et al.*, 1986b). In some species the feeding of compounds such as cholestyramine is also associated with change in hepatic receptor-dependent LDL uptake (Spady *et al.*, 1985a). Two of the most important and universal determinants of plasma LDL-cholesterol concentrations, however, are thought to be ageing and the intake of dietary lipids.

4.2 Effect of ageing

In Western civilizations there is a gradual increase in the plasma LDL-cholesterol level with ageing. When kinetic studies are performed in individuals of varying age it has generally been found that this increase in plasma cholesterol levels is associated with a progressive increase in the LDL production rate and a decrease in the fraction of the LDL pool that is degraded each day, i.e. the fractional catabolic rate. When data such as these are plotted on the appropriate curves (Fig. 5) it is found that the effect of ageing on plasma LDL-cholesterol concentrations is primarily brought about by an increase in production rate, while receptor-dependent transport activity J^m remains relatively constant. In several animal species maintained throughout their life on a low-cholesterol, low-triacylglycerol diet it has also been shown that there is no effect of ageing on receptor number (unpublished data from this laboratory). Taken together, these types of data suggest that ageing *per se* has no effect on receptor-dependent LDL transport and, further, that the progressive increase in plasma LDL-cholesterol concentrations seen in man may be the effect of diet, rather than ageing.

4.3 Effect of various diets

Recent data have clearly demonstrated that when small amounts of cholesterol are added to a lipid-free diet there is progressive loss of receptor-dependent LDL transport in the liver, and a significant increase in the circulating plasma LDL-cholesterol concentration (Spady *et al.*, 1985a). Furthermore, when saturated long-chain triacylglycerols are added to the diet this suppressive effect of dietary cholesterol on LDL receptor activity is augmented and, in addition, there is a marked increase in the LDL-cholesterol production rate. As a consequence of these marked changes in both J^m and J_t, the plasma LDL-cholesterol concentration increases significantly. If, on the other hand, polyunsaturated long-chain triacylglycerols are added to the diet, there is little suppression of LDL receptor activity and the plasma LDL-cholesterol concentration returns toward the normal value (Spady and Dietschy, 1985). Thus the dietary intake of saturated long-chain triacylglycerols has a very significant effect on plasma LDL-cholesterol concentrations by: (i) augmenting the effect of small amounts of dietary cholesterol in suppressing receptor-dependent LDL uptake by the liver; and (ii) markedly increasing the LDL production rate. On the basis of such data, it seems likely that the progressive increase in plasma LDL-cholesterol levels in Western man primarily results from dietary effects rather than the effect of ageing *per se*. For example, groups of patients with severe atherosclerotic heart disease and plasma LDL-cholesterol concentrations in the range 200–250 mg/dl commonly fall near point (c) in Fig. 5. Such patients have therefore lost significant amounts of receptor-dependent LDL transport and have significant overproduction of LDL. This is identical with the situation seen in the experimental animal placed on the same amounts of cholesterol and triacylglycerols found in typical Western diets. Finally, however, it should be emphasized that there is little understanding why different individuals (or experimental animals) placed on the same diet respond differently with respect to these various parameters. Clearly it is extremely important that future research focuses on the causes for this individual variability.

Acknowledgements

Portions of this work were supported by US Public Health Service Research Grants HL-09610 and AM-19329, and by a grant from the Moss Heart Fund.

References

Brown, M. S. and Goldstein, J. L. (1979). Receptor-mediated endocytosis: insights from the lipoprotein receptor system. *Proc. Natl Acad. Sci. USA* **76**, 3330–3337.

Clayman, R. V., Bilhartz, L. E., Spady, D. K., Buja, L. M. and Dietschy, J. M. (1986a). Low density lipoprotein-receptor activity is lost *in vivo* in malignantly transformed renal tissue. *FEBS Lett.* **196**, 87–90.

Clayman, R. V., Bilhartz, L. E., Buja, L. M., Spady, D. K. and Dietschy, J. M. (1986b). Renal cell carcinoma in the Wistar–Lewis rat: a model for studying the mechanisms of cholesterol acquisition by a tumor *in vivo. Cancer Res.* **46**, 2958–2963.

Dietschy, J. M. (1987). In *Atherogenesis and Aging* (ed. S. R. Bates and E. C. Gangloff), pp. 104–122. Springer-Verlag, New York.

Dietschy, J. M. and Spady, D. K. (1986). In *Receptor-Mediated Uptake in the Liver* (ed. H. Greten, E. Windler and U. Beisiegel), pp. 56–65. Springer-Verlag, Berlin.

Koelz, H. R., Sherrill, B. C., Turley, S. D. and Dietschy, J. M. (1982). Correlation of low and high density lipoprotein binding *in vivo* with rates of lipoprotein degradation in the rat. A comparison of lipoproteins of rat and human origin. *J. Biol. Chem.* **257**, 8061–8072.

Meddings, J. B. and Dietschy, J. M. (1986). Regulation of plasma levels of low-density lipoprotein cholesterol: interpretation of data on low-density lipoprotein turnover in man. *Circulation* **74**, 805–814.

Meddings, J. B. and Dietschy, J. M. (1987a). In *Contributions of Chemistry to Health*, Vol. 2 (ed. H. Machleidt), pp. 269–282. VCH Verlag, Frankfurt.

Meddings, J. B. and Dietschy, J. M. (1987b). In *Progress in Clinical Biochemistry and Medicine*, Vol. 5, pp. 1–24. Springer-Verlag, New York.

Spady, D. K. and Dietschy, J. M. (1985). Dietary saturated triacylglycerols suppress hepatic low density lipoprotein receptor activity in the hamster. *Proc. Natl Acad. Sci. USA* **82**, 4526–4530.

Spady, D. K., Bilheimer, D. W. and Dietschy, J. M. (1983). Rates of receptor-dependent and -independent low density lipoprotein uptake in the hamster. *Proc. Natl Acad. Sci. USA* **80**, 3499–3503.

Spady, D. K., Turley, S. D. and Dietschy, J. M. (1985a). Rates of low density lipoprotein uptake and cholesterol synthesis are regulated independently in the liver. *J. Lipid. Res.* **26**, 465–472.

Spady, D. K., Turley, S. D. and Dietschy, J. M. (1985b). Receptor-independent low density lipoprotein transport in the rat *in vivo*. Quantitation, characterization, and metabolic consequences. *J. Clin. Invest.* **76**, 1113–1122.

Spady, D. K., Meddings, J. B. and Dietschy, J. M. (1986a). Kinetic constants for receptor-dependent and receptor-independent low density lipoprotein transport in the tissues of the rat and hamster. *J. Clin. Invest.* **77**, 1474–1481.

Spady, D. K., Stange, E. F., Bilhartz, L. E. and Dietschy, J. M. (1986b). Bile acids regulate hepatic low density lipoprotein receptor activity in the hamster by altering cholesterol flux across the liver. *Proc. Natl Acad. Sci. USA* **83**, 1916–1920.

Spady, D. K., Huettinger, M., Bilheimer, D. W. and Dietschy, J. M. (1987). Role of receptor-independent low density lipoprotein transport in the maintenance of tissue cholesterol balance in the normal and WHHL rabbit. *J. Lipid Res.* **28**, 32–41.

Thomson, A. B. R. and Dietschy, J. M. (1984). In *Handbook of Experimental Pharmacology*, Vol. 70/II (ed. T. Z. Csaky), pp. 165–269. Springer-Verlag, New York.

Turley, S. D. and Dietschy, J. M. (1988). In *The Liver: Biology and Pathobiology* (ed. I. Arias, H. Popper, D. Schachter and D. A. Shafritz). Raven Press, New York.

Westergaard, H., Holtermuller, K. H. and Dietschy, J. M. (1986). Measurement of resistance of barriers to solute transport *in vivo* in rat jejunum. *Am. J. Physiol.* **250**, G727–G735.

3

Recent Advances in the Structure and Biosynthesis of Apolipoproteins B100 and B48

H. B. BREWER, K. HIGUCHI, A. HOSPATTANKAR, J. HOEG and R. E. GREGG

Molecular Disease Branch, National Heart, Lung, and Blood Institute, National Institutes of Health, Bethesda, Maryland, USA

1 Introduction

Apolipoprotein (apo) B plays a pivotal biological role in intercellular transport and cellular delivery of cholesterol. It is the principal structural apolipoprotein on chylomicrons, very low density lipoproteins, intermediate density lipoproteins and low density lipoproteins, and is important in chylomicrons and hepatogenous very low density lipoprotein biosynthesis and secretion. ApoB also functions as the ligand on low density lipoproteins that interacts with the LDL receptor, and initiates absorptive endocytosis and cellular uptake of low density lipoproteins (Brown and Goldstein, 1986).

In human plasma apoB exists as two isoproteins designated apoB48 and apoB100, which can be separated by SDS gel electrophoresis (Kane *et al.*, 1980; Kane, 1983). It has been proposed (Kane *et al.*, 1980; Kane, 1983) that in man apoB100 and apoB48 are synthesized by the liver and intestine respectively. *In vitro* studies with HepG2 and normal hepatocytes have suggested that apoB100 is the principal B apolipoprotein secreted by the human liver (Edge *et al.*, 1985). In contrast, both apoB48- and apoB100-equivalent apolipoproteins have been reported to be secreted by the rat liver, indicating that there is significant interspecies variability of the quantity of apoB48-equivalent apolipoprotein secreted by the liver (Elovson *et al.*, 1981; Wu and Windmuller, 1981; Sparks *et al.*, 1981).

There is no agreement in the literature regarding the apoB isoproteins secreted by the human intestine. Kane and colleagues (Kane *et al.*, 1980, Kane, 1983) have proposed that only apoB48 is secreted from the human intestine. Glickman *et al.* (1986) have reported that foetal organ cultures initially secreted apoB100; however, following the 18th week of gestation, the apoB isoprotein secreted was apoB48. These studies were interpreted as indicating that the apoB isoproteins secreted from the intestine were developmentally regulated. In contrast with these conclusions, Dullaart *et al.* (1986) reported the presence of apoB100 in adult human intestine utilizing monoclonal antibodies specific for apoB100. Recently our laboratory reported (Hoeg *et al.*, 1987) that apoB100 as well as apoB48 were secreted by human organ cultures *in vitro*. In the rat, Lee *et al.* (1984) reported that an apoB100-equivalent apolipoprotein was secreted by the intestine. However, without protease inhibitors, apoB100 was cleaved to an apolipoprotein similar in size to apoB48 when analysed by SDS gel electrophoresis. Other investigators have reported that the apoB48-equivalent isoprotein was the principal apoB isoprotein secreted by the rat intestine (Wu and Windmuller, 1981; Sparks *et al.*, 1981; Krishnaiah *et al.*, 1980).

2 Covalent structure of human apoB100

Major insights into our understanding of the structure and function of apoB100 were achieved by the elucidation of the complete cDNA sequence of apoB100 from overlapping cDNA clones (Law *et al.*, 1986a; Knott *et al.*, 1986; Chen *et al.*, 1986; Cladaras *et al.*, 1986). Human apoB100 mRNA contains 14 121 nucleotides, and mature apoB100 contains 4536 amino acids. ApoB100 contains a signal peptide of 27 amino acids, and the calculated amino acid molecular weight of mature apoB100 is 512 723. ApoB100 contains 20 potential glycosylation sites, and 12 out of a total of 25 cysteine residues are located in the amino terminal regions of the apolipoprotein, providing a potential for a complex globular structure at the amino terminus of the apolipoprotein.

The single gene for apoB is located on chromosome 2 (Law *et al.*, 1985; Higuchi *et al.*, 1987). The apoB gene spans 43 kb (kilobases) and contains 29 exons (Blackhart *et al.*, 1986). A single exon, exon 26, is 7572 bp (base pairs) long, and contains over half of the coding sequence.

3 Covalent structure of human apoB48

As outlined above, apoB48 has been proposed as the major apoB isoprotein secreted by the intestine. Initial studies using amino acid composition, protein

Fig. 1 Northern blot analysis of liver (L) and intestinal (I) poly $(A)^+$ RNA. The blot was hybridized with a nick-translated 5′ apoB cDNA probe.

sequencing and monoclonal antibody analyses (Marcel *et al.*, 1982; Curtis and Edgington, 1982, Hardman and Kane, 1986) were interpreted as indicating that apoB48 was the amino terminal half of apoB100. Studies from our laboratory identified two apoB mRNAs in the human intestine (Law *et al.*, 1985, 1986a,b; Higuchi *et al.*, 1987). A 14.1 kb mRNA was similar to the apoB100 mRNA present in the liver, and a second mRNA, 7.5 kb in length, was of sufficient size to code for apoB48 (Fig. 1). Recently our laboratory (Hospattankar *et al.*, 1987), Chen *et al.* (1987) and Powell *et al.* (1987) have established that human intestinal apoB mRNA contains a premature in-frame translational stop codon that provides a mechanism for the biosynthesis of apoB48. The premature stop codon in intestinal mRNA involves a single base substitution of a "C" to "U" at nucleotide 6538, which converts the codon "CAA" coding for the amino acid glutamine in apoB100, residue 2153, to an in-frame stop codon "UAA" (Fig. 2). Autoradiograms of DNA sequencing gels of a cDNA clone containing the stop codon ("TAA") from human intestine, and a similar region of the coding sequence of human liver apoB100 cDNA

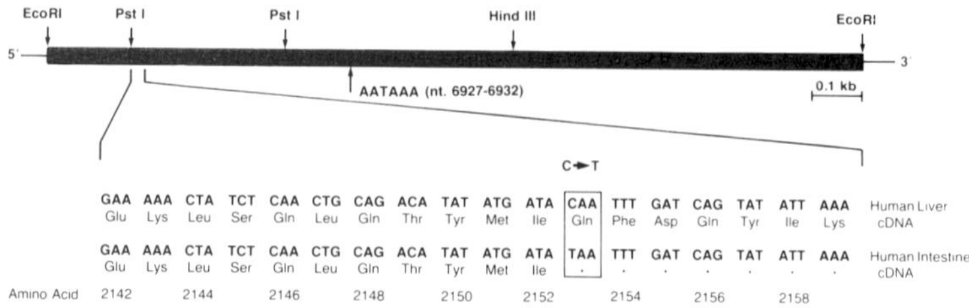

Fig. 2 Restriction enzyme map of 1.5 kb apoB cDNA insert isolated from a human intestinal cDNA library. The region corresponding to amino acids 2142–2159 present in the 14.1 kb in long apoB mRNA is shown in the lower panel. In the human intestine, a single base substitution of a "C" for a "T" in the apoB cDNA introduces a new in-frame stop codon. The introduction of the premature stop codon provides a mechanism for the biosynthesis of apoB48.

containing the "CAA" codon for glutamine at residue 2153, are illustrated in Fig. 3.

The availability of the nucleotide sequence at the in-frame stop codon permitted the synthesis of two 30-base-long synthetic oligonucleotides designated apoB-Stop (5′-ATACTGATCAAATTATATCATATATGTCTG-3′) and apoB-Gln (5′ATACTGATCAAATTGATCATATATGTCTG-3′), which are complementary nucleotides at positions 6523–6552 of the apoB

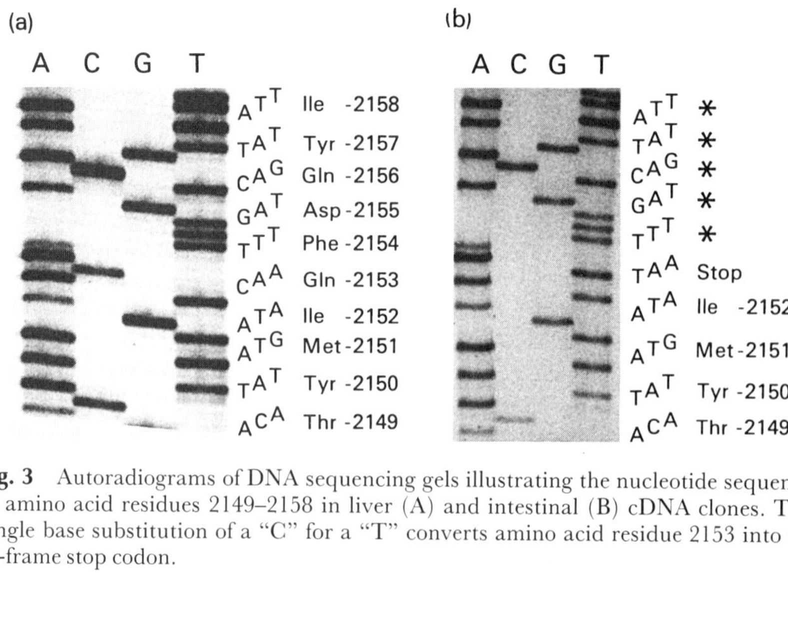

Fig. 3 Autoradiograms of DNA sequencing gels illustrating the nucleotide sequence of amino acid residues 2149–2158 in liver (A) and intestinal (B) cDNA clones. The single base substitution of a "C" for a "T" converts amino acid residue 2153 into an in-frame stop codon.

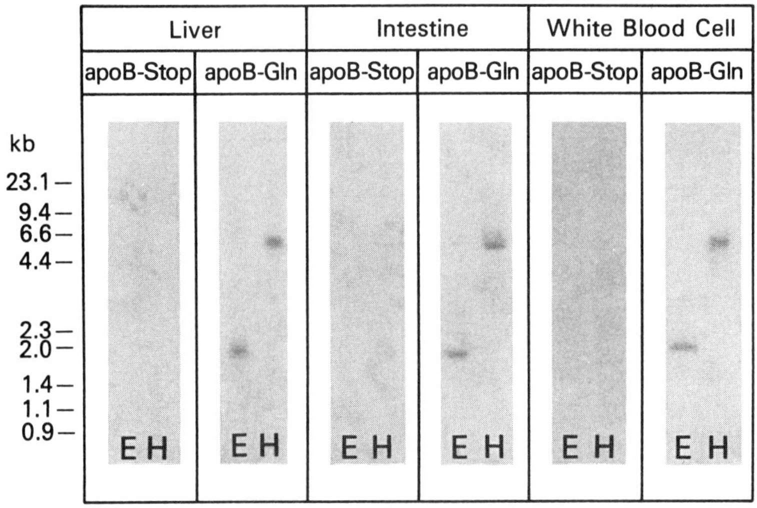

Fig. 4 Southern blot analysis of human genomic DNA isolated from liver, intestine and white blood cells. Genomic DNA was digested with EcoRI(E) and Hind III(H), and the hybridization of the separate fragments was performed with synthetic oligonucleotide probes apoB-Stop and apoB-Gln, which are specific for the stop codon in apoB48 and the glutamine codon present in apoB100 respectively. Molecular-weight markers are shown on the left.

mRNA containing the stop codon ("UAA") and apoB100 glutamine codon ("CAA") respectively. The sequence-specific apoB-Stop and apoB-Gln probes were used to analyse genomic DNA from liver, intestine and leukocytes. Only the apoB-Gln probe hybridized to the genomic DNAs, establishing that the stop codon was not present at the DNA level, and involved a new novel RNA editing mechanism (Fig. 4). The introduction of a premature in-frame stop codon at the RNA level represents a fascinating new mechanism for the biosynthesis of two proteins from a single gene and nuclear RNA. This mechanism may also be used for the editing of mRNA of other genes, and represents a new control mechanism for eukaryotic gene expression.

4 Human intestinal biosynthesis of the B apolipoproteins

The identification of the stop codon and a mechanism for the biosynthesis of apoB48 provided us with the opportunity to reexamine the apoB isoproteins secreted from the human intestine. The apoB isoproteins secreted from the human intestine were initially examined by an analysis of the apoB isoproteins

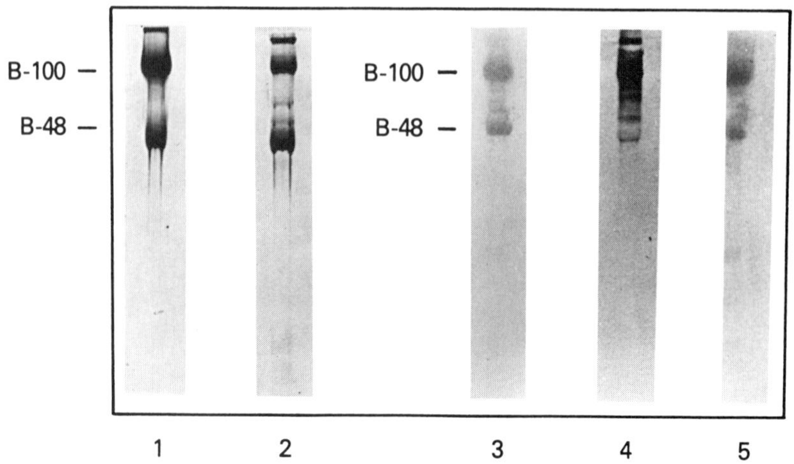

Fig. 5 ApoB isoproteins secreted by intestinal organ cultures *in vitro*. The lipoproteins secreted by the organ cultures were isolated by ultracentrifugation (1.21 g/ml) and analysed by SDS gel electrophoresis and immunoblot analysis utilizing apoB monoclonal antibodies. Lanes 1 and 2 contain apoB100 and apoB48 standards stained with Coomassie Blue, lanes 3 and 5 contain apoB100 and apoB48 standards and intestinal organ culture lipoproteins immunoblotted with a monoclonal antibody that recognizes both apoB100 and apoB48. Lane 4 contains organ culture lipoproteins immunoblotted with a carboxyl terminal apoB100-specific monoclonal antibody.

secreted into the media of intestinal organ cultures *in vitro* (Hoeg *et al.*, 1987) (Fig. 5). The apoB isoproteins were analysed by monoclonal apoB antibodies that were specific for apoB100 as well as antibodies that recognized both apoB48 and apoB100. As illustrated in Fig. 5, apoB100 was readily identified in the media of human intestinal organ cultures, indicating that both apoB48 as well as apoB100 may be secreted from the human intestine.

In order to evaluate further the potential mechanism for the biosynthesis of apoB100 in the human intestine, we examined the apoB mRNA isolated from human intestine by Northern blot analysis utilizing the sequence-specific probes, apoB-Gln and apoB-Stop, which recognize the mRNA coding for apoB100 and apoB48 respectively (Higuchi *et al.*, 1988). Both the 14.1 and 7.5 kb apoB mRNA present in the intestine hybridized to the apoB-Stop probe, indicating that the stop codon was present in both the 14.1 and 7.5 kb apoB mRNAs (Fig. 6). The apoB-Gln probe also hybridized to the 14.1 kb apoB mRNA, indicating that mRNA coding for apoB100 was present in the intestine (Fig. 6). The 14.1 kb mRNA therefore contains a mixture of mRNAs containing the "CAA" codon for apoB100, and the "UAA" stop codon, which codes for apoB48 (Higuchi *et al.*, 1988).

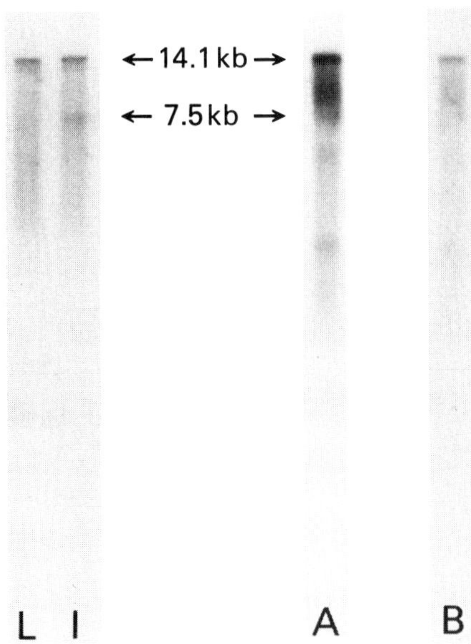

Fig. 6 Northern blot analysis of liver (L) and intestinal (I) poly $(A)^+$ RNA utilizing a 5′ apoB cDNA probe. Intestinal apoB mRNA was also hybridized with the apoB-Stop (A) and apoB-Glyn (B) probes. The apoB-Stop probe hybridized to both the 14.1 and 7.5 kb apoB mRNA. The apoB-Gln probe hybridized to the 14.1 kb apoB mRNA, indicating that the 14.1 kb apoB mRNA contains a mixture of mRNA containing both the "Gln" and "Stop" mRNA codons.

The presence of the apoB mRNA for apoB100 was also directly addressed by analysis of apoB clones in intestinal cDNA libraries. The libraries were screened with the apoB-Stop and apoB-Gln probes. Seven apoB clones were identified that were positive to the apoB-Stop probe, whereas two clones were positive on hybridization with the apoB-Gln probe. The apoB-Gln-positive clones were sequenced and the "CAA" codon for glutamine was identified in both clones. The nucleotide sequences of clones positive for the apoB-Stop (λMDB II-1) and apoB-Gln (λMDB II-3) clones are illustrated in Fig. 7. These results definitively established that the human intestine contains mRNA containing the premature stop codon encoding for apoB48 and mRNA containing the "CAA" codon for glutamine (Higuchi *et al.*, 1988).

A summary of our concept of the biosynthesis of intestinal apoB isoproteins is shown schematically in Fig. 8. A single gene for apoB is present on chromosome 2. A single nuclear RNA is synthesized and some of the mRNA is edited either co- or post-transcriptionally to contain the "UAA" stop codon, the remaining mRNA is unedited and contains the "CAA" codon. Therefore

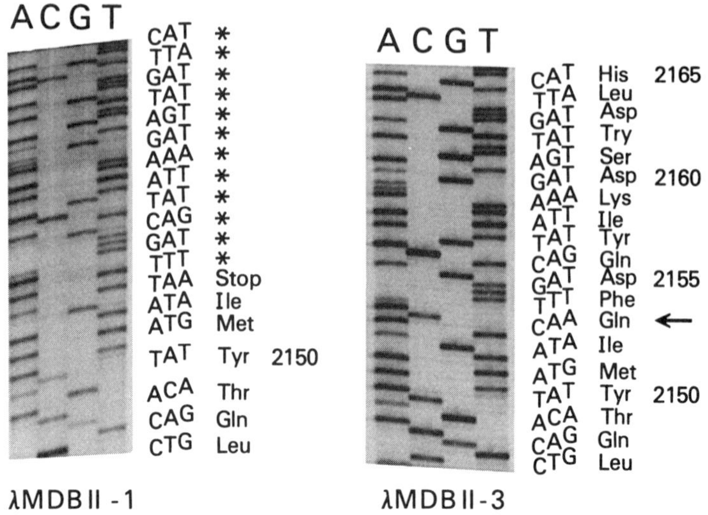

Fig. 7 Autoradiogram of DNA sequencing gels illustrating the cDNA sequence of intestinal clones that were positive to the apoB-Stop (λMDBII-1) and apoB-Gln (λMDBII-3) probes. The intestinal clones contain two separate clones, one containing the stop codon of apoB48 and the other having the "CAA" codon coding for apoB100.

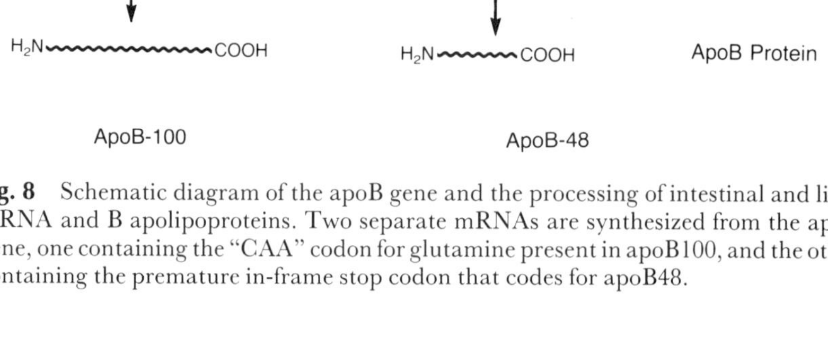

Fig. 8 Schematic diagram of the apoB gene and the processing of intestinal and liver mRNA and B apolipoproteins. Two separate mRNAs are synthesized from the apoB gene, one containing the "CAA" codon for glutamine present in apoB100, and the other containing the premature in-frame stop codon that codes for apoB48.

the enterocyte contains both the "UAA" and "CAA" mRNAs coding for apoB48 and apoB100 respectively. It will be of major interest through future research to determine the factors, including diet, hormones and kinases, that may ultimately determine the percentage of mRNA that is edited to contain the "UAA" stop codon. In addition, the elucidation of the mechanism involved in the editing of the mRNA may provide new insights into the control of apolipoprotein gene expression.

5 Abetalipoproteinaemia

The cloning and structural analysis of the apoB gene has provided an opportunity to evaluate the molecular defect in patients with abetalipoproteinaemia. Abetalipoproteinaemia is an autosomal recessive disease initially described by Bassen and Kornzweig (1950). The clinical manifestations of the disease include ataxia, retinitis pigmentosa, acantocytosis and fat malabsorption (Herbert *et al.*, 1983). Plasma cholesterol and triglycerides are significantly reduced, and chylomicrons, very low density lipoproteins and low density lipoproteins are absent in the plasma (Herbert *et al.*, 1983). The high density lipoproteins are the only plasma lipoproteins present in abetalipoproteinaemia. The characteristic apolipoprotein abnormality is a virtual complete absence of plasma apoB100 and apoB48. A similar dyslipoproteinaemia, hypobetalipoproteinaemia, is also characterized by a deficiency of plasma apoB100 and apoB48, but is clearly distinguished from abetalipoproteinaemia by the reduced plasma levels of apoB in the oligate heterozygotes (Herbert *et al.*, 1983). A third interesting variant of apoB deficiency is normotriglyceridaemic abetalipoproteinaemia, which is characterized by the presence in plasma of chylomicrons, very low density lipoproteins and apoB48, but the absence of low density lipoproteins and apoB100 (Malloy *et al.*, 1981).

The defect in abetalipoproteinaemia has been studied in two independent probands with classical abetalipoproteinaemia (Lackner *et al.*, 1986). Liver tissue was obtained by needle biopsy in one proband, and at post mortem in the second patient. Plasma was analysed for apoB by immunoblot analysis following SDS gel electrophoresis. No apoB isoproteins could be detected following the concentration of one litre of plasma by radioimmunoassay or gel electrophoresis. The apoB gene was evaluated by Southern blot analysis utilizing probes that covered the entire 40 kb gene. No major insertions, deletions or rearrangements were detected in the apoB gene in either patient (Fig. 9). Northern blot analysis of total and poly $(A)^+$ RNA revealed that the apoB mRNA was the same size as apoB mRNA isolated from a control subject (Fig. 10). Dot blot quantitation of hepatic apoB mRNA from the two probands with abetalipoproteinaemia is illustrated in Fig. 11. The apoB mRNA was

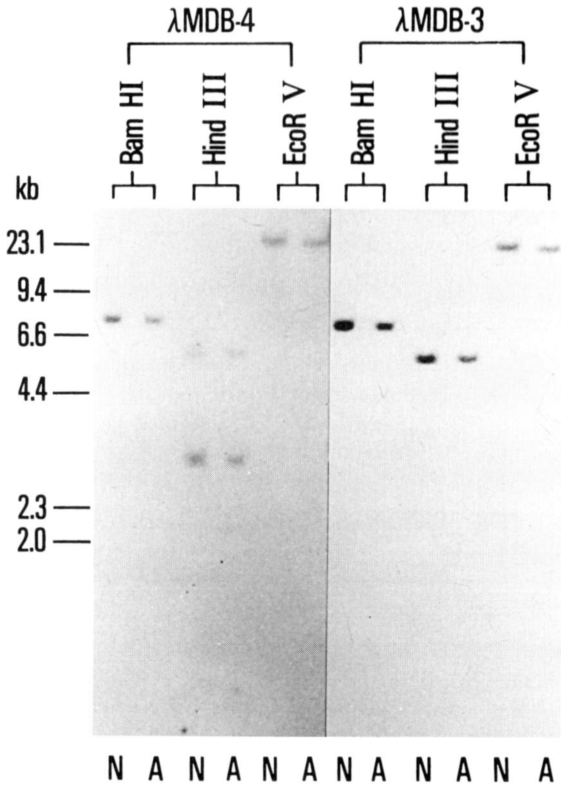

Fig. 9 Representative Southern blot analysis of genomic DNA isolated from a normal control (N) and an abetalipoproteinaemic (A) patient. Results from two different probes, λMDB-3 and λMDB-4, are illustrated. Additional studies were performed utilizing probes that spanned the entire apoB gene.

increased approximately six-fold when compared with the levels of apoB mRNA in three control subjects. The presence of apoB in the cytoplasm of hepatocytes was evaluated by immunocytochemistry. Significant apoB was present in the hepatocyte, indicating that the B apolipoprotein was translated from the apoB mRNA. These combined results have been interpreted as indicating that the defect in abetalipoproteinaemia is due to a defect in transport of apoB out of the hepatocyte (Lackner *et al.*, 1986). The increased level of apoB mRNA in abetalipoproteinaemia may reflect a compensatory response of the apoB gene in the hepatocyte due to failure of feedback of cholesterol entering the cell via the low density lipoprotein–LDL receptor pathway.

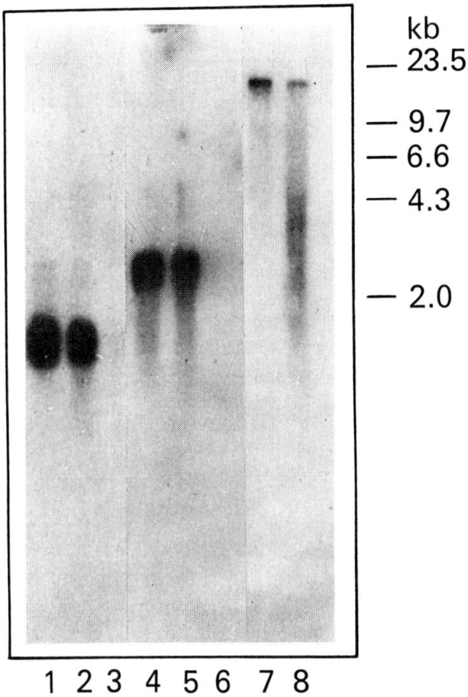

Fig. 10 Northern blot analysis of liver mRNA from a normal control (1, 4, 7) and an abetalipoproteinaemic patient (2, 5, 8). Lanes 3 and 6 were control lanes without DNA. Lanes 1–3, 4–6 and 7, 8 were hybridized with cDNA probes specific for apoA-I, albumin, and apoB100.

6 Summary

During the last year, major advances have developed in our understanding of the covalent structure and function of apoB48 and apoB100. The cloning and structural analysis of human apoB100 represents the culmination of two decades of research on apoB100, research that was often frustrating and difficult owing to the insolubility of apoB100 in aqueous solutions. The use of molecular biology techniques resolved one of the most recalcitrant problems in the lipoprotein field, the covalent structure of apoB100. The elucidation of the premature stop codon mechanism for the biosynthesis of apoB48 is of particular interest since it represents a new novel mechanism for the synthesis of two proteins from a single gene. The modulation of the RNA editing mechanism by diet, hormones and other ligands will be a major focus of research in the future,

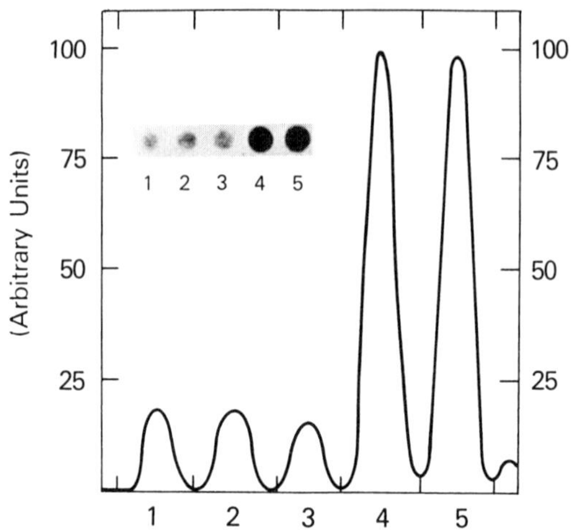

Fig. 11 Dot blot quantitation of hepatic apoB mRNA from three control subjects (1–3) and two probands with abetalipoproteinaemia (4, 5). The inset illustrates the dot blots from the five subjects, and the dot blots scanned with a laser densitometric scanner are illustrated in the lower panel.

and will undoubtedly provide new insights into the control of apolipoprotein gene regulation.

References

Bassen, F. A. and Kornzweig, A. L. (1950). Malformations of the erythrocytes in a case of atypical retinitis pigmentosa. *Blood* **5**, 381.

Blackhart, B. D., Ludwig, E. M., Pierolli, V. R., Caiati, L., Onasch, M. A., Wallis, S. C., Powell, L., Pease, R., Knott, T. J., Chu, M. L., Mahley, R. W., Scott, J., McCarthy, B. J. and Levy-Wilson, B. (1986). Structure of the human apolipoprotein B gene. *J. Biol. Chem.* **261**, 15264–15368.

Brown, M. S. and Goldstein, J. L. (1986). A receptor-mediated pathway for cholesterol homeostasis. *Science* **232**, 34–47.

Chen, S. H., Yang, C. Y., Chen, P. F., Setzer, D., Tanimura, M., Li, W. H., Gotto, A. M. and Chan, L. (1986). The complete cDNA and amino acid sequence of human apolipoprotein B-100. *J. Biol. Chem.* **261**, 12918–12921.

Chen, S. H., Habib, G., Yang, C.-Y., Gu, Z.-W., Lee, B. R., Weng, S.-A., Silberman, S. R., Cai, S.-J, Deslypere, J. P., Rosseneu, M., Gotto, A. M., Li, W. H. and Chan, L. (1987). Apolipoprotein B-48 is the product of a messenger RNA with an organ-specific in-frame stop codon. *Science* **238**, 363–366.

Cladaras, C., Hadzopoulou-Cladaras, M., Nolte, R. T., Atkinson, D. and Zannis, V. I. (1986). The complete sequence and structural analysis of human apolipoprotein B-100: relationship between apoB-100 and apoB-48 forms. *EMBO J.* **5**, 3495–3508.

Curtis, L. K. and Edgington, T. S. (1982). Immunochemical heterogeneity of human plasma apolipoprotein B. I. Apolipoprotein B binding of mouse hybridoma antibodies. *J. Biol. Chem.* **257**, 15213–15221.

Dullaart, R., Speelberg, B., Schuurman, H. J., Milne, R. W., Havekes, L. M., Marcel, Y. L., Geuze, H. J., Hulshof, M. M. and Erkelens, D. W. (1986). Epitopes of apoB100 and B48 in both liver and intestine. *J. Clin. Invest.* **78**, 1379–1404.

Edge, S. B., Hoeg, J. M., Schneider, P. D. and Brewer, H. B. (1985). Apolipoprotein B synthesis in humans: liver synthesizes only apolipoprotein B-100. *Metabolism* **34**, 726–730.

Elovson, J., Huang, Y. O., Baker, N. and Kannan, R. (1981). Apolipoprotein B is structurally and metabolicly heterogeneous in the rat. *Proc. Natl Acad. Sci. USA* **78**, 157–161.

Glickman, R. M., Rogers, M. and Glickman, J. N. (1986). Apolipoprotein B synthesis by human liver and intestine *in vitro*. *Proc. Natl Acad. Sci. USA* **83**, 5296–5300.

Hardman, D. A. and Kane, J. P. (1986). Isolation and characterisation of apolipoprotein B-48. *Meth. Enzym.* **128**, 262–272.

Herbert, P. N., Assmann, G., Gotto, A. M. and Fredrickson, D. S. (1983). In *The Metabolic Basis of Inherited Diseases* (ed. J. B. Stanbury, J. B. Wyngaarden, D. S. Fredrickson, J. L. Goldstein and M. S. Brown), pp. 589–621. McGraw-Hill, New York.

Higuchi, K., Monge, J. C., Lee, N., Law, S. W. and Brewer, H. B. (1987). The human apoB-100 gene: apoB-100 is encoded by a single copy gene in the human genome. *Biochem. Biophys. Res. Commun.* **144**, 1332–1339.

Higuchi, K., Hospattankar, A. V., Law, S. W., Meglin, N., Cortright, J. and Brewer, H. B. (1988). *Proc. Natl Acad. Sci. USA* (in press).

Hoeg, J. M., Svvudov, D. D., Law, S. W., Demosky, J. F., Meng, M. S. Repin, V. S., Smimov, V. N. and Brewer, H. B. (1987). Adult human intestine synthesizes and secretes apolipoprotein B-100. *Atherosclerosis* **7**, 491a.

Hospattankar, A. V., Higuchi, K., Law, S. W., Meglin, N. and Brewer, H. B. (1987). Identification of a novel in-frame translational stop codon in human intestine apoB mRNA. *Biochem. Biophys. Res. Commun.* **148**, 279–285.

Kane, J. P. (1983). Apolipoprotein B: structural and metabolic heterogeneity. *Ann. Rev. Physiol.* **45**, 637–650.

Kane, J. P., Hardman, D. A. and Paulus, H. E. (1980). Heterogeneity of apolipoprotein B: isolation of a new species from human chylomicrons. *Proc. Natl Acad. Sci. USA* **77**, 2465–2469.

Knott, T. J., Pearse, R. J., Powell, L. M., Wallis, S. C., Rall, S. C., Innerarity, T. L., Blackhart, B., Taylor, W. H., Marcel, Y., Milne, R., Johnson, D., Fuller, M., Lusis, A. J., McCarthy, B. J., Mahley, R. W., Levy-Wilson, B. and Scott, J. (1986). Complete protein sequence and identification of structural domains of human apolipoprotein B. *Nature* **323**, 734–738.

Krishnaiah, K. V., Walker, L. F., Borensztajn, J., Schonfeld, G. and Getz, G. S. (1980). Apolipoprotein B variant derived from rat intestine. *Proc. Natl Acad. Sci. USA* **77**, 3806–3810.

Lackner, K. J., Monge, J. C., Gregg, R. E., Hoeg, J. M., Triche, T. J., Law, S. W. and Brewer, H. B. (1986). Analysis of the apolipoprotein B gene and messenger ribonucleic acid in abetalipoproteinaemia. *J. Clin. Invest.* **78**, 1707–1712.

Law, S. W., Lackner, K. J., Hospattankar, A. V., Anchors, J. M., Sakaguchi, A. Y., Naylor, S. L. and Brewer, H. B. (1985). Human apolipoprotein B-100: cloning, analysis of liver mRNA, and assignment of the gene to chromosome 2. *Proc. Natl Acad. Sci. USA* **82**, 8340–8344.

Law, S. W., Grant, S. M., Higuchi, K., Hospattankar, A., Lackner, K., Lee, N. and Brewer, H. B. (1986a). Human liver apolipoprotein B-100 cDNA: complete nucleic acid and derived amino acid sequence. *Proc. Natl Acad. Sci. USA* **83**, 8142–8146.

Law, S. W., Lackner, K. J., Monge, J. C., Hospattankar, A. V., Lee, N., Hoeg, J. M. and Brewer, H. B. (1986b). Cloning of the human apolipoprotein (apo)B: insights on biosynthesis and metabolism of triglyceride rich lipoproteins. *DNA* **5**, 81 (abstract).

Law, S. W., Monge, J. C., Lackner, K. J., Hospattankar, A. V., Grant, S. M., Higuchi, K., Gregg, R. E., Lee, N. and Brewer, H. B. (1986c). In *Cardiovascular Disease 86. Molecular and Cellular Mechanisms and Preventive Treatment. Sixth International Washington Spring Symposium* (ed. L. L. Gallo) (in press).

Lee, D. M., Koren, E., Singh, S. and Mok, T. (1984). Presence of B-100 in rat mesenteric chyle. *Biochem. Biophys. Res. Commun.* **123**, 1149–1156.

Malloy, M. J., Kane, J. P., Hardman, D. A., Hamilton, R. L. and Dalal, K. B. (1981). Normotriglyceridemic abetalipoproteinaemia. Absence of the B-100 apolipoprotein. *J. Clin. Invest.* **67**, 1441–1450.

Marcel, Y. L., Hoegue, M., Theolis, R. and Milne, R. W. (1982). Mapping of antigenic determinants of human apolipoprotein B using monoclonal antibodies against low density lipoproteins. *J. Biol. Chem.* **257**, 13165–13168.

Powell, L. W., Wallis, S. C., Pease, R. J., Edwards, Y. H., Knott, T. J. and Scott, J. (1987). A novel form of tissue-specific RNA processing produces apolipoprotein-B48 in intestine. *Cell* **50**, 831–840.

Sparks, C. E., Hnatiuk, O. and Marsh, J. B. (1981). Hepatic and intestinal contribution of two forms of apolipoprotein B to plasma lipoprotein fractions in the rat. *Can. J. Biochem.* **49**, 693–699.

Wu, A. L. and Windmuller, H. G. (1981). Variant forms of plasma apolipoprotein B. Hepatic and intestinal biosynthesis and heterogeneous metabolism in the rat. *J. Biol. Chem.* **256**, 3615–3618.

4

Apolipoprotein B: A Novel Mechanism for Deriving Two Proteins from One Gene

JAMES SCOTT, SIMON C. WALLIS, RICHARD J. PEASE, TIMOTHY J. KNOTT and LYN POWELL

Division of Molecular Medicine, MRC Clinical Research Centre, Harrow, UK

Summary

Evidence from antibody and peptide mapping, protein sequencing and amino acid composition studies suggests that intestinal apoB48 is colinear with the amino terminal half of hepatic apoB100. To investigate the mechanism of apoB48 production, we examined cDNA clones from human and rabbit small intestine. All clones contained a single C → T base difference from the hepatic sequence, resulting in a translational stop at codon 2153. Amplification by the polymerase chain reaction of cDNA from human and rabbit small intestine, rabbit liver and the human hepatoma cell line HepG2 showed that the stop codon was only present in intestinal mRNA. Enterocyte genomic DNA did not contain the stop codon. We suggest that a co- or post-transcriptional C → U change may result in the production of apoB48, which represents the amino terminal 2152 amino acids of apoB100. This is the first example of tissue specific modification of a single mRNA nucleotide resulting in two different proteins from the same primary transcript.

1 Introduction

Apolipoprotein (apo) B circulates in the blood in two closely related forms as obligatory constituents of the plasma lipoproteins (Kane, 1983). ApoB100 (molecular weight 512 kilodaltons (kD)) is synthesized in the liver and is necessary for the assembly of very low density lipoproteins (VLDL), the

HYPERLIPIDAEMIA AND ATHEROSCLEROSIS
ISBN 0.12.675645-7

vehicles for the transport of endogenously synthesized triglyceride. It is also the ligand that mediates the clearance of low density lipoprotein (LDL) cholesterol from the circulation by the LDL receptor pathway (Brown and Goldstein, 1986). The other form of apoB is synthesized by the intestine and designated apoB48 on the centile system because it is roughly half the size of apoB100. It is essential for the chylomicron formation and the absorption and transport of dietary cholesterol and triglyceride.

The entire amino acid sequence of apoB100 has been deduced from cDNA clones (Knott *et al.*, 1986a; Cladaras *et al.*, 1986; Law *et al.*, 1986; Yang *et al.*, 1986; Olofsson *et al.*, 1987), and intron–exon organization of the apoB gene has been determined (Blackhart *et al.*, 1986; Carlsson *et al.*, 1986; Higuchi *et al.*, 1987; Wagener *et al.*, 1987). Human apoB100 mRNA is 14 121 nucleotides in length and encodes a 4563 amino acid precursor from which a 27 residue signal peptide is cleaved. The corresponding gene spans only 43 kilobases (kb) and comprises 29 exons. Over half of the coding sequence is carried by the 7572 base pair (bp) exon 26.

Available evidence from antibody and peptide mapping, protein sequencing and amino acid composition studies suggests that apoB48 represents the amino terminal half of apoB100 (Hardman and Kane, 1986; Marcel *et al.*, 1987; Olofsson *et al.*, 1987). Several lines of evidence predict the region of apoB100 in which the apoB48 molecule is likely to end. Epitopes for monoclonal antibodies against apoB have been mapped on apoB100/β-galactosidase fusion proteins and proteolytic fragments of apoB100 (Knott *et al.*, 1986a; Marcel *et al.*, 1987). All monoclonal antibodies mapping to the amino terminal half of apoB100 also react with apoB48. A further group do not recognize apoB48 (Knott *et al.*, 1986a; Marcel *et al.*, 1987) and have been localized to the carboxy terminal half of apoB100. There are no apoB48-specific monoclonal antibodies. Furthermore apoB48 does not interact with the LDL receptor (Hui *et al.*, 1984), and the LDL receptor binding domain of apoB100 resides in the carboxy terminal one-third of the protein (Knott *et al.*, 1986a; Marcel *et al.*, 1987). These results therefore point to apoB48 being colinear with the amino terminal half of apoB100 and imply that it will terminate between residues 1700 and 2600. This is consistent with the observed size of apoB48 on SDS–polyacrylamide gels, assuming that it has a similar glycosylation pattern to apoB100 (Knott *et al.*, 1986a; Yang *et al.*, 1986). In addition, the amino acid composition of apoB48 is similar to that of apoB100 between residues 1 and approximately 2200 (Hardman and Kane, 1986). Therefore the carboxy terminal of apoB48 is likely to be within exon 26 (7572 bp) of the apoB gene.

Three mechanisms may explain the origin of apoB48.

(1) ApoB100 and apoB48 could be encoded by different genes. This has

been largely excluded by the analysis of the gene structure (Blackhart *et al.*, 1986; Carlsson *et al.*, 1986; Higuchi *et al.*, 1987; Wagener *et al.*, 1987). Further strong evidence that both apoB proteins are products of a single gene is provided by the work of Young *et al.* (1986), who demonstrated that the same protein polymorphism was present in both apoB100 and apoB48 in 23 subjects examined.

(2) ApoB48 may be produced by co-translational or post-translational proteolytic processing of apoB100. In support of this, monoclonal antibodies have been used to demonstrate apoB100-specific epitopes in human intestinal cells, and a large form of apoB is reported to be secreted into intestinal lymph and processed to a form similar in size to apoB48 in the rat. However, pulse-chase and polysome run-off translation experiments provide no evidence of proteolytic processing (Reuben and Elovson, 1985; Demmer *et al.*, 1986; Glickman *et al.*, 1986).

(3) Differential processing of a primary nuclear RNA transcript could produce distinct mRNAs, coding for apoB100 and apoB48 in the liver and intestine respectively. Several groups have reported northern blots showing two apoB mRNAs in the small intestine; an abundant 14.5 kb mRNA and an mRNA of approximately 7.0 kb that hybridizes with 5′ but not 3′ apoB100 cDNA probes (Deeb *et al.*, 1985; Mehrabian *et al.*, 1985; Cladaras *et al.*, 1986; Olofsson *et al.*, 1987). However, the detection of the small transcript has been inconsistent, and this has led to the suggestion that it may be a degradation product of the larger mRNA (Mehrabian *et al.*, 1985).

In this study we set out to investigate the molecular basis for the production of apoB48 by examining clones from human and rabbit small intestinal cDNA libraries and comparison of these with the sequences of hepatic cDNAs and genomic DNA.

2 Results

2.1 ApoB cDNA

From maps of monoclonal antibodies, the region between 5 and 8 kb from the 5′ end of the mRNA was delineated as the predicted end of apoB48 (Fig. 1).

Clones covering the entire 14.1 kb coding region were isolated from a human mid-jejunal cDNA library using probes from the whole length of apoB100 cDNA. Detailed restriction mapping of cDNA clones failed to demonstrate any differences, apart from previously identified common polymorphisms (Blackhart *et al.*, 1986), between the hepatic (Knott *et al.*,

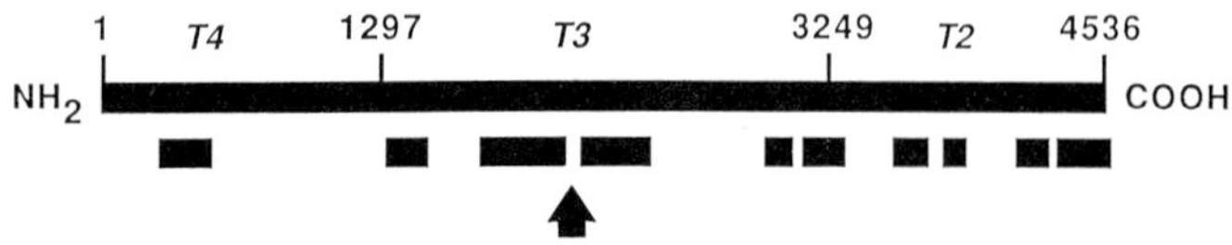

Fig. 1 Epitope map of monoclonal antibodies binding to apoB. The predicted end of apoB48 is indicated by the arrow. Boxes to the left of the arrow represent epitopes common to apoB100 and apoB48, and to the right of this arrow are epitopes for monoclonal antibodies that are specific for apoB100. The sizes of the thrombin cleavage products T4, T3 and T2 of apoB100 are shown. (Cardin *et al.*, 1984.)

1986b) and intestinal mRNA except in the region where we predict apoB48 to end. In all 10 intestinal cDNA clones (Fig. 2a) that included nucleotide 6666 of the apoB100 mRNA sequence an in-frame stop codon (TAA) was found after codon 2152. Amino acid 2153 is glutamine (CAA) in all five published apoB100 cDNA sequences and in all three published gene sequences. In addition, three of the human intestinal cDNA clones from this region were polyadenylated at different positions downstream of the termination codon (Table 1). This confirms the presence of a 7 kb apoB mRNA species in human

Table 1 Positions of potential polyadenylation signals.

	Sequence		Position of of Poly (A)	
Human clone				10 ↓ 20 ↓ 30 ↓
Hu 1	ACCAAA	9 bp	6910	gatacaagaaaaactgcagcagcttaagag
Hu 2	AATAAA	19 bp	7080	aacacTTTGTTataaatcTTaTTGGGaTT
Hu 3	TATAAA	24 bp	7121	gagaaaatcaatgccttcagagccaaagtc
Rabbit clone				10 ↓ 20 ↓ 30 ↓
Rab 1 + 2	AATTAA	17 bp	6774	atcatatccGTGcacatTTAATTaaatcaa
Rab 3	AATTAA	15 bp	6815	taTTTGTTTaTTGaagctaTTGaTTTTaac
Rab 4	AATAAA	19 bp	7080	aatacTTTGTTataaataTTaTTGaaaaTT

The positions of the potential polyadenylation signals relative to the site of polyadenylation in the human and rabbit cDNA clones are shown. There are three different hexamers that may act as polyadenylation signals in addition to the canonical AATAAA. One of these, AATTAA, has been previously recognized as a functional hexamer (Birnstiel *et al.*, 1985). The other two (Hu 1 and Hu 3) have not been previously implicated in polyadenylation. However, the only other sequences 5′ to these sites that could be used as signals for polyadenylations are AACAAA (61 bp 5′ of the site used in Hu 1) and AATAAA (60 bp 5′ of Hu 3). Polyadenylation can occur 42 bp downstream of a polyadenylation signal (Kessler *et al.*, 1987). Sequences within the 30 bp 3′ to the polyadenylation site, possibly involved in polyadenylation, are in capital letters. These include an inverted repeat TTAATT of the polyadenylation signal in the rabbit clones polyadenylated at position 6774. "G/T cluster" sequences implicated by Birnstiel *et al.* (1985) are also marked. Hu 1 and Hu 3 do not possess any homologous inverted repeats or G/T sequences 3′ to the polyadenylation site.

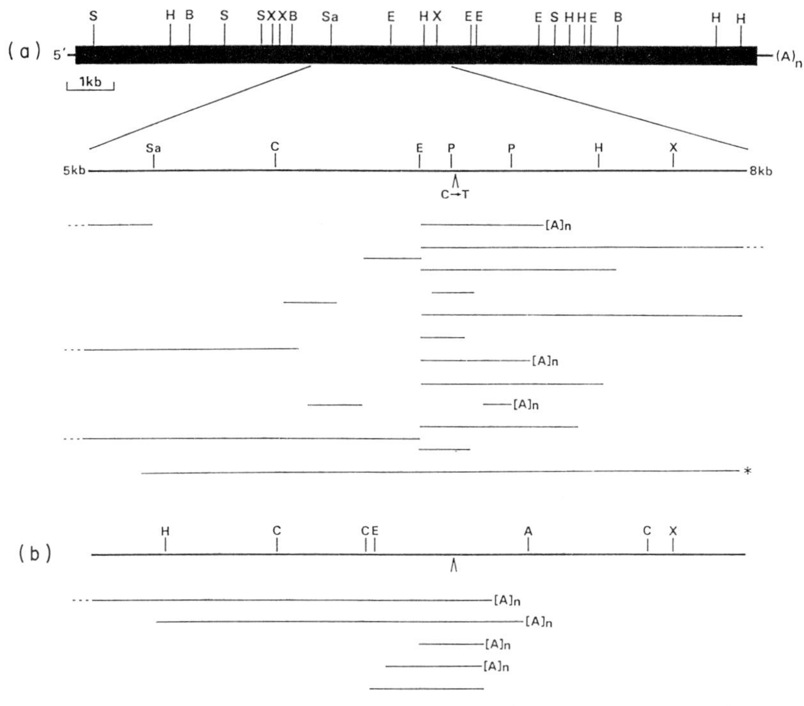

Fig. 2 (a) Restriction map of apoB cDNA. Abbreviations: A, AccI; Sa, SalI; H, HindIII; B, BamHI; X, XbaI; S, SstI; E, EcoRI; C, ClaI; P, PstI. The region between 5 and 8 kb is expanded. The position of the C to T change resulting in the introduction of the in-frame stop codon is marked with an arrow. The cDNA clones that were isolated, mapped and sequenced from the first human jejunal library are shown, including the three with poly (A) tails. The single large clone from the second small intestinal library is marked with an asterisk. (b) Restriction map of rabbit small intestinal cDNA clones. The position of the stop codon is indicated by the arrow. (From Powell *et al.* (1987) *Cell* **50**, 831–840.)

intestine. The remaining cDNA clones were not polyadenylated and contained sequences extending up to 1.4 kb downstream of the stop codon (Fig. 2a).

To eliminate the possibility of cloning artefacts or of mutation in this subject, we examined clones from a different human jejunal library and from a rabbit small intestinal library (Hunziker *et al.*, 1986); the rabbit is also known to produce both the 14.5 kb and the 7 kb apoB mRNAs (Cladaras *et al.*, 1986). The stop codon was present at the same position in the only cDNA clone isolated from the second human intestinal library that carried sequences in the region of interest (Fig. 2a). In the rabbit all six small intestinal cDNA clones (Fig. 2b) from the comparable region also contained a stop codon (TAA) replacing the normal glutamine codon (CAA) at the identical position. Poly

```
2088    LeuGlyLysLeuProGlnGlnAlaAsnAspTyrLeuAsnSerPheAsnTrpGluArgGln
6471    CTGGGAAAACTCCCACAGCAAGCTAATGATTATCTGAATTCATTCAATTGGGAGAGACAA

1471    CTGGGAAAACTCCCACAGCAAGTTAATGATTATCTGAGTACATTCAATTGGGAGAGACAA
491     LeuGlyLysLeuProGlnGlnValAsnAspTyrLeuSerThrPheAsnTrpGluArgGln

2108    ValSerHisAlaLysGluLysLeuThrAlaLeuThrLysLysTyrArgIleThrGluAsn
6531    GTTTCACATGCCAAGGAGAAACTGACTGCTCTCACAAAAAAGTATAGAATTACAGAAAAT

1531    GTTTCCAGTGCCAAGGAGAAACTAACTACTTTCACAAAAAATTATAAAATTACAGAGAAT
511     ValSerSerAlaLysGluLysLeuThrThrPheThrLysAsnTyrLysIleThrGluAsn

2128    AspIleGlnIleAlaLeuAspAspAlaLysIleAsnPheAsnGluLysLeuSerGlnLeu
6591    GATATACAAATTGCATTAGATGATGCCAAAATCAACTTTAATGAAAAACTATCTCAACTG

1591    GATATACAAACTGCATTGGATAATGCCAAAATCAACTTAAATGAAAAACTGTCTCAACTT
531     AspIleGlnThrAlaLeuAspAsnAlaLysIleAsnLeuAsnGluLysLeuSerGlnLeu

2148    GlnThrTyrMetIle***
6651    CAGACATATATGATATAATTTGATCAGTATATTAAAGATAGTTATGATTTACATGATTTG

1651    CAGACATATGTGATATAATTTGATCAGTATATTAAAGATAATTTTGATCTACATGATTTT
551     GlnThrTyrValIle***

6711    AAAATAGCTATTGCTAATATTATTGATGAAATCATTGAAAAATTAAAAAGTCTTGATGAG

1717    AAAATAGCTATAGCTAGTATTATAGATCAAATCATGGAAAAATTAAAAATTCTTGATGAA


6771    CACTATCATATCCGTGTAAATTTAGTAAAAACAATCCATGATCTACATTTGTTTATTGAA

1777    CGTTATCATATCGGTGCACATTTAATTAAATCAATCCATAATTTATATTTGTTTATTGAA
           *                                       *
6831    AATATTGATTTTAACAAAAGTGGAAGTAGTACTGCATCCTGGATTCAAAATGTGGATACT

1837    GCTATTGATTTTAACAAAATTGGAAGTAGTACTGCATCTTGGATTCAAAATGTGGATACC

                          *
6891    AAGTACCAAATCAGAATCCAGATACAAGAAAAACTGCAGCAGCTTAAGAGACACATACAG

1897    AAGTATCAAGTCAGAATCTGGATACAAGAAATATTGCAACAGTTTAAGACACAGATTCAG

6951    AATATAGACATCCAGCACCTAGCTGGAAAGTTAAAACAACACATTGAGGCTATTGATGTT

1957    AATACAAACATCCCATACCTGGCTGAAAAACTGAAACAACAGATTGAGGCTATTGATGTC

7011    AGAGTGCTTTTAGATCAATTGGGAACTACAATTTCATTTGAAAGAATAAATGATGTTCTT

2017    AGAGTGCTTTTAGATCAATTGAGAACTACAATTCCATTTCGTATAATAAAGGACATTATT

                *                                         *
7071    GAGCATGTCAAACACTTTGTTATAAATCTTATTGGGGATTTTGAAGTAGCTGAGAAAATC

2077    GAACATTTCAAATACTTTGTTATAAATATTATTGAAAATTTTGAAGTAATTGACAAAATC
                *
```

Fig. 3 Comparison of the DNA and protein sequence from the human and rabbit small intestine cDNA. The human nucleotide sequence starts at position 6741 (amino acid 2088). 3 kb of rabbit sequence has been determined. The numbering of the homologous rabbit sequence starts at one; the displayed sequence begins at 491. Amino acid differences are underlined for the rabbit. The positions at which poly (A) tails were added are marked (*); see also Table 1. (From Powell *et al.* (1987) *Cell* **50**, 831–840.)

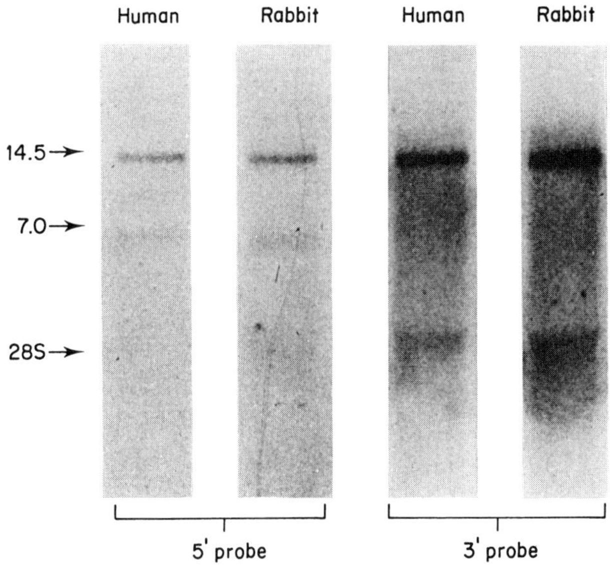

Fig. 4 Northern blots of human and rabbit total intestinal RNA. Lanes 1 (human) and 2 (rabbit) were hybridized with a probe containing the 5′ 520 bp of apoB100 cDNA. Lanes 3 (human) and 4 (rabbit) were hybridized with a 2 kb fragment containing the 3′ end of the apoB100 cDNA. The 14.5 kb and 7 kb intestinal apoB mRNAs and the position of 28S ribosomal RNA are arrowed. (From Powell *et al.* (1987) *Cell* **50**, 831–840.)

(A) tails were also found in the rabbit clones, but the sites of polyadenylation were different from those occurring in the human intestine (Table 1). A comparison of the rabbit sequence to that of the human (Fig. 3) shows 85.8% homology between nucleotides 5000–8000 and 78.7% homology at the protein level. The DNA sequence conservation increases to 90% between nucleotides 6566–6766 spanning the stop codon.

Northern blot analysis of intestinal mRNA from both rabbit and human tissue (Fig. 4) confirms the presence of two apoB messages. Hybridization with probes derived from the 3′ half of apoB100 detects a single species of approximately 14.5 kb, equivalent to the 14 121 base message characterized from the liver cDNA libraries (Knott *et al.*, 1986b). However, hybridization with probes from the 5′ end of apoB100, the region encoding apoB48, detects the large message and a smaller, 7 kb, species.

Owing to the small size of the intestinal cDNA clones, it is not certain that those lacking a poly (A) tail derive from the 14.5 kb transcript. It is important to determine whether the 14.5 kb mRNA contains the stop codon and encodes apoB48 or whether it encodes apoB100. To study this, the relevant mRNA

Table 2 Oligodeoxynucleotide used for amplification and differential screening.

			Position of 5′ nucleotide
BSTOP	TACTGATCAAATTATATCA	19mer.	6679
BGLN	TACTGATCAAATTGTATCA	19mer.	6679
PCR5	CTGAATTCATTCAATTGGGAGAGACAAG	28mer.	6504
PCR8	CGGATATATAGTGCTCATCAAGAC	25mer.	6784
PCR9	GCACGGATATCATAACGTTCATC	23mer.	6787
PCR10	CCATGATTTGATCTATAATACTAG	24mer.	6747
PCR11	CCAATCAGAAATGTAGGTGACAAG	24mer.	7787

sequences were enzymatically amplified by the polymerase chain reaction (PCR) (Saiki *et al.*, 1985) and screened with synthetic oligonucleotides designed to detect the single C to T base change.

RNA was isolated from terminal ileum from a third human subject, rabbit liver, rabbit jejunum, and the hepatoma cell line HepG2 (known to produce apoB100). First strand cDNA synthesis was primed either with oligo (dT) or synthetic oligonucleotides PCR9 and PCR11 (Table 2). Use of oligo (dT) and PCR9 ensures that sequences from both the 14.5 and 7.0 kb mRNAs are represented in the cDNA, whereas PCR11 directs synthesis of cDNA exclusively from the large transcript. Second strand synthesis was completed by the method of Gubler and Hoffmann (1983), and amplification was performed using specific primers as shown in Fig. 5. The amplified segment (281 bp)

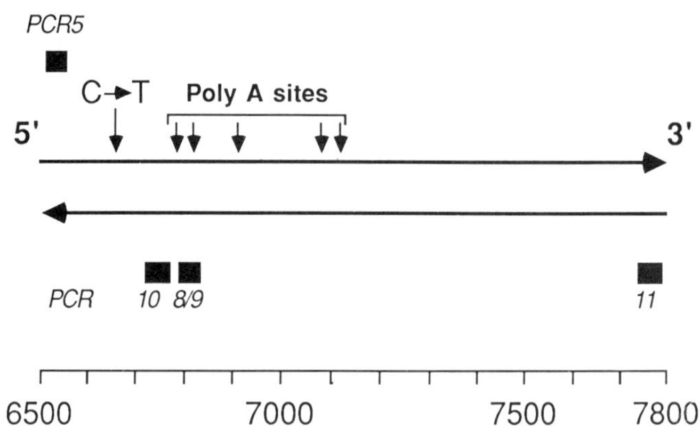

Fig. 5 Polymerase chain reaction. The positions of oligonucleotides (Table 2) used to amplify intestinal genomic and cDNA and to prime cDNA synthesis are shown. The position of the C to T change and polyadenylation sites (Table 1) are shown.

spans nucleotides 6504 to 6784 of the human mRNA and a corresponding region of the rabbit message. Amplified cDNAs were run on agarose gels then dried down and hybridized sequentially with oligonucleotide BGLN (TACTGATCAAATTGTATCA), which is specific for DNA containing a C at position 6666, and a second oligonucleotide, BSTOP (TACTGATCAAATTATATCA), which is specific for DNA containing the stop codon. Hybridization and washing conditions for both oligonucleotides were determined empirically (Fig. 6). In addition, serial 1 : 10 dilutions of the PCR reactions were dot-blotted onto Zetaprobe membranes (Fig. 6). HepG2 and rabbit liver cDNA PCR only hybridized with oligonucleotide BGLN. Rabbit small intestine cDNA PCR hybridized strongly with BSTOP oligonucleotide and only weakly with BGLN oligonucleotide. Human terminal ileum cDNA PCR hybridized strongly with BSTOP and very weakly with BGLN.

These observations indicate that both the 14.5 kb and 7.0 kb mRNAs from human ileum produce mainly apoB48 and very little, if any, apoB100. The same is true of rabbit jejunum. No transcripts containing the stop codon can be detected using this method in the RNA from rabbit liver or the human hepatoma cell line HepG2.

2.2 *ApoB gene*

One explanation for these results is that the apoB gene is duplicated such that one gene copy carrying the CAA sequence is transcribed in the liver and the second copy with the TAA sequence is transcribed in the small intestine. To examine the possibility that there may be two apoB genes, Southern blots of human genomic DNA were hybridized with a range of flanking and internal gene probes (Fig. 7). Each digest gives hybridizing fragments that are unique. Probes that detect the hypervariable region 3′ to the apoB gene (Knott *et al.*, 1986c) reveal only two alleles in each individual. The conclusion must be that either there is a very large duplication unit (>50 kb) undergoing extensive gene conversion or there is only one apoB gene.

2.3 *Exon shuffling is not involved in the production of apoB 48*

An alternative explanation for the appearance of a stop codon in intestinal message is duplication of part or the whole of exon 26 coupled with tissue-specific exon shuffling. Probes taken from each end of exon 26 and from the region containing the stop codon hybridize to unique fragments on Southern

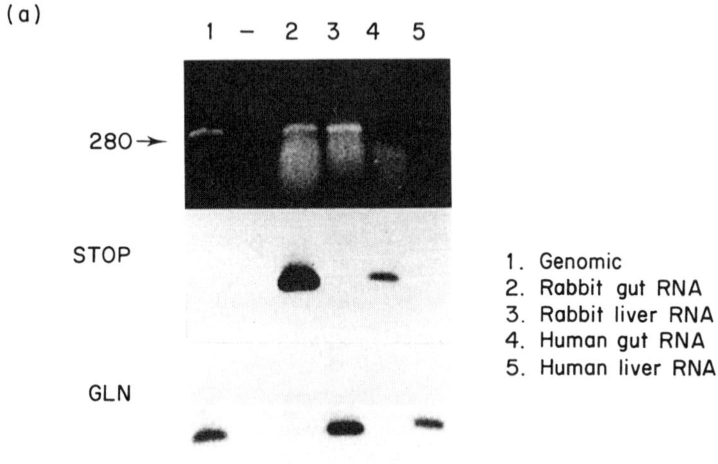

Fig. 6 (a) 1% agarose gel of cDNA and enterocyte genomic DNA PCR reactions. Lane 1, rabbit enterocyte amplified genomic DNA. Lane 2, rabbit small intestine PCR9 primed. Lane 3, rabbit liver total RNA PCR9 primed. Lane 4, human terminal ileum poly $(A)^+$ PCR11 primed. Lane 5, HepG2 poly $(A)^+$ oligo (dT) primed. Human cDNA was amplified with PCR5 and PCR8. Rabbit cDNA and enterocyte genomic DNA were amplified with PCR5 and PCR10. The intense ethidium staining at the bottom of the gel is due to the carrier tRNA. The specifically amplified segment is approximately 280 bp long. Southern blot of gel hybridized sequentially with BSTOP (−) and BGLN (+). Lane 1, rabbit enterocyte amplified genomic DNA. Lane 2, rabbit small intestine PCR9 primed cDNA. Lane 3, rabbit liver PCR9 primed cDNA. Lane 4, human terminal ileum PCR11 primed cDNA. Lane 5, HepG2 oligo (dT) primed cDNA. Exposure time was 12 hours, with an intensifying screen at −70°C. (b) Dot blot of PCR reactions hybridized with BGLN (+) or BSTOP (−). From top to bottom the samples are: pα20C plasmid; rabbit small intestinal cDNA containing T at 6666; pSB9 plasmid; human genomic subclone with C at 6666; rabbit enterocyte genomic DNA; human terminal ileum cDNA primed with PCR11; human terminal ileum cDNA primed with oligo (dT); HepG2 cDNA primed with oligo (dT). Exposure time was 6 hours, with an intensifying screen at −70°C. (c) Discriminating washing conditions: digests of pα20C (T,STOP) and pSB9 (C,GLN) were transferred to Zetaprobe membranes and strips were hybridized with oligonucleotide BSTOP or BGLN at 42°C and washed at room temperature in (6×) SSC until background was minimal. Then the strips were incubated for 10 minutes at the temperatures shown and exposed at room temperature for 2 hours. (From Powell *et al.* (1987) *Cell* **50**, 831–840.)

(b)

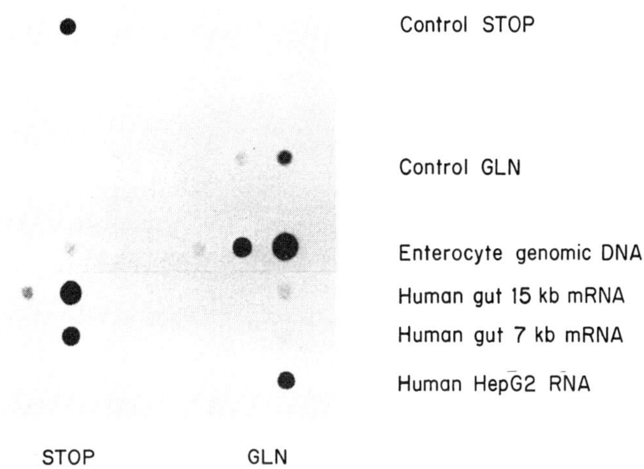
Control STOP
Control GLN
Enterocyte genomic DNA
Human gut 15 kb mRNA
Human gut 7 kb mRNA
Human HepG2 RNA
STOP
GLN

(c)

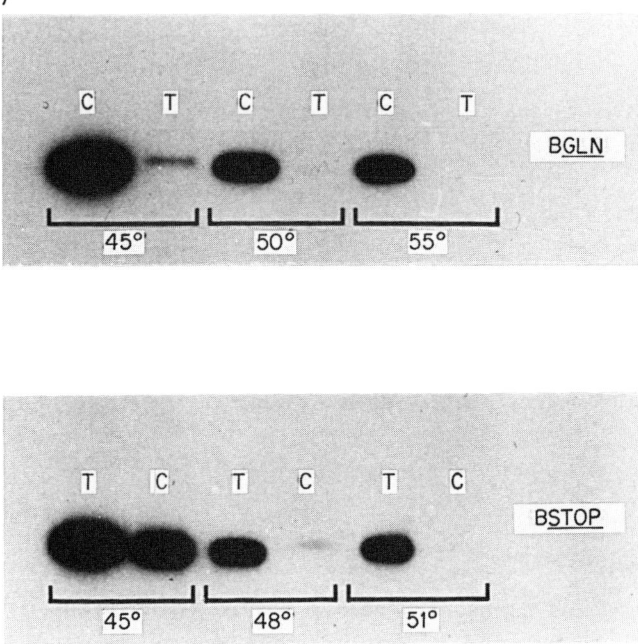
C
T
C
T
C
T
BGLN
45°
50°
55°
T
C
T
C
T
C
BSTOP
45°
48°
51°

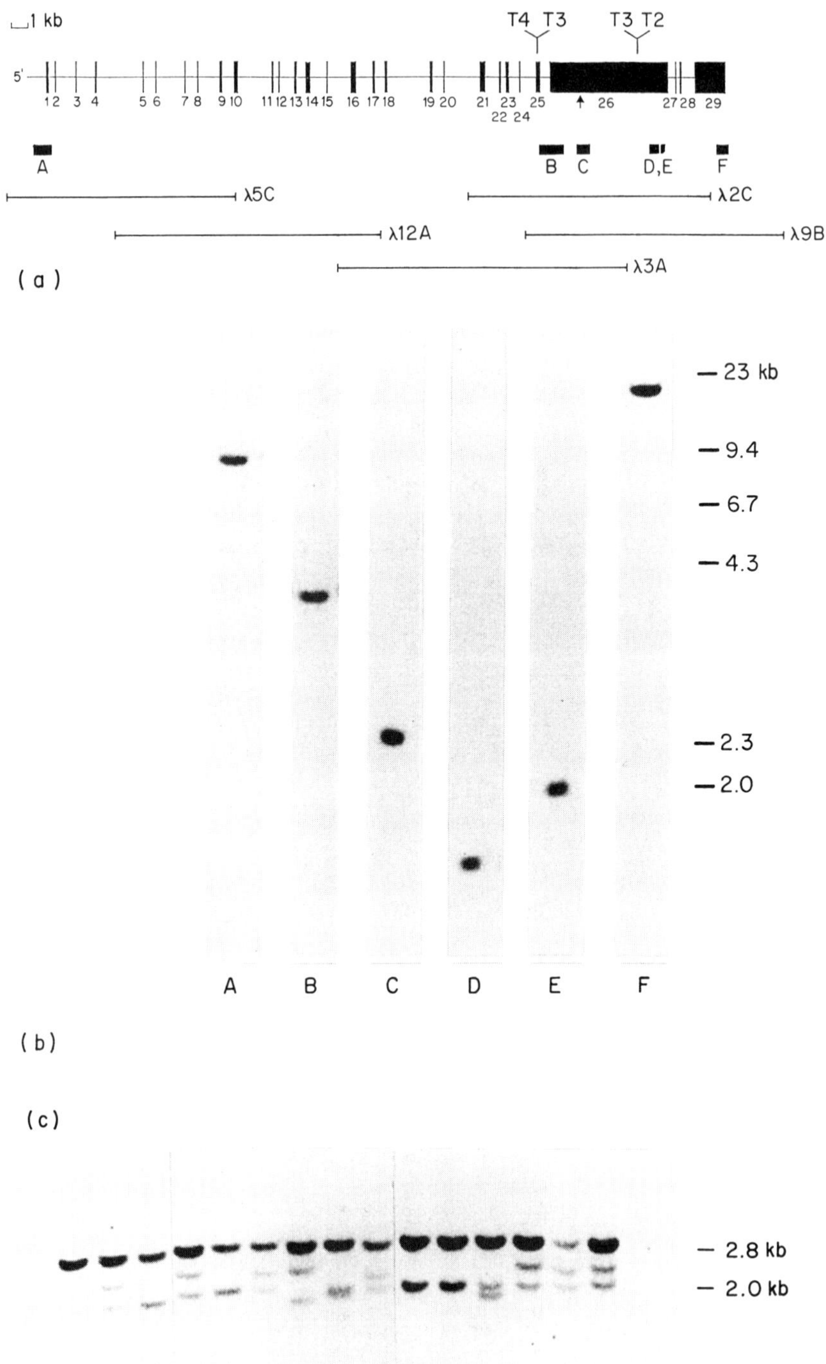
1 kb
T4 T3
T3 T2
5'
1 2 3 4 5 6 7 8 9 10 11 12 13 14 15 16 17 18 19 20 21 23 25 26 27 28 29
22 24
A
B C D,E F
λ5C
λ2C
λ12A
λ9B
λ3A
(a)
23 kb
9.4
6.7
4.3
2.3
2.0
A B C D E F
(b)
(c)
2.8 kb
2.0 kb

blots of human genomic DNA (Fig. 7). Exon 26 has been sequenced at least five times in its entirety from genomic clones by our own group and others (unpublished results and Blackhart *et al.*, 1986; Carlsson *et al.*, 1986; Wagener *et al.*, 1987). There is no evidence for duplication either of exon 26 or for small segments of it that might participate in alternative splicing. In the absence of gene duplication or exon shuffling, it is necessary to invoke either somatic mutation or RNA modification as mechanisms for the production of apoB48.

To investigate the possibility of somatic mutation of the apoB gene in intestinal tissue, we carried out localized amplification of a 280 bp region spanning the stop codon, using as the template rabbit enterocyte DNA. Enterocytes were prepared by the method of Peters and Shio (1976) and their purity was assessed by electron microscopy (Fig. 8a). At least 70% of the cell population had brush borders. The region was amplified using synthetic oligomers and the reaction run on an agarose gel. The 280 bp band was isolated and, after trimming the ends with Mung Bean nuclease, cloned into the Bluescript vector pKS+. One hundred colonies were picked, gridded on filters and screened with labelled oligonucleotides. Twelve hybridizing colonies were identified. Plasmid DNA was prepared from these clones, linearized with restriction enzymes (Fig. 8b) and blotted. Dot blots of uncloned amplified DNA were also prepared. Differential hybridization was carried out using the synthetic oligonucleotide probes specific for either C or T at position 6666 as described previously. Only the C-specific oligonucleotide hybridizes to the 12 intestinal genomic clones (Fig. 8c, d). Further analysis of these clones by DNA sequencing confirmed the presence of only the CAA codon in enterocyte genomic DNA. When dot blots of PCR-amplified enterocyte genomic DNA were hybridized with the BSTOP and BGLN oligonucleotides the signal obtained with BGLN was at least 100-fold greater than that obtained with BSTOP (Fig. 6c).

Fig. 7 (a) Intron–exon organization of the human apoB gene. The predicted end of apoB48 in exon 26 is indicated by the arrow. The sites of thrombin cleavage in the protein are shown. The solid bars indicate fragments used to probe genomic Southerns (see (b) and (c)). (b) Genomic Southern blots showing hybridization to unique restriction fragments flanking the apoB gene, exon 26 and the region containing the termination codon at nucleotide 6666. Human genomic DNA was digested, fractionated on agarose and transferred to nitrocellulose for hybridization with oligolabelled probes (see (a)). All lanes are EcoRI digests. (c) A 350 bp fragment containing the 3′ untranslated region and flanking sequences of the gene that detects 2 alleles of the 3′ hypervariable region. The length polymorphisms in the hypervariable region of 15 different individuals are shown after MspI digestion. The size differences are generally with ±200 bp. (From Powell *et al.* (1987) *Cell* **50**, 831–840.)

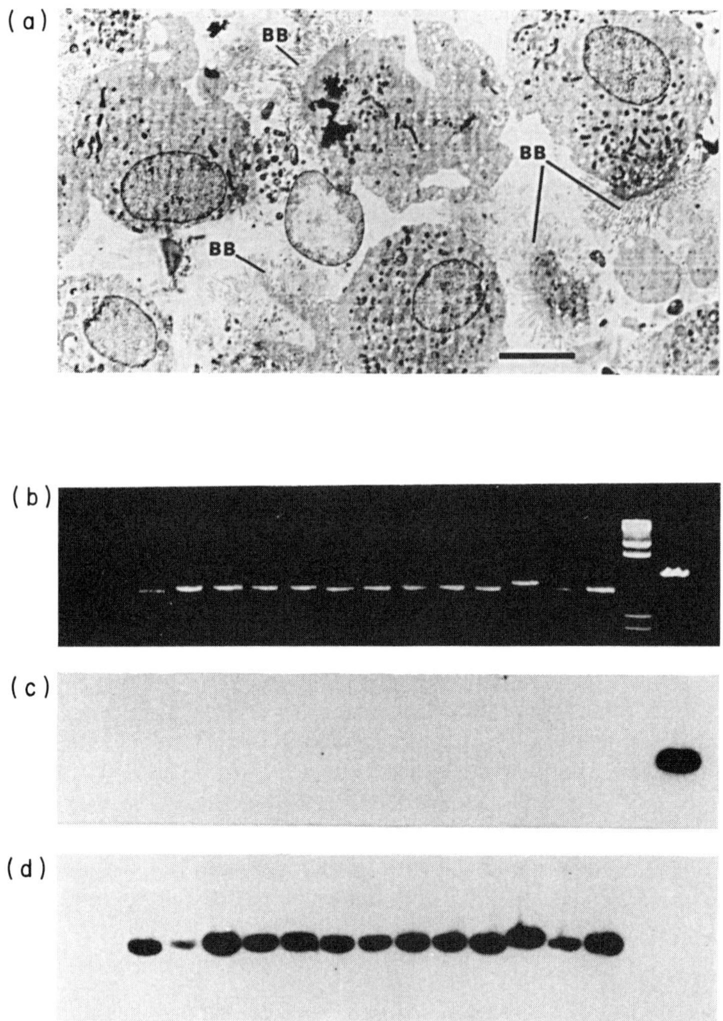

Fig. 8 (a) Electron micrograph of a rabbit enterocyte preparation used as the source of genomic DNA for PCR amplification. Brush borders (BB) are indicated. The scale bar represents 5 μm. (b) Ethidium bromide stained agarose gel of PCR amplified, genomic DNAs cloned in Bluescript pKS+. Plasmid DNA prepared by the boiling method (Holmes and Quigley, 1981) was linearized with HindIII, electrophoresed on 1% agarose and blotted on to nitrocellulose. (1) Cloned, human leukocyte DNA amplified with PCR5 and PCR8. (2)–(13) Twelve rabbit enterocyte clones. Amplification was with PCR5 and PCR9. (14) Markers; Lambda DNA digested with HindIII. (15) Plasmid pα20c; a 1.7 kb rabbit intestinal cDNA carrying the stop codon cloned in pUC18. (c) Gel (b) blotted and hybridized with oligonucleotide BSTOP and washed as described in the legend to Fig. 6. Only the rabbit intestinal cDNA control plasmid hybridizes with TAA. (d) The same filter re-hybridized with oligonucleotide BGLN, showing that human leukocyte and rabbit enterocyte DNA contain the CAA sequence. This was confirmed by DNA sequencing. (From Powell *et al.* (1987) *Cell* **50**, 831–840.)

3 Discussion

To examine the mechanism of formation of intestinal apoB, we compared the nucleotide sequences of human and rabbit intestinal cDNAs and genomic DNA with human hepatic cDNA. In human intestinal cDNA there is an in-frame TAA triplet at codon 2153, whereas in the hepatic cDNAs and in the gene codon 2153 is glutamine (CAA). This same change is present in rabbit intestinal cDNA. This observation is confirmed by differential hybridization to amplified cDNA and genomic DNA of labelled oligonucleotides containing either TAA or CAA. There is no likelihood that the stop codon in intestinal cDNA arose either as a result of a systematic reverse transcriptase error or as a polymerase chain reaction artefact, because CAA is found in amplified HepG2 cDNA. Our study predicts that apoB48 is identical with the amino terminal 2152 amino acids of apoB100 with a molecular weight (before glycosylation) of 240.8 kD. This is in very close agreement with the findings of Innerarity and colleagues (personal communication). These workers used antibodies and peptide mapping to predict that the carboxy terminus of human apoB48 would be within five residues of amino acid 2151.

The observations reported here could be explained by the presence of two apoB genes, one of which was expressed in the small intestine and the other in the liver. If this is the case then the duplication must be perfect and encompass the whole gene and flanking sequence. Sequence analysis reveals only a few base differences between the intestinal cDNAs and our published hepatic cDNA sequence (Knott *et al.*, 1986b), and these are consistent with polymorphic variations seen amongst liver cDNA clones derived from several individuals (Cladaras *et al.*, 1986; Law *et al.*, 1986; Yang *et al.*, 1986; Olofsson *et al.*, 1987). Furthermore, all genomic clones fit precisely into one linear map (Blackhart *et al.*, 1986; Carlsson *et al.*, 1986; Higuchi *et al.*, 1987; Wagener *et al.*, 1987). Another explanation would be the differential or cryptic splicing of an intestine-specific exon containing the stop codon. Both these possibilities have been eliminated by the use of flanking sequence and intragenic probes that identify only single bands of genomic Southerns, by fine restriction mapping of cloned genomic DNA and by determining the nucleotide sequence of the entire gene (Ludwig *et al.*, 1987). Specifically, there is no duplication of exon 26, which contains the stop codon, and no direct repeats, which might represent alternative exons. Furthermore, enzymatic amplification of the relevant region of intestinal DNA followed by DNA sequencing and differential oligonucleotide hybridization shows that no stop codon is encoded in the rabbit genome. In the absence of gene duplication or exon shuffling, the conclusion must be that the stop codon arises as a result of co- or post-transcriptional RNA editing involving a single C to U substitution.

Our results show that both distal human and proximal rabbit small intestine contain 7 kb and 14.5 kb apoB mRNAs. Sequencing of intestinal cDNAs from both species indicates the presence of a TAA at codon 2153 in every clone examined. It was important to establish whether all the 14.5 kb transcripts contain the stop codon and are translated into apoB48 or whether most contain the glutamine codon and produce apoB100. To address this issue, we have amplified both specifically primed intestinal cDNA (from a position chosen to exclude all the poly (A) addition sites in Table 1 and encompass only the large mRNA) and oligo (dT) primed cDNA. We find evidence for only low levels of the glutamine codon in intestinal mRNA. The most straightforward conclusion is that both intestinal mRNAs encode apoB48.

Although our data predict that adult small intestine synthesizes predominantly apoB48, the work of Glickman *et al.* (1986) demonstrated that both apoB100 and apoB48 are produced by the human jejunum in organ cultures of tissue taken late in gestation. However, they agree that only apoB48 is produced by this tissue in the adult. These authors performed pulse chase studies, but were not able to establish definitively that apoB48 was produced by post- or co-translational proteolytic cleavage. Recent studies have shown that the colonic carcinoma cell line CaCo2, which behaves like foetal small intestine, produces mainly apoB100 and a small quantity of apoB48 (Hughes *et al.*, 1987). These observations suggest that intestinal cells may be pluripotent with respect to apoB48 production until relatively late in development.

In human and rabbit intestine a proportion of the mRNAs are polyadenylated downstream of the stop codon at sites that follow canonical and non-canonical poly (A) additional signals, whereas in human liver no small mRNA has been observed and no stop codon found. This suggests that polyadenylation and editing may be coupled.

Developmentally regulated, tissue-specific substitution of a single nucleotide in mRNA leading to different gene products is unprecedented. The closest analogy to this situation occurs in trypanosomes, where it has been demonstrated that additional nucleotides are inserted into transcripts by an RNA editing mechanism (Benne *et al.*, 1986; Feagin *et al.*, 1987). We cannot speculate what the mechanism might be, but it appears to be highly specific. Analogies may be found in the processing of primary nuclear transcripts and in the modified bases that are found in tRNA. Whatever the explanation for these intriguing observations, it seems unlikely that they are unique to the intestine; they may have more general biological implications.

Acknowledgements

The authors wish to thank Kokila Chotai for technical assistance; Drs Hunziker, Spiess, Semenza and Lodish for the gift of the rabbit small intestine cDNA library; Roland Bartsch for terminal ileum RNA; Madeline Nobbs for EM work; and Lesley Sargeant for preparation of the manuscript.

References

Benne, R., Van Den Burg, J., Brakenhoff, J., Sloof, P., Van Boom, J. H. and Tromp, M. C. (1986). Major transcript of the frameshifted CoxII gene from trypanosome mitochondria contains four nucleotides that are not encoded in the DNA. *Cell* **46**, 819–826.

Birnstiel, M. L., Busslinger, M. and Strub, K. (1985). Transcription termination and 3′ processing: the end is in site! *Cell* **41**, 349–359.

Blackhart, B. D., Ludwig, E. M., Pierotti, V. R., Caiati, L., Onasch, M. A., Wallis, S. C., Powell, L., Pease, R., Knott, T. J., Chu, M.-L., Mahley, R. W., Scott, J., McCarthy, B. J. and Levy-Wilson, B. (1986). Structure of the human apolipoprotein B gene. *J. Biol. Chem.* **261**, 15364–15367.

Brown, M. S. and Goldstein, J. L. (1986). A receptor mediated pathway for cholesterol homeostasis. *Science* **232**, 34–47.

Cardin, A. D., Witt, K. R., Chao, J., Margolius, H. S., Donaldson, V. H. and Jackson, R. L. (1984). Degradation of apolipoprotein B-100 of human plasma low density lipoproteins by tissue and plasma kallikreins. *J. Biol. Chem.* **259**, 8522–8528.

Carlsson, P., Darnfors, C., Olofsson, S.-O., and Bjursell, G. (1986). Analysis of the human apolipoprotein B gene; complete structure of the B74 region. *Gene* **49**, 29–51.

Cladaras, C., Hadzopoulou-Cladaras, M., Nolte, R. T., Atkinson, D. and Zannis, V. I. (1986). The complete sequence and structural analysis of human apolipoprotein B100: relationship between apoB100 and apoB48 forms. *EMBO J.* **5**, 3495–3507.

Deeb, S. S., Motulsky, A. G. and Albers, J. J. (1985). A partial cDNA clone for human apolipoprotein B. *Proc. Natl Acad. Sci. USA* **82**, 4983–4986.

Demmer, L. A., Levin, M. S., Elovson, J., Reuben, M. A., Lusis, A. J. and Gordon, J. I. (1986). Tissue-specific expression and developmental regulation of the rat apolipoprotein B gene. *Proc. Natl Acad. Sci. USA* **83**, 8102–8106.

Feagin, J. E., Jasmer, D. P. and Stuart, K. (1987). Developmentally regulated addition of nucleotides within apocytochrome b transcripts in *Trypanosoma brucei*. *Cell* **49**, 337–345.

Glickman, R. M., Rogers, M. and Glickman, J. N. (1986). Apolipoprotein B synthesis by human liver and intestine *in vitro*. *Proc. Natl Acad. Sci. USA* **83**, 5296–5300.

Hardman, D. A. and Kane, J. P. (1986). Isolation and characterisation of apolipoprotein B48. *Meth. Enzymol.* **128**, 262–272.

Higuchi, K., Monge, J. C., Lee, N., Law, S. W. and Brewer, H. B. (1987). ApoB100 is encoded by a single copy gene in the human genome. *Biochem. Biophys. Res. Commun.* **144**, 1332–1339.

Holmes, D. S. and Quigley, M. (1981). A rapid boiling method for the preparation of bacterial plasmids. *Anal. Biochem.* **114**, 193–197.

Hughes, T. E., Sasak, W. V., Ordovas, J. M., Forte, T. M., Lamon-Fava, S. and Schaefer, E. J. (1987). A novel cell line (CaCo-2) for the study of intestinal lipoprotein synthesis. *J. Biol. Chem.* **262**, 3762–3767.

Hui, D. Y., Innerarity, T. L., Milne, R. W., Marcel, Y. L. and Mahley, R. W. (1984). Binding of chylomicron remnants and β VLDL to hepatic and extra-hepatic lipoprotein receptors: a process independent of apolipoprotein B48. *J. Biol. Chem.* **259**, 15060–15068.

Hunziker, W., Spiess, M., Semenza, G. and Lodish, H. F. (1986). The sucrose–isomaltase complex: primary structure, membrane-orientation and evolution of a stalked intrinsic Brush Border protein. *Cell* **46**, 227–234.

Jones, A. L., Hradek, G. T., Hornick, C., Renaud, G., Windler, E. and Havel, R. J.

(1984). Uptake and processing of remnants of chylomicrons and VLDL by rat liver. *J. Lipid. Res.* **25**, 1151–1158.

Kane, J. P. (1983). Apolipoprotein B: structural and metabolic heterogeneity. *Ann. Rev. Physiol.* **45**, 637–650.

Kessler, M. M., Westhafer, M. A., Carson, D. D. and Nordstrom, J. L. (1987). Polyadenylation at a cryptic site in the pBR322 portion of pSV2-neo: prevention of its utilization by the SV40 late poly (A) signal. *Nucl. Acids Res.* **15**, 631–642.

Knott, T. J., Pease, R. J., Powell, L. M., Wallis, S. C., Rall, S. C., Innerarity, T. L., Blackhart, B., Taylor, W. H., Marcel, Y., Milne, R., Johnson, D., Fuller, M., Lusis, A. J., McCarthy, B. J., Mahley, R. W., Levy-Wilson, B. and Scott, J. (1986a). Complete protein sequence and identification of structural domains of human apolipoprotein B100. *Nature* **323**, 734–738.

Knott, T. J., Wallis, S. C., Powell, L. M., Pease, R. J., Lusis, A. J., Blackhart, B., McCarthy, B. J., Mahley, R. W., Levy-Wilson, B. and Scott, J. (1986b). Complete cDNA and derived protein sequence of human apolipoprotein B100. *Nucl. Acids Res.* **14**, 7501–7504.

Knott, T. J., Wallis, S. C., Pease, R. J., Powell, L. M. and Scott, J. (1986c). A hypervariable region 3′ to the human apolipoprotein B gene. *Nucl. Acid. Res.* **14**, 9215–9216.

Law, S. W., Grant, S. M., Higuchi, K., Hospattankar, A., Lackner, K., Lee, N. and Brewer, H. B. (1986). Human liver apolipoprotein B100 cDNA: complete nucleic acid and derived amino acid sequence. *Proc. Natl Acad. Sci. USA* **83**, 8142–8146.

Ludwig, E. H., Blackhart, B. D., Pierotti, V. R., Caiati, L., Fortier, C., Knott, T. J., Scott, J., Mahley, R. W., Levy-Wilson, B. and McCarthy, B. J. (1987). DNA sequence of the human apolipoprotein B gene. *DNA*, in press.

Marcel, Y. L., Innerarity, T. L., Spilman, C., Mahley, R. W., Protter, A. A. and Milne, R. W. (1987). Mapping of human apolipoprotein B antigenic determinants. *Arteriosclerosis* **7**, 166–175.

Mehrabian, M., Schumaker, V. N., Fareed, G. C., West, R., Johnson, D. F., Kirchgessner, T., Lin, H.-C., Wang, X., Ma, Y., Mendiaz, E. and Lusis, A. J. (1985). Human apolipoprotein B: identification of cDNA clones and characterisation of mRNA. *Nucl. Acids Res.* **13**, 6937–6953.

Olofsson, S.-O., Bjursell, G., Boström, K., Carlsson, P., Elovson, J., Protter, A. A., Reuben, M. A. and Bondjers, G. (1987). Apolipoprotein B; structure, biosynthesis and role in the lipoprotein assembly process. *Atherosclerosis* **68**, 1–17.

Peters, T. J. and Shio, H. (1976). Analytical subcellular fractionation studies on rat liver and on isolated jejunal enterocytes with special reference to the separation of lysosomes, peroxisomes and mitochondria. *Clin. Sci. Mol. Med.* **50**, 355–366.

Reuben, M. A. and Elovson, J. (1985). Biosynthesis of apolipoprotein B in rat liver and intestine. Federation of American Societies for Experimental Biology. 69th annual meeting Anaheim, California, 21–26 April, p. 1455.

Saiki, R. K., Scharf, S., Faloona, F., Mullis, K. B., Horn, G. T., Erlich, H. and Arnheim, V. (1985) Enzymatic amplification of β-globin gene sequences and restriction site analysis for diagnosis of sickle cell anemia. *Science* **230**, 1350–1354.

Wagener, R., Pfitzner, R. and Stoffel, W. (1987). Studies on the organization of the human apolipoprotein B100 gene. *Biol. Chem. Hoppe-Seyler* **368**, 419–425.

Yang, C.-Y., Chen, S.-H., Gianturco, S. H., Bradley, W. A., Sparrow, J. T., Tanimura, M., Li, W.-H., Sparrow, D. A., DeLoof, H., Rosseneu M., Lee, F.-S., Gu, Z.-W., Gotto, A. M. and Chan, L. (1986). Sequence, structure, receptor-binding domains and internal repeats of human apolipoprotein B100. *Nature* **323**, 738–742.

Young, S. G., Bertics, S. J., Scott, T. M., Dubois, B. W., Curtiss, L. K. and Witztum, J. L. (1986). Parallel expression of the MB19 genetic polymorphism in apoprotein B100 and apoprotein B48. *J. Biol. Chem.* **261**, 2995–2998.

5

Regulation of the ApoB100 Cascade

SHLOMO EISENBERG
Department of Medicine B, Hadassah University Hospital, Jerusalem, Israel

1 The VLDL→IDL→LDL cascade

Precursor–product relationships between lipoprotein particles have been suspected to constitute part of the physiology of the lipoprotein system as early as 1958 (Gitlin *et al.*, 1958). Definite evidence for lipoprotein conversion processes along the apoB100 cascade, however, was not obtained until the nature of the major apolipoproteins (A-I, A-II, B, C's and E) had been elucidated. The initial studies were carried out in human subjects injected with VLDL labelled with [^{125}I]apoproteins B and C (Bilheimer *et al.*, 1972; Eisenberg *et al.*, 1972, 1973). Labelled apoC was shown to distribute between VLDL and HDL by an exchange mechanism already 10 minutes after the injection and to decay from plasma in parallel. The behaviour of the apoB moiety of the VLDL was distinctly different, and all of the apoB remained associated with the VLDL. With time, however, labelled apoB disappeared from the VLDL density range and appeared first at the plasma density fraction of 1.006–1.019 g/ml (designated as intermediate density lipoprotein or IDL) and later, in LDL. In normolipidaemic people most of the labelled apoB was found in IDL 6–12 hours after the injection of [^{125}I]VLDL, and in LDL 12–14 hours after the injection. Thus metabolic precursor–product relationships were established between VLDL, IDL and LDL.

The role of lipoprotein lipase (LPL) as the major enzyme responsible for the VLDL to LDL conversion was established when subjects were injected with [^{125}I]VLDL and 10 minutes later, with heparin (Eisenberg *et al.*, 1973). Within minutes of the release of endothelial-bound lipases into the bloodstream, the large-sized triglyceride-rich VLDL particles were lipolysed,

HYPERLIPIDAEMIA AND ATHEROSCLEROSIS
ISBN 0.12.675645-7

labelled apoB moved to the dense VLDL particle populations and IDL, and labelled apoC were transferred to HDL. The further transfer of [^{125}I]apoB to LDL, occurred much later. Experiments carried out *in vitro*, first with post-heparin plasma (Eisenberg and Rachmilewitz, 1975) and later with purified bovine milk LPL (Deckelbaum, 1979; Eisenberg and Olivecrona, 1979), conclusively showed that lipase action was sufficient to produce IDL-like and even LDL-like particles from VLDL. An important finding was the demonstration that along the cascade one and only one product particle is generated from each precursor particle. Thus the maximum number of LDL particles generated is determined by the number of VLDL particles secreted from the liver (Eisenberg, 1976a,b).

Several other events operating along the cascade were elucidated by our studies. Analysis of the turnover data (Berman *et al.*, 1978), as well as direct measurements (Eisenberg *et al.*, 1973) demonstrated a continuous interconversion of large-sized and less-dense particles to smaller-size and denser particles. Within the VLDL and IDL density range, apoC molecules are deleted from the particles in proportion to the decrease of their surface area, leaving all of the apoB and some or most of the apoE molecules associated with the particle (Eisenberg, 1976a,b). ApoE appears to be deleted at the later stages of the cascade. In LDL, apoB is the only protein. This changing apoprotein profile could conceivably direct the large particles to interactions with lipoprotein lipases, while the smaller particles would interact avidly with cellular receptors, predominantly the apoB,E (LDL) receptor (Eisenberg and Levy, 1975).

A role for the hepatic lipase in conversion of small VLDL and IDL particles to LDL has been originally suggested by us (Eisenberg and Levy, 1975). Recently conducted experiments have supported this suggestion (Goldberg *et al.*, 1982). Observations in human patients with specific deficiencies of either lipoprotein lipase or hepatic lipase help in more exact delineation of the role that the two enzymes play along the cascade. In the former patients (LPL deficient), small amounts of LDL of abnormal structure and composition can be identified (unpublished observations), but the conversion of VLDL to LDL is minimal and is greatly delayed. In the latter patients, LDL levels can be normal, but excess of IDL and VLDL is found (Breckenridge *et al.*, 1982). Together with the *in vitro* studies, these findings indicate that *in vivo* both enzymes participate in the VLDL delipidation pathway. LPL is essential for VLDL triglyceride hydrolysis, and when absent, hepatic lipase activity alone cannot cause conversion of substantial amounts of VLDL to LDL. The hepatic lipase, when present, appears to play a role in IDL metabolism, but this action can be mediated also by LPL, although at a lower efficiency.

2 The origin of HDL

Loss of surface constituents is an obligatory part of the VLDL to LDL delipidation process. Analysis of VLDL and LDL particles shows that as much as 70–80% of the proteins, phospholipid and free cholesterol molecules present in an average VLDL particle (MW 20×10^6) must be excluded when one LDL (MW 2.5×10^6) is formed (Eisenberg, 1980). We suggested that these surface constituents provide a major source of the HDL system and proposed two mechanisms by which LPL action on triglyceride-rich lipoproteins affects HDL. The first pathway is release of surface fragments composed of apoproteins, phospholipids and free cholesterol from lipolysed VLDL (and chylomicrons). Such fragments can be found in the HDL density range when VLDL is lipolysed by endothelial bound (Chajek and Eisenberg, 1978) or unassociated LPL (Eisenberg and Olivecrona, 1979) in the absence of HDL. By electron microscopy, these surface remnants appear as discoidal structures, very similar to nascent HDL found in perfused rat liver (Hamilton *et al.*, 1976). When apoA-I is present, the surface remnants are substrates for the enzyme lecithin cholesterol acyltransferase (LCAT), and with displacement of the hydrophobic cholesteryl ester molecules to the core of the bilayer, they become spherical, HDL_3 particles. This route is followed by chylomicron surface remnants that contain apoA-I. Indeed, in patients lacking HDL (Herbert *et al.*, 1978) or LCAT (Glomset *et al.*, 1975), surface remnants accumulate in plasma shortly after a fatty meal. The second pathway involves assimilation of surface constituents released from lipolysed triglyceride-rich lipoproteins by existing HDL_3 particles. Under *in vitro* conditions, HDL_3 was shown to serve as an excellent acceptor for phospholipids, apoproteins and free cholesterol molecules generated during VLDL lipolysis (Patsch *et al.*, 1978). These lipid-enriched HDL_3 have been transformed to HDL_2-like particles, and we indicated that if acted upon by LCAT, true HDL_2 may be formed from HDL_3. As discussed elsewhere (Eisenberg, 1984), this pathway provides a physiological basis for regulation of HDL subpopulation distribution and for the strong and significant relationships that are constantly found between HDL levels—in particular HDL_2—and the lipoprotein lipase system. It is of special interest to note that in the rat an apoE-rich HDL population exists normally (designated HDL_1) and that HDL conversions *in vivo* can be followed along an HDL_3 to HDL_2 to HDL_1 axis (Gavish *et al.*, 1987).

3 Effects of lipid transfer proteins on the cascade

Transfers of triglycerides and cholesteryl esters between lipoproteins are reactions mediated by a specific protein that take place in the plasma of humans and several animal species (Tall, 1986). The most significant consequences of lipid transfer reactions on the cascade are related to the enrichment of VLDL with cholesteryl esters. For example, in hypertriglyceridaemia when lipid transfer reactions are excessive, the VLDL is enriched with cholesteryl esters (and free cholesterol) and has a low content of triglycerides. Under these conditions, LDL (and HDL) are poor in cholesteryl esters (and free cholesterol), enriched with triglycerides and proteins, and are smaller and denser than normally (Eisenberg *et al.*, 1984). These abnormalities are proportional to the degree of hypertriglyceridaemia and revert towards normal when triglyceride-lowering therapy (with bezafibrate) is initiated. In the VLDL range, the lighter and larger subfraction (VLDL-I) is affected to the greatest degree, while VLDL-III is affected the least (Oschry *et al.*, 1985; Eisenberg, 1985). The implications of these findings for the metabolism of VLDL are of great significance. It appears that the content of cholesteryl esters in VLDL-I (and perhaps part of the VLDL-II fraction) is much larger than that found in normal LDL (Oschry *et al.*, 1985). Since mechanisms that remove cholesteryl esters from VLDL do not exist in human plasma, the cholesteryl-ester-rich VLDL particles cannot possibly complete the cascade and must be removed from the plasma as VLDL remnants. Such particles are potentially atherogenic.

The effects of lipid transfer on LDL and HDL are described in detail elsewhere (Eisenberg, 1984; Kleinman *et al.*, 1985). For the sake of completeness, however, it should be mentioned that cholesteryl ester : triglyceride heteroexchange, followed by hydrolysis of transferred triglycerides, regulates HDL subpopulation distribution and has major effects on LDL : cell interactions and on plasma and cellular cholesterol metabolism (Kleinman *et al.*, 1985).

4 Regulation of lipoprotein metabolism along the cascade

The concept that catabolism of some VLDL and/or IDL particles prior to the formation of LDL is a process responsible for regulation of LDL synthesis, originates from studies in rats. In this species 80–90% of the VLDL-apoB is taken up by the liver at the stage of small VLDL or IDL and does not contribute to the LDL pool (Eisenberg and Rachmilewitz, 1973a, b). This finding suggested that removal of intermediate particles (also called VLDL remnants) by a receptor-specific pathway is responsible for the paucity of LDL in the rat, while in humans all, or most of the VLDL particles complete the cascade (Eisenberg, 1976; Eisenberg and Levy, 1975). Subsequent analysis of human turnover studies suggested that direct catabolism of VLDL remnants occurs also in the human, and that as much as 50% of the VLDL particles may be removed from the plasma compartment before reaching the stage of LDL (Kesäniemi *et al.*, 1985).

The metabolic basis responsible for liver catabolism of VLDL remnants and IDL is not clear. Observations in human subjects with familial hypercholesterolaemia and in Watanabe Hereditable Hyperlipidaemic rabbits suggested that apoB,E receptors are also responsible for the catabolism of VLDL remnants and IDL (Brown and Goldstein, 1986). Other pathways, however, have not been ruled out. Regardless of mechanism, it appears that small VLDL and IDL particles may follow either the cascade route, or the irreversible catabolism route. It has been established that functional apoE (E-3, E-4) molecules are responsible for interaction of VLDL (and IDL) particles with apoB, E receptors (Mahley and Innerarity, 1983). Quantitatively, in order to serve as efficient regulators of the apoB100 cascade, the VLDL remnants and the IDL must have very high affinity towards the apoB, E receptor or other catabolic receptors. Indeed, in rabbits, apoB/apoE containing VLDL or IDL particles have been shown to disappear from plasma at an extremely rapid rate, compatible with the above assumption (Yamada *et al.*, 1986). A similar situation appears to exist in rats. The behaviour of human lipoproteins in human systems, however, has not been thoroughly investigated. We found recently that human IDL particles containing 2–3 moles of apoE per mole of apoB interact with apoB, E receptors on either fibroblasts or HepG2 cells with an affinity similar to that of LDL and that their proteolytic degradation is about one-half that of LDL (Friedman *et al.*, 1986). With VLDL preparations, cell interaction is barely detectable when the lipoproteins are isolated from normolipidaemic subjects and is minimal for lipoproteins from hyperlipidaemic subjects. Addition of exogenous recombinant or plasmatic apoE-3 increased VLDL : cell interactions many fold and doubled IDL : cell interactions (Eisenberg *et al.*, 1987). Yet, even with addition of apoE-3, the catabolic rates of VLDL or IDL are less, or similar to those of LDL. More studies are evidently needed to elucidate the mechanism(s) responsible for direct degradation of VLDL remnants and IDL in the human. The findings so far do not support the notion that in humans as much as 50% of the VLDL particles can be catabolized prior to the formation of LDL unless specific non-apoB, E receptors are involved with this process or if unknown factors, that are not present in the cell culture system, are operative *in vivo*.

5 Conclusion and perspectives

Figure 1 depicts the behaviour of apoB100-containing lipoproteins along the cascade. As is illustrated, VLDL synthesis, VLDL conversions and irreversible degradation of VLDL remnants and IDL determine the number of LDL

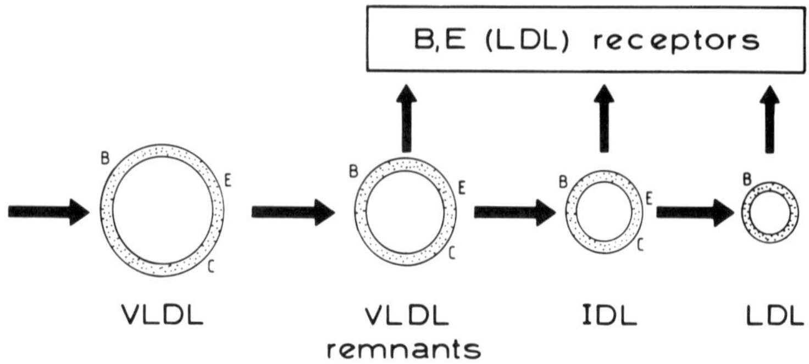

Fig. 1 Regulation of lipoprotein metabolism along the apoB100 cascade. The number of lipoprotein particles at each stage is determined by the number of secreted VLDL particles, rates of VLDL and IDL conversions, fraction of VLDL remnants and IDL that are irreversibly catabolized and the activity of LDL receptors. Hence LDL levels are determined by VLDL secretion, VLDL and IDL remnants catabolism and LDL clearance.

particles formed. Together with LDL degradation rates, this metabolic process therefore regulates plasma LDL levels. However, the mechanism responsible for regulation of metabolism of apoB100 lipoproteins is largely unknown. In addition the basis for completely different behaviour of remnants and IDL observed between species has not been elucidated. Questions such as the nature of receptors other than the apoB, E (LDL) receptor that may be involved with remnant catabolism or the specific physical and chemical alteration of lipoprotein particles that cause accelerated cellular catabolism have not been answered. Even more importantly, the atherogenic potentialities of different lipoproteins that are generated along the cascade have not been elucidated. These, and many other aspects of the physiology and pathophysiology of the apoB100 cascade should and probably will form a focus of intense scientific investigation during the coming decade.

References

Berman, M., Eisenberg, S., Hall, M., Levy, R. I., Bilheimer, D. W., Phair, R. D. and Goebel, R. H. (1978). Metabolism of apoB and apoC apoproteins in man: Kinetic studies in normal and hyperlipoproteinemic subjects. *J. Lipid Res.* **19**, 38–56.

Bilheimer, D. W., Eisenberg, S. and Levy, R. I. (1972). The metabolism of very low density lipoprotein proteins. I. Preliminary *in vitro* and *in vivo* observations. *Biochim. Biophys. Acta* **260**, 212–221.

Breckenridge, W. C., Little, J. A., Alaupovic, P., Wang, C. S., Kuksis, A., Kakis, G. F.,

Lindgren, F. and Gardiner, G. (1982). Lipoprotein abnormalities associated with a familial deficiency of hepatic lipase. *Atherosclerosis* **45**, 161–179.

Brown, M. S. and Goldstein, J. L. (1986). A receptor-mediated pathway for cholesterol homeostatis. *Science* **232**, 34–47.

Chajek, T. and Eisenberg, S. (1978). Very low density lipoprotein. Metabolism of phospholipids, cholesterol, and apolipoprotein C in the isolated perfused rat heart. *J. Clin. Invest.* **61**, 1654–1665.

Deckelbaum, R. J., Eisenberg, S., Fainaru, M., Barenholz, Y. and Olivecrona, T. (1979). *In vitro* production of human plasma low density lipoprotein-like particles. A model for very low density lipoprotein catabolism. *J. Biol. Chem.* **254**, 6079–6087.

Eisenberg, S. (1976a). Lipoprotein metabolism and hyperlipidemia. *Atherosclerosis Rev.* **1**, 23–60.

Eisenberg, S. (1976b). Metabolism of very low density lipoprotein. *Lipoprotein Metabolism* (ed. H. Greten) pp. 32–43. Springer-Verlag, Heidelberg.

Eisenberg, S. (1980). Plasma lipoproteins interconversion. *Ann. NY Acad. Sci.* **346**, 30–47.

Eisenberg, S. (1984). High density lipoprotein metabolism (review). *J. Lipid Res.* **25**, 1017–1058.

Eisenberg, S. (1985). Preferential enrichment of large-sized very low density lipoprotein populations with transferred cholesteryl esters. *J. Lipid Res.* **26**, 487–494.

Eisenberg, S. and Levy, R. I. (1975). Lipoprotein metabolism. *Adv. Lipid Res.* **13**, 1–90.

Eisenberg, S. and Olivecrona, T. (1979). Very low density lipoprotein. Fate of phospholipids, cholesterol and apolipoprotein C during lipolysis *in vitro*. *J. Lipid Res.* **20**, 614–623.

Eisenberg S. and Rachmilewitz, D. (1973a). Metabolism of rat plasma very low density lipoprotein. I. Fate in circulation of the whole lipoprotein. *Biochim. Biophys. Acta* **326**, 378–390.

Eisenberg S. and Rachmilewitz, D. (1973b). Metabolism of rat plasma very low density lipoprotein. II. Fate in circulation of apoprotein subunits. *Biochim. Biophys. Acta* **326**, 391–405.

Eisenberg S. and Rachmilewitz, D. (1975). Interaction of rat plasma very low density lipoprotein with lipoprotein lipase-rich (post-heparin) plasma. *J. Lipid Res.* **16**, 341–351.

Eisenberg, S., Bilheimer, D. W. and Levy, R. I. (1972). The metabolism of very low density lipoprotein proteins. II. Studies on the transfer of apoproteins between plasma lipoproteins. *Biochim. Biophys. Acta* **280**, 94–106.

Eisenberg, S., Bilheimer, D. W., Lindgren, F. T. and Levy, R. I. (1973). On the metabolic conversion of human plasma very low density lipoprotein to low density lipoprotein. *Biochim. Biophys. Acta* **326**, 361–377.

Eisenberg, S., Gavish, D., Oschry, Y., Fainaru, M. and Deckelbaum, R. J. (1984). Abnormalities in very low, low and high density lipoproteins in hypertriglyceridemia. Reversal towards normal with bezafibrate treatment. *J. Clin. Invest.* **74**, 470–482.

Eisenberg, S., Friedman, G. and Vogel, T. (1987). Enhanced metabolism of normolipidemic human plasma very low density lipoprotein in cultured cells by exogenous recombinant apoE-3. Submitted for publication.

Friedman, G., Gavish, D. and Eisenberg, S. (1986). Metabolism of human intermediate and low density lipoproteins by cultured HepG2 cells (abstract). *Arteriosclerosis* **6**, 590a.

Gavish, D., Oschry, Y. and Eisenberg, S. (1987). *In vivo* conversion of human HDL_3 to HDL_2 and apoE-rich HDL_1 in the rat: Effects of lipid transfer protein. *J. Lipid Res.* **28**, 257–267.

Gitlin, D., Cornwall, D. G., Nakasato, D., Oncley, J. L., Hughes, W. L. and Janeway, C. A. (1958). Studies on the metabolism of plasma proteins in the nephrotic syndrome. II. The lipoproteins. *J. Clin. Invest.* **37**, 172–184.

Glomset, J. A., Norum, K. R., Nichols, A. V. *et al.* (1975). Plasma lipoproteins in familial lecithin : cholesterol acyltransferase deficiency. *Scand. J. Clin. Lab. Invest.* **35**, Suppl. 142, 1–55.

Goldberg, I. R., Le, N. A., Paterniti, J. L., Ginsberg, H. N., Lindgren, F. T. and Brown, W. V. (1982). Lipoprotein metabolism during acute inhibition of hepatic triglyceride lipase in the cynomolgus monkey. *J. Clin. Invest.* **70**, 1184–1192.

Hamilton, R. L., Williams, M. C., Fielding, C. J. and Havel, R. J. (1976). Discoidal bilayer structure of nascent high density lipoproteins from perfused rat liver. *J. Clin. Invest.* **58**, 667–680.

Herbert, P. N., Forte, T., Heinen, R. J. and Fredrickson, D. S. (1978). Tangier disease: one explanation of lipid storage. *N. Engl. J. Med.* **299**, 519–521.

Kesäniemi, Y. A., Belz, W. F. and Grundy, S. M. (1985). Comparison of metabolism of apolipoprotein B in normal subjects, obese patients, and patients with coronary heart disease. *J. Clin. Invest.* **76**, 586–595.

Kleinman, Y., Eisenberg, S., Oschry, Y., Gavish, D., Stein, O. and Stein, Y. (1985). Defective metabolism of hypertriglyceridemic low density lipoprotein in cultured human skin fibroblasts. *J. Clin. Invest.* **75**, 1796–1803.

Kleinman, Y., Schonfeld, G., Gavish, D., Oschry, Y. and Eisenberg, S. (1987). Hypolipidemic therapy modulates expression of apolipoprotein B epitopes on low density lipoproteins. Studies in mild to moderate hypertriglyceridemic patients. *J. Lipid Res.* **28**, 540–548.

Mahley, R. W. and Innerarity, T. L. (1983). Lipoprotein receptors and cholesterol homeostasis. *Biochim. Biophys. Acta* **737**, 197–222.

Oschry, Y., Olivecrona, T., Deckelbaum, R. J. and Eisenberg, S. (1985). Is hypertriglyceridemic very low density lipoprotein a precursor of normal low density lipoproteins? *J. Lipid Res.* **26**, 158–167.

Patsch, J. R., Gotto, A. M., Olivecrona, T. and Eisenberg, S. (1978). Formation of high density $lipoprotein_2$-like particle during lipolysis of very low density lipoprotein *in vitro*. *Proc. Natl Acad. Sci. USA* **75**, 4519–4523.

Tall, A. R. (1986). Plasma lipid transfer proteins. *J. Lipid Res.* **27**, 361–367.

Yamada, N., Shames, D. M., Stoudemire, J. B. and Havel, R. J. (1986). Metabolism of lipoproteins containing apolipoprotein B100 in blood plasma of rabbits: heterogeneity related to the presence of apolipoprotein E. *Proc. Natl Acad. Sci. USA* **83**, 3479–3483.

6

Cholesterol Absorption Regulates Cholesterol Metabolism and Within-Population Variation of Serum Cholesterol

T. A. MIETTINEN and Y. A. KESÄNIEMI

Second Department of Medicine, University of Helsinki, and Department of Medicine, University of Oulu, Finland

1 Introduction

A high serum cholesterol level, or more specifically a high low density lipoprotein (LDL) cholesterol, is linked causally with development of atheromatous artery disease, especially coronary heart disease. Thus, from the preventive and therapeutic point of view, it is important to know what the actual reasons for the increased LDL cholesterol levels are and what effective dietary and pharmacological measures lower these raised concentrations. The between-population variation of the serum LDL cholesterol level is mainly due to differences in the diet. Thus a diet high in saturated animal fat, cholesterol and calories maintains a high serum cholesterol content. Accordingly, dietary recommendations directed to populations as a whole or even to individuals to lower the serum cholesterol levels include reduction of calories, fat, especially animal fat, and cholesterol (Consensus Conference, 1985). In a high-cholesterol country this type of diet was shown to reduce serum cholesterol by about a quarter, even in a rural population (Ehnholm *et al.*, 1982). Most of this effect is due to changes in quantity and quality of dietary fatty acids, but, in addition, a reduction in dietary cholesterol intake can evidently have some serum cholesterol lowering effect (Grundy *et al.*, 1988).

Inhibition of cholesterol absorption artificially, for instance with plant sterols (Grundy *et al.*, 1969), AOMA (surfomer, Monsanto) (Crouse *et al.*, 1982), sucrose polyester (Crouse and Grundy, 1979) or in particular neomycin (Miettinen, 1979; Sedaghat *et al.*, 1975), results in a decrease in the serum

HYPERLIPIDAEMIA AND ATHEROSCLEROSIS
ISBN 0.12.675645-7

cholesterol level and enhanced cholesterol synthesis. Similarly, a decrease in dietary cholesterol intake reduces the amount of absorbed cholesterol. This is most likely compensated for by enhanced cholesterol synthesis, yet serum cholesterol may be lowered. However, altered cholesterol absorption is not consistently associated with changes in the serum cholesterol level, as is illustrated by cholesterol feeding experiments in which serum cholesterol is found to increase inconsistently. Furthermore, a benzodiazepine derivative that effectively reduced cholesterol absorption had no effect on serum cholesterol, even though neomycin, which caused exactly similar cholesterol malabsorption and compensatory changes in sterol metabolism in the same patients, markedly lowered serum total, LDL and HDL cholesterol (Miettinen and Kesäniemi, 1986). Obviously, causal association between cholesterol absorption and the regulation of serum cholesterol levels are not yet understood.

Knowledge of factors regulating the within-population variation of the serum cholesterol concentration is quite meagre. Recent comparative studies have indicated that within a population the subjects with the highest decile of serum cholesterol have low fractional catabolic rates but high production rates of LDL apoprotein B (apoB), while in the subjects within the lowest decile the fractional catabolic rates are high and production rates are low (International Collaborative Study Group, 1986). This does, in fact, suggest that the receptor-mediated catabolism of LDL apoB is an important regulator of the serum cholesterol level within the population when the receptors are up-regulated and down-regulated in subjects with low and high serum cholesterol respectively. Our preliminary studies have suggested that this regulation takes place through cholesterol absorption, which, in turn, is regulated by genetically determined apoE polymorphism (Kesäniemi *et al.*, 1987). Therefore this chapter will deal with the role of cholesterol absorption in the regulation of cholesterol metabolism and serum cholesterol variation, and with the relationship between cholesterol absorption and apoE polymorphism.

2 Cholesterol absorption efficiency in a random population

Previous preliminary studies indicated that in a normal population the absorption efficiency of dietary cholesterol, measured by the double-isotope technique or plasma plant sterol contents, was clearly higher in subjects with a high serum cholesterol level than in those with a low cholesterol level (Kesäniemi and Miettinen, 1987). Furthermore, cholesterol synthesis as evaluated by the sterol balance technique or, in particular, by the serum contents of cholesterol precursors, was low in subjects with effective cholesterol absorption and high when the absorption efficiency was low. Since these preliminary studies indicated that cholesterol absorption might regulate the within-population variation of serum cholesterol, a random fifty-year-old male population was recruited for closer investigations.

Altogether 87 out of 300 invited volunteered. They were advised to use their normal diet and they kept a seven-day food record for determination of dietary fat, cholesterol and calorie intakes. Fractional cholesterol absorption was measured with the double-label continuous feeding method from a three-day stool collection (Crouse and Grundy, 1978). This method was also used for quantitation of faecal bile acids and neutral sterols. Cholesterol synthesis was obtained as the difference between faecal steroids of cholesterol origin and dietary cholesterol. Total intestinal cholesterol flux was obtained by dividing faecal neutral sterols by the fractional absorption of cholesterol. Total flux minus dietary cholesterol is equivalent to the endogenous cholesterol flux, mainly as a result of biliary secretion, but may include some cholesterol of mucosal origin. In addition to total lipid and lipoprotein analysis, non-cholesterol sterols were quantitated, including cholestanol, the plant sterols campesterol and sitosterol, and the cholesterol precursors lathosterol and desmosterol. Serum plant sterols and cholestanol concentrations reflect closely cholesterol absorption efficiency (Miettinen *et al.*, 1987a, Tilvis and Miettinen, 1986). The cholesterol precursor sterol levels are related to cholesterol synthesis (Miettinen, 1985), and the concentrations of these sterols exhibit a highly significant correlation with hepatic HMG-CoA reductase activity (Björkhem *et al.*, 1987).

In this population the mean of total plasma cholesterol was 6.5 ± 1.2 mmol/l, with a range from 3.7 to 9.9 mmol/l. The respective LDL-cholesterol values were 4.5 ± 1.0 and 2.8 and 7.0 mmol/l. The range for triglycerides was 0.54–7.67 mmol/l and for HDL cholesterol 0.75–2.28 mmol/l.

In an experimental study an increase of dietary cholesterol from 172–310 to 787–918 mg/day caused a small decrease in fractional cholesterol absorption (McNamara *et al.*, 1987). This is in contrast with other studies, which demonstrate that fractional absorption is not decreased until excessively large doses are fed (Kudchodkar *et al.*, 1973, Maranhao and Quintao, 1983; Quintao *et al.*, 1971). In our population study the fractional cholesterol absorption varied from 0.25 to 0.74, and it was unrelated to dietary cholesterol (range 191–1033 mg/day) or even to total intestinal cholesterol flux (range 714–3170 mg/day). This would mean that within the physiological limits of long-term cholesterol intake the fraction of absorbed cholesterol was constant at any level of intestinal cholesterol content. Thus the higher the absorption efficiency or the more cholesterol entering the intestinal lumen from diet or bile, the higher was the amount of absorbed dietary, total and biliary cholesterol ($r = 0.568–0.840$, $p < 0.001$). This indicates that in the normal population the efficiency of cholesterol absorption strongly regulates the amount of absorbed cholesterol.

3 Cholesterol absorption and metabolism

In the light of these results we must understand the cholesterol elimination in faeces and cholesterol synthesis at different absorption efficiencies under normal baseline conditions. Analysis revealed that the higher the fractional absorption, the less cholesterol remained to be excreted in faeces (Miettinen *et al.*, 1987a, b). This negative association was statistically significant for total faecal steroids ($r = -0.483$), total endogenous steroids ($r = -0.383$) and endogenous neutral sterols ($r = -0.338, p < 0.01$), but not quite for faecal bile acids ($r = -0.242$). Similar associations were obtained for absorbed dietary cholesterol, indicating that an increase in dietary cholesterol absorption by 1 mg/kg per day reduced faecal elimination of cholesterol from endogenous sources by about 1 mg/kg per day. This would suggest that the body cholesterol pool ought to increase by 2 mg/kg per day unless cholesterol synthesis was reduced. Cholesterol synthesis, measured with the sterol balance technique, was negatively correlated with the fractional absorption ($r = -0.496$) or the absorbed amount of dietary cholesterol ($r = -0.643$). In fact, the regression equation ($y = 1.98x + 15.75$) indicated that an increase of dietary cholesterol absorption by 1 mg/kg per day would reduce cholesterol synthesis by about 2 mg/kg per day. Extrapolating further, cholesterol synthesis would be zero at a dietary cholesterol absorption of about 8 mg/kg per day, and on a cholesterol-free diet cholesterol synthesis would be about 16 mg/kg per day. In our series, the mean of absorbed dietary cholesterol was 2.9 mg/kg per day and that of cholesterol synthesis 10.0 mg/kg per day when only one of the subjects showed a positive sterol balance. It is interesting to note that in a cholesterol feeding experiment (1350 mg of crystalline cholesterol/day), which included normocholesterolaemic and hypercholesterolaemic subjects, diminished cholesterol synthesis was the main intervening mechanism (Maranhao and Quintao, 1983).

4 Serum non-cholesterol sterols and cholesterol metabolism

The concentration of the non-cholesterol sterols in serum also appears to be strongly related to the cholesterol absorption efficiency in this random male population. Thus the cholesterol precursors desmosterol and lathosterol were significantly negatively correlated both with fractional and absolute absorption of dietary cholesterol (r ranged from -0.356 to -0.497) and positively with cholesterol synthesis ($r = 0.382$ and 0.379) measured with the sterol balance technique (Miettinen *et al.*, 1987a). On the other hand, cholestanol and the plant sterols campesterol and sitosterol exhibited positive correlations with both fractional and absolute absorption of dietary cholesterol (r ranged from 0.288 to 0.424) and negative ones with cholesterol synthesis ($r = -0.300$ and -0.422). The determination of these non-cholesterol sterols is rapid and convenient from non-saponifiable serum lipids by gas–liquid chromatography on a capillary column (Miettinen, 1985; Miettinen and Koivisto, 1983). The measurement of serum cholestanol, cholesterol precursor sterols and plant sterols gives valuable information on cholesterol absorption and synthesis for baseline recording in population studies. It is not known at the moment whether cholesterol feeding affects the level of these sterols.

5 Cholesterol feeding

Our baseline studies above indicated that within the normal dietary cholesterol intake (mean 486 ± 165 mg/day) the absorbed dietary cholesterol did not activate cholesterol elimination but inhibited it proportionately in faeces as bile acid plus neutral sterols. All of the subjects, except one, absorbed dietary cholesterol clearly less than would be theoretically necessary (8 mg/kg per day) to bring cholesterol synthesis to zero. Exceeding this limit, which would be about 1 g/day of cholesterol in the diet, ought to change cholesterol elimination. Otherwise, excessively absorbed cholesterol would accumulate with the body. Earlier cholesterol feeding experiments have actually revealed in some subjects an increase in re-excretion of cholesterol as neutral sterols and in others as bile acids (Lin and Connor, 1980; Maranhao and Quintao, 1983; Quintao *et al.*, 1971). Thus, on the basis of these and our own observations (Miettinen, 1988), it appears that faecal cholesterol elimination follows a U-shaped curve as a function of dietary cholesterol intake, i.e. elimination decreases until synthesis reaches zero, followed by variable increase as bile acids or neutral sterols are excreted to avoid excessive cholesterol accumulation. Interindividual variation appears to be large and studies over a sufficient period of time are lacking.

6 Cholesterol absorption and serum cholesterol

The effects of cholesterol feeding on serum cholesterol concentrations appear to be variable. Serum cholesterol has been reported to increase most consistently when the baseline intake has been low, while virtually no effect is seen when cholesterol is added to normal diet containing about 400–500 mg of cholesterol (Grundy *et al.*, 1988). In our studies an addition of 1 g of cholesterol to the diet to bring the final intake to about 1.5 g/day resulted in a significant increase in cholesterol elimination as bile acids and neutral sterols. Serum cholesterol concentrations increased insignificantly, the change being proportional to the starting level (Miettinen, 1988). On the other hand, in our other unpublished study, cholesterol feeding to vegetarians on a low baseline cholesterol intake increased dietary cholesterol absorption by about 330 mg/day (5 mg/kg per day) and resulted in a significant increase in serum total, LDL and HDL cholesterol levels. Other studies have indicated that the response of serum cholesterol concentration to a modest dietary cholesterol intake added to a low baseline cholesterol intake is positively correlated with total and HDL_2 cholesterol levels and negatively with habitual cholesterol intake (Katan and Beynen, 1987).

The question now arises as to whether dietary cholesterol-induced reduction in cholesterol synthesis, proportional to cholesterol absorption efficiency, is a strong enough compensatory factor to keep serum cholesterol unrelated to cholesterol absorption in the normal population. A plot of fractional cholesterol absorption (Table 1) against serum lipids revealed positive correlations with total, LDL and HDL cholesterol levels. This indicated that the cholesterol absorption efficiency significantly regulated serum cholesterol under normal dietary conditions. Further studies indicated that the plasma kinetics of LDL apoB was related to cholesterol absorption, synthesis and serum concentration. Thus turnover studies of LDL apoB showed that the fractional catabolic rate of apoB was negatively associated with the LDL-cholesterol level and cholesterol absorption, measured either isotopically or with the plant sterol and cholestanol levels. This parameter was correlated positively with choles-

Table 1 Relationship of apoE polymorphism and cholesterol absorption efficiency with different parameters of cholesterol metabolism.

Parameter	E2 $n = 5$	E4 $n = 11$	r-value[a]	Absorption
LDL-cholesterol (mmol/1)	100	212*	0.671*	0.343*
LDL-apoB (mg/dl)	100	192*	0.671*[b]	0.595*[b]
Fractional catabolic rate of apoB (pools/day)	100	63*	−0.715*[b]	−0.338*[b]
Production rate of apoB (mg/kg per day)	100	115	0.265[b]	0.445*[b]
Cholesterol absorption (%)	100	132*	0.474*	1.000
Campesterol (μmol/mol cholesterol)	100	152*	0.370*	0.426*
Cholesterol synthesis (mg/kg per day)	100	72	−0.298*	−0.483*
Lathosterol (mmol/mol cholesterol)	100	72*	−0.526*	−0.497*
Bile acid synthesis (mg/kg per day)	100	121	−0.146	−0.207

[a]Correlation of each individual's lipid value with his apoE phenotype when E2/2 = 1, E2/3 = 2, E2/4 = 3, E3/3 = 4, E3/4 = 5 and E4/4 = 6.

[b]Studied in 35 subjects; values of E2 subjects were set to 100 and those of the E4 cases normalized to this.

*Significant ($p < 0.05$) difference or correlation.

terol synthesis, especially when evaluated with the serum levels of cholesterol precursors. The production rate of LDL-apoB, on the other hand, had correlations opposite to that of the fractional catabolic rate of apoB. The findings can be interpreted, according to current opinion on cholesterol transport (Brown and Goldstein, 1986), as indicating that a high cholesterol absorption efficiency overloads the liver with cholesterol, which, in turn, down-regulates cholesterol synthesis and LDL apoB/E receptors, resulting in increased LDL-cholesterol concentration. The mechanism behind the increase in HDL-cholesterol due to dietary cholesterol is not known at present.

7 ApoE polymorphism and cholesterol metabolism

The apoprotein E4 allele is known to be associated with high serum LDL-cholesterol, while subjects with the E2 phenotype have usually low serum cholesterol level or type III dyslipoproteinaemia (Ehnholm *et al.*, 1986; Mahley, 1985). The high cholesterol absorption efficiency of subjects in the highest decile of the serum cholesterol concentration prompted us to relate the cholesterol absorption efficiency to the apoE phenotype, which is known to show a unique distribution among the Finns (Ehnholm *et al.*, 1986). The preliminary findings actually indicated that the subjects with a high serum cholesterol level and a high cholesterol absorption might have apoE4 phenotypes and correspondingly a low cholesterol synthesis (Kesäniemi *et al.*, 1987). The distribution of different apoE phenotypes was in the present population of 87 men as follows: E2/2 6%, E3/2 6%, E2/4 3%, E3/3 58%, E3/4 24% and E4/4 9%. As shown in Table 1, LDL-cholesterol and LDL-apoB concentrations were about twice as high in the subjects with apoE4 as in those with the E2 allele. The values in the E3/3 subjects fell in between. It can also be seen that when one moves from the E2 to the E4 subjects, cholesterol absorption gradually increases, cholesterol and bile acid synthesis correspondingly decreases, and catabolism of LDL apoB is impaired and its production, if anything, is enhanced.

It is interesting to note that, according to our preliminary unpublished studies, the cholesterol absorption efficiency of E3/4 subjects with familial hypercholesterolaemia was higher than that of E3/3 subjects. Serum total and LDL-cholesterol levels were correspondingly insignificantly higher and cholesterol synthesis lower. It should be noted, however, that if our normal male population had included familial hypercholesterolaemia patients or if these patients were included in that population, the associations of parameters for sterol metabolism or of apoE phenotype with the parameters of serum lipoproteins would have disappeared because LDL-apoB receptor deficiency (Brown and Goldstein, 1986) increases the LDL-cholesterol levels of these subjects above those of the normal subjects. It is tempting to suggest on the basis of our findings that in the normal male population the subjects with the apoE4 allele absorb cholesterol effectively, overloading hepatocytes with absorbed cholesterol. This, in turn, would down-regulate cholesterol synthesis (indicated by sterol balance and serum precursor sterol data) and LDL-apoB receptors (shown by low fractional catabolic rates), resulting through impaired hepatic uptake of LDL-apoB at high LDL cholesterol concentration. On the other hand, in the subjects with apoE2 allele the associations are mainly opposite to those in the subjects with the apoE4 allele.

ApoE polymorphism alone does not appear to explain the relationship between serum cholesterol and cholesterol absorption. Thus in the subjects with the apoE3/3 phenotype, cholesterol absorption efficiency and serum plant sterol levels were still significantly negatively associated with cholesterol synthesis measured with the sterol balance technique or serum lathosterol ($r = -0.409, p < 0.01$ and $r = -0.598, p < 0.001$ respectively) and positively with the serum total ($p < 0.05$) and LDL ($p < 0.01$) cholesterol levels. Other confounding factors may contribute to this relationship. However, a stepwise multifactorial analysis, including absorption efficiency, obesity and dietary plant sterols, cholesterol and saturation index of dietary fat revealed that cholesterol absorption efficiency alone explained the variation in serum cholesterol or lipoprotein levels. The findings clearly indicate that cholesterol absorption efficiency significantly regulates cholesterol metabolism and the within-population variation of serum cholesterol even when the apoE phenotype is standardized.

References

Björkhem, I., Miettinen, T., Reihner, E., Ewerth, S., Angelin, B. and Einarsson, K. (1987). Correlation between serum levels of some cholesterol precursors and activity of HMG-CoA reductase in human livers. *J. Lipid Res.* **28**, 1137–1143.

Brown, M. S. and Goldstein, J. L. (1986). A receptor-mediated pathway for cholesterol homeostasis. *Science* **232**, 34–47.

Consensus Conference (1985). Lowering blood cholesterol to prevent heart disease. *J. Am. Med. Assoc.* **253**, 2080–2086.

Crouse, J. R. and Grundy, S. M. (1978). Evaluation of a continuous isotope feeding method for measurement of cholesterol absorption in man. *J. Lipid Res.* **19**, 967–971.

Crouse, J. R. and Grundy, S. M. (1979). Effects of sucrose polyester on cholesterol metabolism in man. *Metabolism* **28**, 994–1000.

Crouse, J. R., Grundy, S. M. and Johnson, J. H. (1982). Effects of AOMA on cholesterol metabolism in man. *Metabolism* **31**, 733–739.

Ehnholm, C., Huttunen, J. K., Pietinen, P., Leino, U., Mutanen, M., Kostiainen, E., Pikkarainen, J., Dougherty, R., Iacono, J. and Puska, P. (1982). Effect of diet on

serum lipoproteins in a population with a high risk of coronary heart disease. *N. Engl. J. Med.* **307**, 850–855.
Enholm, C., Lukka, M., Kuusi, T., Nikkilä, E. and Utermann, G. (1986). Apolipoprotein E polymorphism in the Finnish population: gene frequencies and relation to lipoprotein concentrations. *J. Lipid Res.* **27**, 227–235.
Grundy, S. M., Ahrens, E. H. and Davignon, J. (1969). The interaction of cholesterol absorption and cholesterol synthesis in man. *J. Lipid Res.* **10**, 304–315.
Grundy, S. M., Barrett-Connor, E., Rudel, L., Miettinen, T. and Spector, A. (1988). *Am. J. Clin. Nutr.* (in press).
International Collaborative Study Group (1986). Metabolic epidemiology of plasma cholesterol. Mechanisms of variation of plasma cholesterol within populations and between populations. *Lancet* **ii**, 991–996.
Katan, M. B. and Beynen, A. C. (1987). Characteristics of human hypo- and hyperresponders to dietary cholesterol. *Am. J. Epidemiol.* **125**, 387–399.
Kesäniemi, Y. A. and Miettinen, T. A. (1987). Cholesterol absorption efficiency regulates plasma cholesterol level in the Finnish population. *Eur. J. Clin. Invest.* **17**, 391–395.
Kesäniemi, Y. A., Ehnholm, C. and Miettinen, T. A. (1987). Intestinal cholesterol absorption efficiency in man is related to apoprotein E phenotype. *J. Clin. Invest.* **80**, 578–581.
Kudchodkar, B. J., Sodhi, H. S. and Horlick, L. (1973). Absorption of dietary cholesterol in man. *Metabolism* **22**, 155–163.
Lin, D. S. and Connor, W. E. (1980). The long term effects of dietary cholesterol upon the plasma lipids, lipoproteins, cholesterol absorption, and the sterol balance in man: the demonstration of feedback inhibition of cholesterol biosynthesis and increased bile acid excretion. *J. Lipid Res.* **21**, 1042–1052.
McNamara, D. J., Kolb, R., Parker, T. S., Batwin, H., Samuel, P., Brown, C. D. and Ahrens, E. H. (1987). Heterogeneity of cholesterol homeostasis in man. Response to changes in dietary fat quality and cholesterol quantity. *J. Clin. Invest.* **79**, 1729–1739.
Mahley, R. W. (1985). Atherogenic lipoproteins and coronary artery disease: concepts derived from recent advances in cellular and molecular biology. *Circulation* **72**, 943–948.
Maranhao, R. C. and Quintao, E. C. R. (1983). Long term steroid metabolism balance studies in subjects on cholesterol-free and cholesterol-rich diets: comparison between normal and hypercholesterolemic individuals. *J. Lipid Res.* **24**, 167–173.
Miettinen, T. A. (1979). Effects of neomycin alone and in combination with cholestyramine on serum cholesterol and fecal steroids in hypercholesterolemic subjects. *J. Clin. Invest.* **64**, 1485–1493.
Miettinen, T. A. (1985). In *Proceedings of the NATO Meeting. Coordinate Regulation of Cholesterol Metabolism Santa Fe, USA* (ed. A. Sanghvi), pp. 87–106.
Miettinen, T. A. (1988). *Am. J. Clin. Nutr* (in press).
Miettinen, T. A. and Kesäniemi, Y. A. (1986). Inhibition of cholesterol absorption with unaltered plasma lipoprotein levels. *Abstracts of Ninth International Symposium on Drugs Affecting Lipid Metabolism, Florence, Italy*, p. 113.
Miettinen, T. A. and Koivisto, P. (1983). In *Bile Acids and Cholesterol in Health and Disease* (ed. G. Paumgartner, A. Stiehl and W. Gerok), pp. 183–187. MTP, Lancaster.
Miettinen, T. A., Kesäniemi, Y. A. and Tilvis, R. S. (1987a). Dietary cholesterol absorption regulates cholesterol metabolism and serum cholesterol within population. *Circulation* **76**, IV-36.

Miettinen, T. A., Tilvis, R. and Kesäniemi, Y. A. (1987b). Regulation of cholesterol metabolism by cholesterol absorption. *Clin. Res.* **35**, 625A.

Quintao, E., Grundy, S. M. and Ahrens, E. H. (1971). Effects of dietary cholesterol on the regulation of total body cholesterol in man. *J. Lipid Res.* **12**, 233–247.

Sedaghat, A., Samuel, P., Crouse, J. P. and Ahrens, E. H. (1975) Effects of neomycin on absorption, synthesis, and/or flux of cholesterol in man. *J. Clin. Invest.* **55**, 12–21.

Tilvis, R. S. and Miettinen, T. A. (1986). Serum plant sterols and their relation to cholesterol absorption. *Am. J. Clin. Nutr.* **43**, 92–97.

7

Therapeutic Mobilization of Tissue Cholesterol

G. R. THOMPSON, M. KANO and J. KOIZUMI
MRC Lipoprotein Team, Hammersmith Hospital, London, UK

1 Introduction

All regression studies are based on the premise that cholesterol is an important constituent of atheromatous plaques which can be mobilized by measures that create a reverse concentration gradient between the extravascular and intravascular pools of cholesterol. Such measures include diets and drugs that reduce steady-state concentrations of low density lipoproteins (LDL) in plasma, and procedures such as plasma exchange that intermittently induce more marked decreases in LDL. By decreasing cholesterol influx, these measures presumably reduce the rate of accumulation of cholesterol within lesions and thus arrest their rate of progression, as has been observed in patients whose raised LDL levels have been lowered by cholestyramine (Levy *et al.*, 1984) and plasma exchange (Thompson *et al.*, 1980).

An alternative approach is to attempt to directly promote cholesterol efflux by increasing the concentration of acceptor particles in the blood and interstitial fluid. In essence this involves the oral administration of drugs that increase the concentration of HDL in plasma or the intravenous administration of HDL or HDL analogues such as phospholipid liposomes. Recent evidence suggests that pharmacological regimens that raise HDL cholesterol as well as lower LDL cholesterol can result in actual regression of atherosclerotic lesions (Blankenhorn *et al.*, 1987). However, there is a dearth of experimental data as to which of these twin actions is the more effective. In an attempt to answer this question, we have undertaken two separate series of studies in rabbits, both cholesterol-fed and spontaneously hypercholesterolaemic.

HYPERLIPIDAEMIA AND ATHEROSCLEROSIS
ISBN 0.12.675645-7

2 Extracorporeal removal of LDL cholesterol

Plasma exchange results in gradual regression of xanthomata in patients with familial hypercholesterolaemia, indicating mobilization of cholesterol that had previously accumulated in skin and tendons (Thompson *et al.*, 1980). Additional evidence was obtained by pre-labelling patients with radioactive cholesterol and showing rises in the specific activity of total or HDL cholesterol after plasma exchange, due to influx of higher specific activity cholesterol from tissues into plasma (Thompson *et al.*, 1975; Thompson, 1981). In view of the putative role of HDL in the transport of cholesterol from the extravascular compartment into plasma (Miller, 1984) and the inverse correlation between HDL cholesterol and coronary heart disease (Rhoads *et al.*, 1976; Castelli *et al.*, 1977), removal of HDL during plasma exchange is potentially deleterious. This can be avoided, however, by instead perfusing plasma through an affinity column that selectively removes LDL but not HDL, a process termed LDL apheresis. We have attempted to compare the cholesterol-mobilizing properties of these two procedures in Watanabe Hereditable Hyperlipidaemic (WHHL) rabbits, an animal model of familial hypercholesterolaemia (Kano *et al.*, 1987).

2.1 Comparison of plasma exchange and LDL apheresis in WHHL rabbits

Female WHHL rabbits were classified as heterozygotes or homozygotes according to their serum cholesterol levels while on a normal diet; those with a value above 100 mg/dl at 3 months were regarded as homozygotes, the remainder as obligate heterozygotes. The former remained on a normal diet, but heterozygotes had the cholesterol content of their diet increased to 0.2% for 4 months prior to the start of the study. Only heterozygotes with cholesterol levels that rose into the homozygote range were used.

Each rabbit received an intravenous injection of cholesterol, 100–600 μCi, at 15–22 days before undergoing plasma exchange or LDL apheresis. Preliminary studies had shown that the specific activity of cholesterol in the plasma of a normocholesterolaemic New Zealand White rabbit became lower than that of skin, adipose tissue, muscle and red blood cells by 2–3 weeks after the injection of [^{3}H]cholesterol.

Prior to undertaking plasma exchange, blood was obtained from New Zealand White rabbits for preparation of lipoprotein-deficient plasma. Plasma was separated and ultracentrifuged at 55 000 rpm in a Beckman 70 Ti rotor for 40 hours after adjusting the density to 1.215 with solid KBr. The infranatant was dialysed, sterilized by Millipore filtration and kept at 4°C until use.

Lipoprotein-deficient plasma prepared in this manner had a cholesterol content of 3–4 μg/ml.

During plasma exchange and LDL apheresis rabbits were anaesthetized and heparinized. These procedures were performed in a manner similar to that described by Yokoyama *et al.* (1984). Blood was obtained from an artery in one ear and returned via a vein in the opposite ear, at a flow rate of 6–10 ml/min. During plasma exchange plasma was removed and replaced with an equivalent volume of lipoprotein-deficient plasma, whereas during LDL apheresis plasma was perfused through an LA 01 column (Kanegafuchi Chemical Industry Ltd, Osaka, Japan), containing dextran sulphate linked to cellulose, and then returned. These columns have the capacity to bind 10 to 12 mg cholesterol per ml, as VLDL and LDL, but do not bind HDL (Yokoyama *et al.*, 1985).

Blood samples were obtained for determination of the concentration and specific activity of total and HDL cholesterol in plasma, and also the concentration of total and HDL phospholipid. HDL was obtained by adding 0.4% phosphotungstic acid and 2 mM $MgCl_2$ to plasma immediately after this had been separated from fresh blood samples at 4°C (Burstein and Scholnick, 1973) followed by centrifugation and filtration of the turbid supernatant (Warnick and Albers, 1978).

2.1.1 Changes in plasma cholesterol

The effects of plasma exchange and LDL apheresis were compared in two similar groups of rabbits, each comprising four homozygotes and two cholesterol-fed heterozygotes.

Mean values of serum total and HDL cholesterol were similar in the two groups before each procedure, although levels tended to be higher in cholesterol-fed heterozygotes than in homozygotes. Percentage decreases in total cholesterol were slightly greater after plasma exchange than after LDL apheresis (66% versus 59%). As expected, the percentage decrease in HDL cholesterol was much more marked after plasma exchange (62%) than after LDL apheresis (28%).

Sequential changes in total and HDL cholesterol during the week after each procedure showed that the greater decrease in total cholesterol after plasma exchange was followed by a faster rate of rebound than after LDL apheresis (58 mg/dl per day versus 32 mg/dl per day). In contrast, although HDL cholesterol fell less after LDL apheresis, the subsequent rise above baseline on Day 5 exceeded that seen after plasma exchange (27% versus 8%) (Fig. 1). Rises in HDL cholesterol concentration after each procedure, expressed as the difference between immediate post-procedure and subsequent peak values, correlated well with preceding decreases both in total and HDL cholesterol.

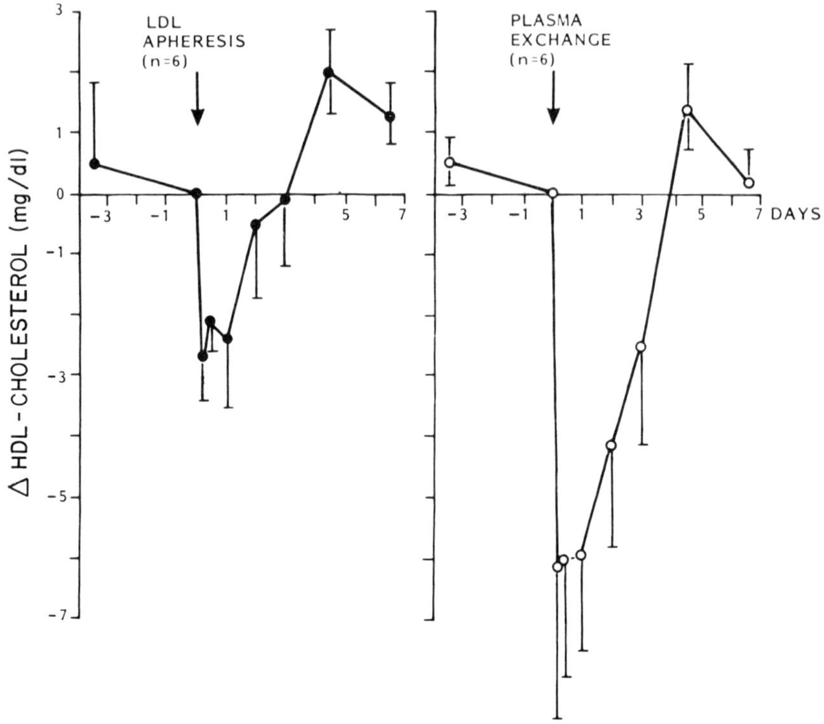

Fig. 1 Changes in HDL cholesterol after LDL apheresis and plasma exchange, expressed as mean ± SE relative to pre-exchange values, including the average level during the week before each procedure. (Reproduced from Kano *et al.* (1987) by permission of the American Heart Association.)

2.1.2 Changes in HDL specific activity and composition

Changes in the specific activities of total and HDL cholesterol in plasma are illustrated in Fig. 2. The specific activity of HDL cholesterol became higher than that of total cholesterol during the first few days after injection of [^{3}H]cholesterol, then declined but rose briefly after LDL apheresis. A similar but even more marked rise occurred after plasma exchange, as shown in Fig. 3. The rise in the relative specific activity of HDL cholesterol was evident within 2–6 hours, reaching a maximum at 24 hours. In contrast, the relative specific activity of total cholesterol showed a slight decrease during the 6 hours after each procedure.

Changes in HDL composition occurred after both plasma exchange and LDL apheresis. Baseline HDL composition differed markedly between

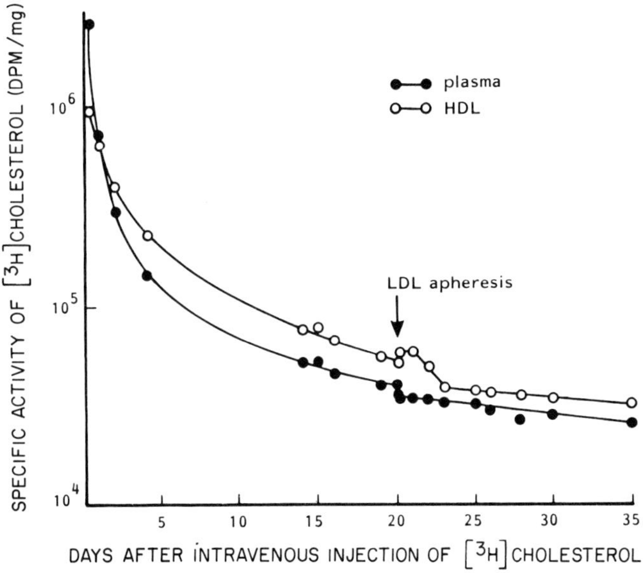

Fig. 2 Effect of LDL apheresis on specific activity of plasma total and HDL cholesterol in a homozygous WHHL rabbit injected with [^{3}H]cholesterol 21 days previously. (Reproduced from Kano *et al.* (1987) by permission of the American Heart Association.)

homozygotes and cholesterol-fed heterozygotes, and this, rather than the type of procedure undergone, was the major determinant of subsequent changes in composition. The mass ratio of cholesterol/phospholipid in baseline HDL was much higher in cholesterol-fed heterozygotes (0.49) than in homozygotes (0.18). This decreased on the first and second days after plasma exchange or LDL apheresis, the change being more marked in cholesterol-fed heterozygotes. Changes in this ratio on Day 1 were negatively correlated with changes in HDL specific activity ($r = -0.68$); ratios returned to their initial values 3–5 days after either procedure.

2.1.3 Role of HDL in cholesterol mobilization

Administration of radioactive cholesterol has long been used to label tissue cholesterol in both humans (Chobanian and Hollander, 1960) and experimental animals (Moutafis and Myant, 1976). Radioactivity in plasma equilibrates rapidly with cholesterol in liver and red cells, more slowly with fat and muscle, and least rapidly with the arterial intima. By waiting long enough, it is possible to ensure that all tissues other than brain will have a higher specific activity

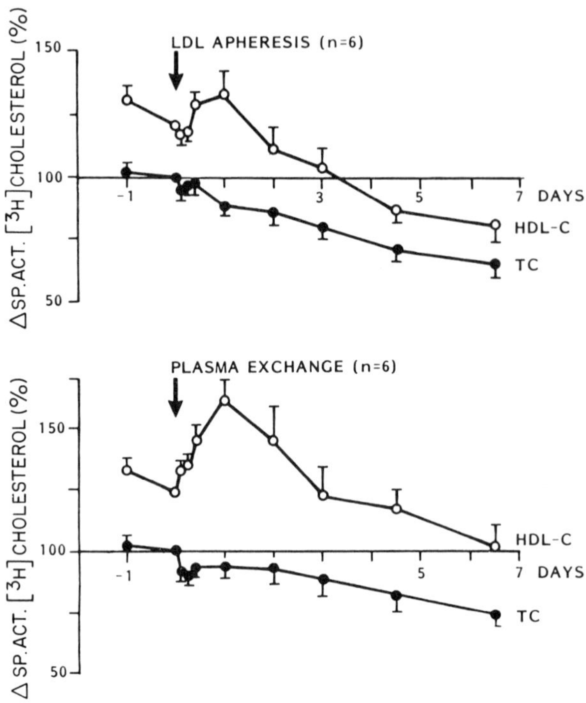

Fig. 3 Change in relative specific activities (means ± SE) of total cholesterol (TC) and HDL cholesterol (HDL-C) after LDL apheresis and plasma exchange, expressed as a percentage of the specific activity of total cholesterol immediately before each procedure. (Reproduced from Kano *et al.* (1987) by permission of the American Heart Association.)

than plasma. Any subsequent rise in plasma specific activity must indicate movement of cholesterol from tissues due either to exchange or net transfer. If the rise follows manouevres that do not entail the introduction into plasma of unlabelled cholesterol then it can be assumed to indicate net transfer rather than exchange. This phenomenon was observed in WHHL rabbits both after plasma exchange with lipoprotein-deficient plasma, which contains only very small amounts of cholesterol, and after LDL apheresis, suggesting that both procedures caused a net efflux of tissue cholesterol into plasma. Rises in HDL specific activity, which were maximal at 24 hours, were more marked after plasma exchange than after LDL apheresis, presumably reflecting the greater reduction of the intravascular pool of HDL. However, it is unlikely that much of the mobilized cholesterol came from arteries, since turnover of cholesterol there is so much slower than in most other tissues, including xanthomata (Jagannathan *et al.*, 1974; Bhattacharyya *et al.*, 1976). The rise in HDL specific activity during the 2 days after each procedure was accompanied by a reduction in the cholesterol/phospholipid ratio of HDL. Both findings are compatible with the entry into plasma of HDL derived from the extravascular compartment, in that the HDL of peripheral lymph has a higher phospholipid content than HDL in plasma (Sloop *et al.*, 1983) and has been reported to be the major acceptor of free cholesterol derived from tissues (Reichl *et al.*, 1980).

On the basis of this evidence, plasma exchange seems comparable to LDL apheresis in its ability to promote efflux of tissue cholesterol, despite the loss of HDL entailed. These findings, together with clinical studies showing the effectiveness of plasma exchange in inducing regression of xanthomata, suggest that extracorporeal removal of HDL does not impair cholesterol mobilization. Conceivably the ensuing increase in HDL turnover might even be beneficial in this context. It would be of interest to assess whether manouevres which reduce HDL cholesterol by decreasing HDL synthesis rather than by stimulating turnover have any adverse effect on cholesterol mobilization.

3 Intravenous administration of HDL analogues

An alternative or possibly complementary approach to extracorporeal reduction of LDL as a means of stimulating mobilization of tissue cholesterol is to increase the concentration of HDL-like, acceptor particles in plasma. The major constituents of HDL are apoA-I and phosphatidylcholine. Complexes of HDL apoproteins, mainly apoA-I, and phosphatidylcholine promote the efflux of free cholesterol from cells *in vitro*, including cultured arterial smooth muscle cells (Stein and Stein, 1973; Stein *et al.*, 1975). Intravenous infusion of phospholipids into animals with experimentally induced atheroma appears to influence the latter favourably (Friedman *et al.*, 1957; Adams *et al.*, 1967), but the effectiveness of this approach is limited by the rapidity with which phospholipid vescicles are cleared from plasma (Dewailly *et al.*, 1976). If apoA-I/phosphatidylcholine complexes were to be cleared at a slower rate, comparable with that of native HDL particles (Malmendier *et al.*, 1983), this could be advantageous in the context of therapeutic attempts to mobilize tissue cholesterol. We have therefore examined the properties *in vitro* and behaviour after injecting into rabbits of complexes of human apoA-I or apoHDL with phospholipid and have compared them with those of Lipostabil, a commercial preparation of phospholipid designed for intravenous use.

3.1 Preparation and properties of apoA-I phosphatidylcholine complexes

HDL was obtained by sequential precipitation of human plasma with phosphotungstate and magnesium chloride (Burstein and Scholnick, 1973). The HDL was then delipidated and apoA-I was isolated by chromatographing delipidated HDL on DEAE-sepharose CL-6B (Malmendier *et al.*, 1979). The apoA-I was then dissolved in sodium deoxycholate and mixed with Lipostabil (5% polyunsaturated phosphatidylcholine in 4% deoxycholate, Natterman) in a mass ratio of 1:3, the deoxycholate being removed subsequently by dialysis. The mixture was then chromatographed on Sepharose CL-6B and the apoA-I phosphatidylcholine complexes were sterilized by Millipore filtration.

Human apoA-I/phosphatidylcholine complexes showed a single peak on Sepharose CL-6B gel chromatography, which eluted ahead of HDL, indicating a slightly larger particle size. Analysis of the combined fractions comprising the main peak showed a mass ratio of phosphatidylcholine:apoA-I: deoxycholate of 2.25:1:0.26.

The fractional catabolic rate of human apoA-I/phosphatidylcholine complexes and human HDL labelled with ^{125}I or ^{131}I apoA-I were measured in normal rabbits. The fractional catabolic rate values of apoA-I/phosphatidylcholine complexes and HDL were 2.05 per day and 1.61 per day respectively, suggesting fairly similar rates of removal. Plasma obtained 4 hours after injection of apoA-I/phosphatidylcholine complexes and HDL showed sharp peaks of radioactivity, with elution profiles similar to those observed prior to injection.

When apoA-I/[^{14}C]phosphatidylcholine complexes were incubated with normolipidaemic rabbit plasma *in vitro*, 60% and 75% of the added [^{14}C]phosphatidylcholine and mass of phospholipid respectively were initially recovered in HDL after phosphotungstate–$MgCl_2$ precipitation. With Lipostabil less phospholipid was initially recovered in HDL, despite similar incubation conditions, but the proportion of labelled phospholipid association with HDL gradually increased, as did phospholipid mass.

The distribution of the apoA-I/[^{14}C]phosphatidylcholine complexes and apoA-I/[^{14}C]phosphatidylcholine-labelled Lipostabil after incubation with rabbit plasma was also analysed by single discontinuous density gradient ultracentrifugation. This showed that the density of the apoA-I/phosphatidylcholine complexes was similar to HDL throughout, whereas the pre-incubation density of Lipostabil was similar to LDL. However, during the 3 hours incubation of Lipostabil the distribution of radioactivity progressively shifted from the LDL to the HDL region of the gradient.

3.1.1 Single infusions of human apoA-I/phosphatidylcholine complexes and Lipostabil into rabbits

When 100 mg of phospholipid in the form of apoA-I/phosphatidylcholine complexes or Lipostabil were infused into normal rabbits there were increases in plasma and HDL phospholipids and in total cholesterol at 60 minutes in both instances, with little change in HDL cholesterol (Figs. 4 and 5). Most of the rise in plasma phospholipid after apoA-I/phosphatidylcholine complexes was attributable to a rise in HDL phospholipid, but less than 50% of the increment after Lipostabil was localized to HDL. In both instances plasma and HDL phospholipids returned to near basal levels within 6 hours.

Taken together, these data suggest that apoA-I/phosphatidylcholine complexes resembled HDL more closely in their physical and metabolic properties than does Lipostabil.

3.2 Effects of apoHDL/phosphatidylcholine complexes on cholesterol efflux

For experiments requiring large quantities of complexes it was preferable to prepare apoHDL/phosphatidylcholine complexes rather than apoA-I/phosphatidylcholine complexes, owing to the losses involved in purification of apoA-I. *In vitro* studies or those involving single injections were undertaken using human apoHDL, but those involving repeated injections were performed with rabbit apoHDL. Both types of complexes were of similar size and had a mass ratio of phosphatidylcholine to protein of approximately 2 : 1 (Fig. 6).

Six cholesterol-fed heterozygous WHHL rabbits were injected with [^{3}H]cholesterol and then infused 4 weeks later with human apoHDL/phosphatidylcholine complexes (100 mg protein, 200 mg phosphatidylcholine) or Lipostabil (200 mg phosphatidylcholine) or an equivalent volume of saline. The pattern of changes in total and HDL phospholipid concentrations in plasma were similar to those observed in normolipidaemic rabbits injected with apoA-I/phosphatidylcholine complexes or Lipostabil or saline (see Fig. 4). However, total cholesterol levels decreased after apoHDL/phosphatidylcholine and Lipostabil, whereas HDL cholesterol increased after apoHDL/phosphatidylcholine complexes but decreased after Lipostabil. Reciprocal changes in the specific activity of HDL cholesterol were observed, as shown in Fig. 7. These findings are difficult to interpret, but do not suggest any influx of high specific activity tissue cholesterol into plasma after apoHDL/phosphatidylcholine complexes had been infused. Since the rise in the specific

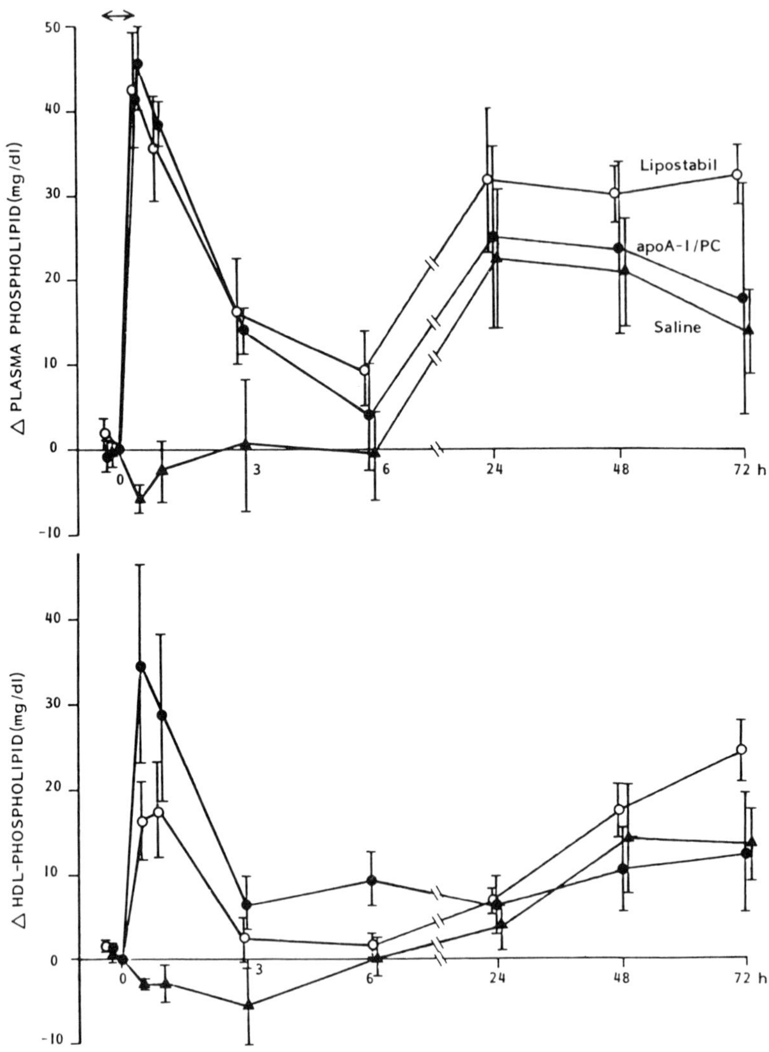

Fig. 4 Changes in plasma and HDL phospholipid in New Zealand White rabbits after infusing human apoA-I/phosphatidylcholine complexes (100 mg phospholipid), Lipostabil (100 mg phospholipid) or saline. The animals were re-fed after 6 hours. Mean ± SE of 4 animals in each group.

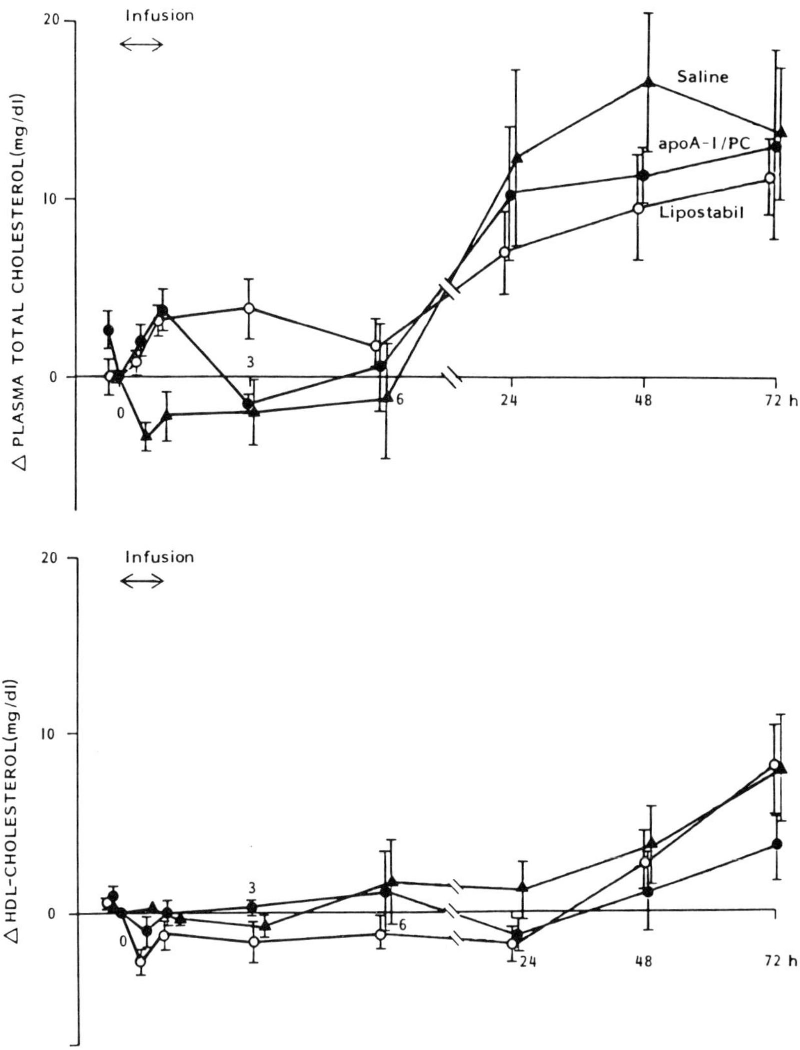

Fig. 5 Changes in plasma and HDL cholesterol in New Zealand White rabbits after infusing human apoA-I/phosphatidylcholine complexes (100 mg phospholipid), Lipostabil (100 mg phospholipid) or saline. Conditions as in Fig. 4.

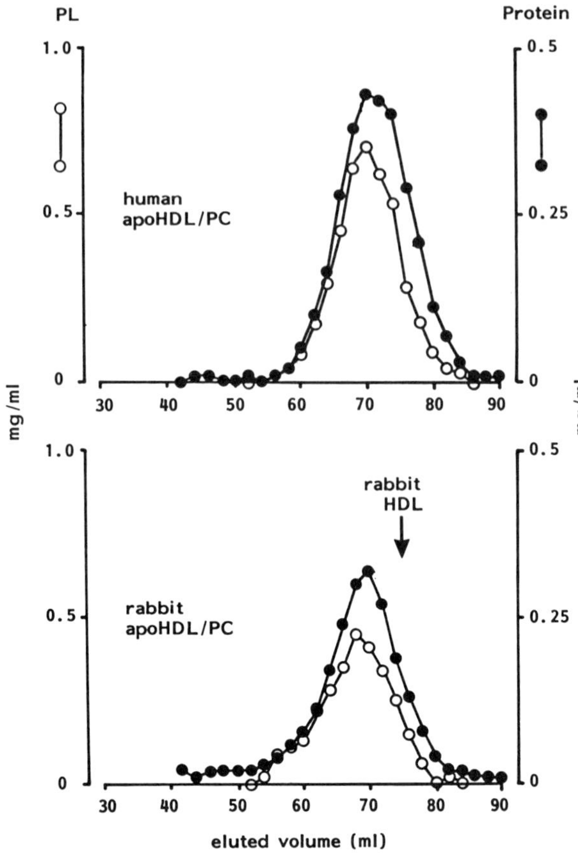

Fig. 6 Elution profiles of human and rabbit apoHDL/phosphatidylcholine complexes on Sepharose CL-6B column.

activity of HDL cholesterol after Lipostabil was mirrored by a corresponding decrease in its concentration, it too is unlikely to represent net influx of tissue cholesterol.

3.2.1 Aortic perfusion in vitro

Aortas of heterozygous WHHL rabbits that had been maintained on a 0.5% cholesterol diet for 44–240 days were perfused *in vitro* (Boyer and Davies, 1978). The aortic perfusate was prepared by the addition of KCl, calcium gluconate, glucose and Na_2CO_3 to 4.5% human albumin solution and was gassed with 5% CO_2, 95% O_2. The aorta was washed with 50 ml of chilled

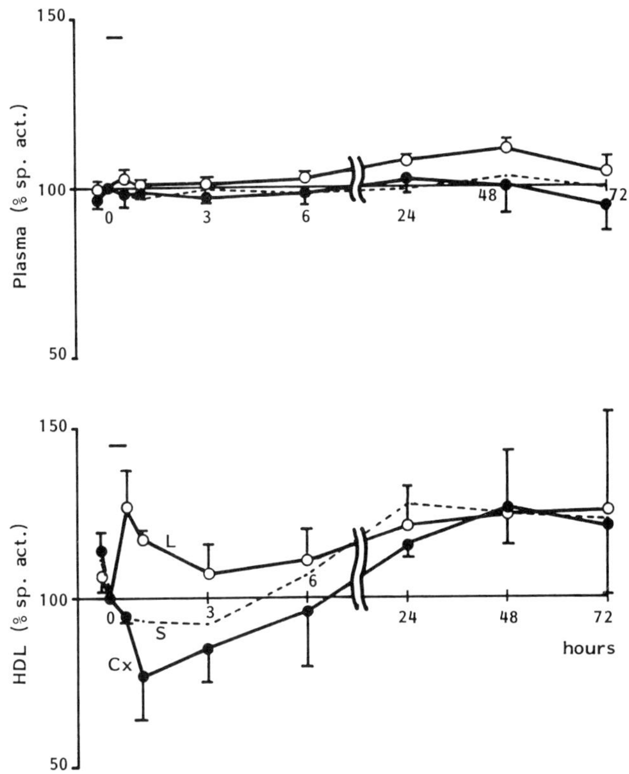

Fig. 7 Changes in relative specific activities of plasma and HDL cholesterol after infusing apoHDL/phosphatidylcholine complexes (Cx), Lipostabil (L) or saline (S) into cholesterol-fed WHHL heterozygotes. Rabbits were fasted for the first 6 hours, then re-fed. The period of infusion is shown by the horizontal bars.

saline and recirculated with 15 ml of perfusate, which was discarded. Three further perfusions were then carried out sequentially during each of which 10 ml of perfusate was recirculated with constant gassing for 40 minutes at 37°C, 90 mmHg mean pressure. During periods I and III the effects of adding 0.6 mg/ml of human apoHDL/phosphatidylcholine complex plus 50 μl/ml of an LCAT-rich fraction of plasma were compared with the control period II, during which the perfusate contained no additives. At the end of the perfusion the aorta was washed and then opened longitudinally. The inner layer, containing intima and media, was peeled off (Wolinsky and Daly, 1970), then homogenized with NH_4OH containing 0.2% Triton X. After extraction with chloroform : methanol (Folch *et al.*, 1957) total cholesterol in homogenate and perfusate was measured by GLC. The increase of cholesterol in the perfusate was calculated by subtracting the amount of cholesterol present before the perfusion.

Preliminary studies showed that the cholesterol content of the perfusate increased most during the first perfusion period and was dependent upon the wet weight and cholesterol content of each individual aorta perfused. To correct for these influences, cholesterol efflux was expressed as the ratio of the increment in the cholesterol content of the perfusate during periods I or III, when human apoHDL/phosphatidylcholine complexes and/or an LCAT-containing fraction of plasma were added to the perfusate, to the increment during the control period II, when the perfusate contained no additives. It was found that the highest ratios occurred when apoHDL/phosphatidylcholine complexes and an LCAT fraction were both added to the perfusate, whereas either of these alone or apoHDL/phosphatidylcholine complex plus heat-inactivated LCAT fraction did not promote efflux to a greater extent than perfusate without additives.

3.2.2 Effect of repeated injections of rabbit apoHDL/phosphatidylcholine complexes on aortic atherosclerosis

Rabbit apoHDL/phosphatidylcholine complexes were prepared in a similar manner to human apoHDL/phosphatidylcholine complexes. Homozygous WHHL rabbits, which were 4-month-old siblings, were kept on a normal diet whereas New Zealand White rabbits were fed a 1% cholesterol diet for 8 weeks, then switched to a normal diet. One group of cholesterol-fed New Zealand White rabbits was killed to assess severity of aortic atherosclerosis after the 8 weeks of 1% cholesterol feeding. The remaining three groups of New Zealand White rabbits and three pairs (1 male, 1 female) of homozygous WHHL rabbits were injected with rabbit apoHDL/phosphatidylcholine complexes (50 mg protein : 100 mg phosphatidylcholine), Lipostabil (100 mg phospholipid) or saline (10 ml) weekly for 8 weeks and then killed and their aortas removed. Each aorta was cut longitudinally and 2 mm wide transverse strips of intima and media were excised at 2 cm intervals. These strips were frozen and stored and the remainder of the aorta was fixed in 10% formalin for staining with Oil Red O (Drury and Wallington, 1967). The aortic strips were homogenized with NH_4OH containing 0.2% Triton X, for measurement of total cholesterol, protein and DNA content (Donkersloot *et al.*, 1972).

Plasma cholesterol changes in the two strains of rabbits are shown in Fig. 8. Values rose during the period of the 1% cholesterol diet in the New Zealand White rabbits and then gradually returned to basal levels when this was discontinued. No obvious differences were seen between the three treatment groups of WHHL rabbits (lower panel, Fig. 8). Nor were any obvious changes

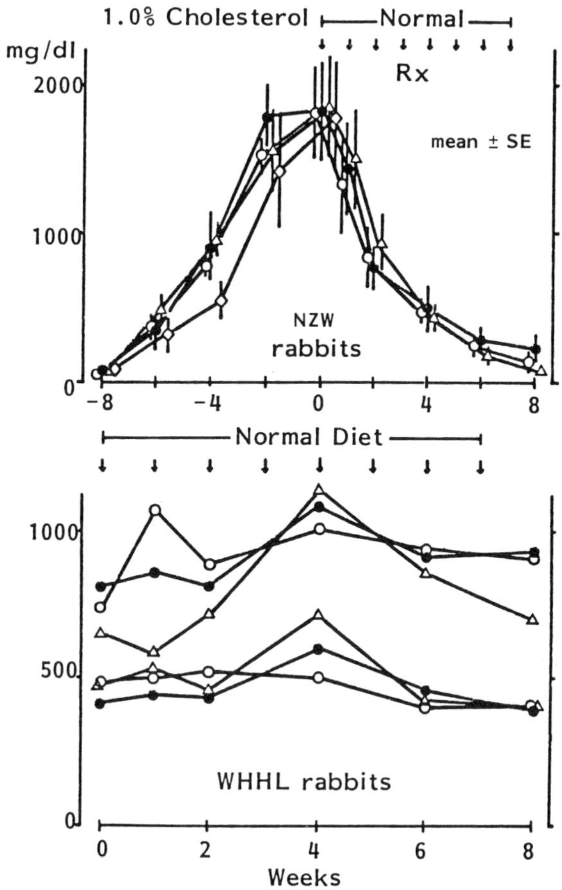

Fig. 8 Plasma total cholesterol values in cholesterol-fed New Zealand White rabbits (3 per group, upper panel) and in individual homozygous WHHL rabbits (lower panel). The arrows indicate injections of rabbit apoHDL/phosphatidylcholine complexes (●), Lipostabil (○) or saline (△).

observed in HDL cholesterol or phospholipid levels among the WHHL rabbits (Fig. 9).

Examination of the Oil Red O stained aortas showed considerable variation within each group, but no obvious differences between the groups. Staining was more intense in cholesterol-fed New Zealand White rabbits (Fig. 10) than in WHHL rabbits (Fig. 11). The cholesterol content of the aortas of WHHL rabbits revealed no consistent differences between the three treatment groups (Table 1).

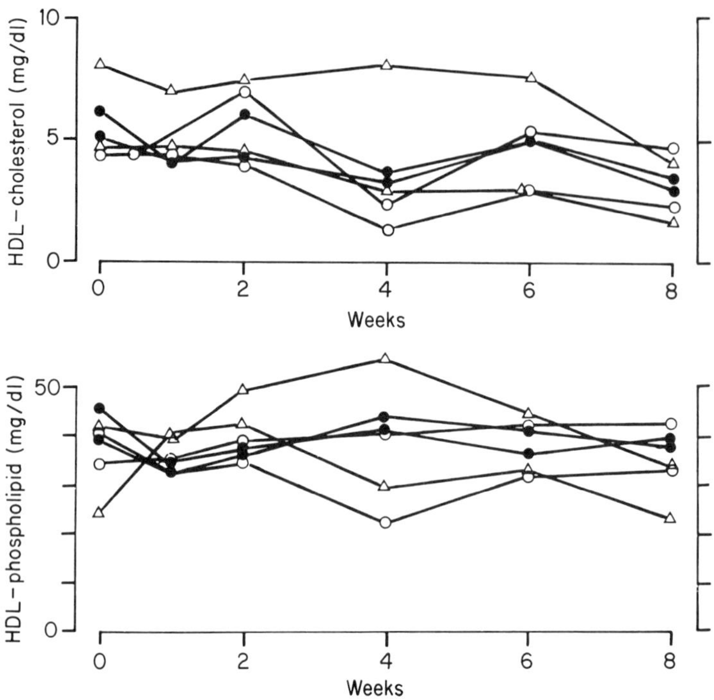

Fig. 9 HDL cholesterol and phospholipid levels in WHHL rabbits receiving weekly injections of apoHDL/phosphatidylcholine complexes (●), Lipostabil (○) or saline (△).

Table 1 Cholesterol content of inner aorta.

No.	Treatment	Cholesterol (mg/mg protein)	Cholesterol (mg/mg DNA)
1	apoHDL/phosphatidylcholine	0.033	0.69
2	apoHDL/phosphatidylcholine	0.106	1.93
3	Lipostabil	0.089	1.84
4	Lipostabil	0.079	1.63
5	Saline	0.057	0.86
6	Saline	0.105	1.95

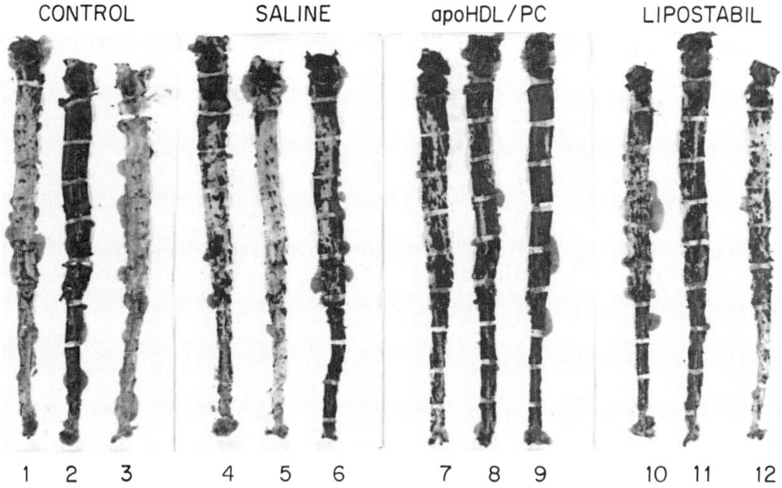

Fig. 10 Oil Red O stained aortas from cholesterol-fed New Zealand White rabbits.

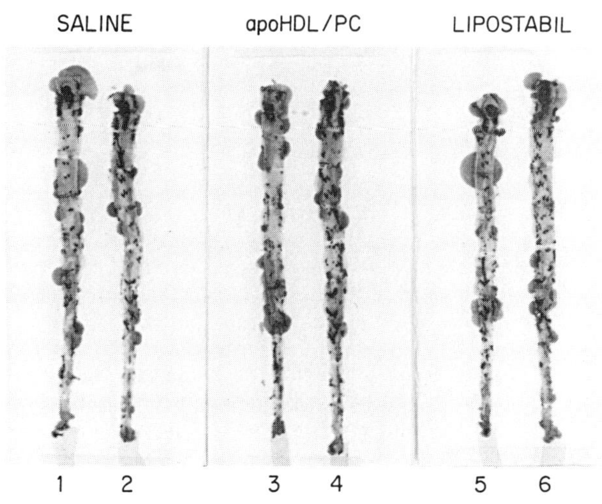

Fig. 11 Oil Red O stained aortas from homozygous WHHL rabbits.

3.2.3 Cholesterol acceptor properties of apoHDL/phosphatidylcholine complexes

Stein and Stein (1973) showed that the ability of phospholipids to act as acceptors of cholesterol from cells *in vitro* could be enhanced by first complexing the phospholipid with apoHDL. These workers later showed removal by apoHDL/phosphatidylcholine complexes of cholesterol from aortic smooth muscle cells (Stein *et al.*, 1975). During the present studies there was some evidence that addition of apoHDL/phosphatidylcholine complexes and LCAT to the perfusion medium promoted efflux of cholesterol from the aorta of hypercholesterolaemic rabbits, but the effect of Lipostabil was not tested because it was considered that its high concentration of deoxycholate would damage the endothelium and spuriously increase the cholesterol content of the perfusate.

Administration of intravenous Lipostabil has been claimed to induce regression of atherosclerosis *in vivo* (Adams *et al.*, 1967). However, we could find no evidence of this when either Lipostabil or rabbit apoHDL/phosphatidylcholine complexes were administered repeatedly to rabbits with spontaneous or diet-induced hypercholesterolaemia. This negative result may simply have been a reflection of the severity of the atherosclerosis, the inadequacy of the amounts infused or the short duration of treatment. It leaves unanswered the question of whether administration of HDL analogues can promote sufficient mobilization of cholesterol in the arterial wall to be therapeutically useful. On the evidence presented here, however, it would seem that for clinical purposes extracorporeal removal of LDL provides a more effective means of mobilizing tissue cholesterol than does infusion of HDL analogues.

References

Adams, C. W. M., Abdulla, Y. H., Bayliss, O. B. and Morgan, R. S. (1967). Modification of aortic atheroma and fatty liver in cholesterol-fed rabbits by intravenous injection of Saturnher and polyunsaturated lecithins. *J. Path. Bact.* **94**, 77–87.

Bhattacharyya, A. K., Connor, W. E., Mausof, F. A. and Flatt, A. E. (1976). Turnover of xanthoma cholesterol in hyperlipoproteinemia patients. *J. Clin. Lab. Med.* **87**, 503–518.

Blankenhorn, D. H., Nessin, S. A., Johnson, R. L., Sanmarco, M. E., Azen, S. P. and Cashin-Hemphill, L. (1987). Beneficial effects of combined colestipol–niacin therapy on coronary atherosclerosis and coronary venous bypass grafts. *J. Am Med. Assoc.* **257**, 3233–3240.

Boyer, D. E. and Davies, P. F. (1978). Effect of concentration of perfusing free fatty acid on arterial lipid synthesis in perfused normal and atherosclerotic rabbit aortas. *Atherosclerosis* **13**, 409–419.

Burstein, M. and Scholnick, H. R. (1973). Lipoprotein–polyanion–metal interactions. *Adv. Lipid. Res.* **11**, 67–108.

Castelli, W. P., Doyle, J. T., Gordon, T. *et al.* (1977). HDL cholesterol and other lipids in coronary heart disease. The cooperative lipoprotein phenotyping study. *Circulation* **55**, 767–772.

Chobanian, A. V. and Hollander, W. (1960). Body cholesterol metabolism in man. 1. The equilibration of serum and tissue cholesterol. *J. Clin. Invest.* **41**, 1732–1737.

Dewailly, P., Decoopman, E., Desreumaux, C. and Fruchart, J. C. (1976). Plasma removal of intravenous essential phospholipids in man. In *Phosphatidylcholine* (ed. H. Peeters), pp. 80–86. Springer-Verlag, Berlin.

Donkersloot, J. A., Robrish, S. A. and Krichevsky, M. I. (1972). Fluorometric determination of deoxyribonucleic acid in bacteria with ethidium bromide. *Appl. Microbiol.* **24**, 179–183.

Drury, P. A. B. and Wallington, E. A. (1967). *Lipids in Carteton's Histological Technique*, 4th edn, pp. 291–304. Oxford University Press, New York.

Folch, J., Lees, M. and Sloane Stanley, G. H. (1957). A simple method for the isolation and purification of total lipids from animal tissues. *J. Biol. Chem.* **226**, 497–509.

Friedman, M., Byers, S. O. and Rosenman, R. H. (1957). Resolution of aortic atherosclerotic infiltration in the rabbit by phosphoatide infusion. *Proc. Soc. Exp. Biol. Med.* **95**, 586–588.

Jagannathan, S. N., Connor, W. E., Baker, W. H. and Bhattacharyya, A. K. (1974). The turnover of cholesterol in human atherosclerotic arteries. *J. Clin. Invest.* **54**, 366–377.

Kano, K., Koizumi, J., Jadhav, A. and Thompson, G. R. (1987). Plasma exchange and low density lipoprotein apheresis in Watanabe Heritable Hyperlipidemic Rabbits. *Arteriosclerosis* **7**, 256–261.

Levy, R. I., Brensike, J. F., Epstein, S. E., Kelsey, S. F., Passamani, E. R., Richardson, J. M., Loh, I. K., Stone, N. J., Aldrich, R. F., Battaglini, J. W., Moriarty, D. J., Fisher, M. L., Friedman, L. F., Friedewald, W. and Detre, K. M. (1984). The influence of changes in lipid values induced by cholestyramine and diet on progression of coronary artery disease: results of the NHLBI type II coronary intervention study. *Circulation* **69**, 325–337.

Malmendier, C. L., Christophe, J. and Ameryckx, J. P. (1979). Separation and partial characterization of new apoproteins from human plasma high density lipoproteins. *Clin. Chem. Acta* **99**, 167–176.

Malmendier, C. L., Delcroix, C. and Ameryckx, J. P. (1983). *In vivo* metabolism of human apoprotein A-I-phospholipid complexes. Comparison with human high density lipoprotein–apoprotein A-I metabolism. *Clin. Chem. Acta* **131**, 201–210.

Miller, N. E. (1984). Current concepts of the role of HDL in reverse cholesterol transport. In *Clinical and Metabolic Aspects of High-Density Lipoproteins* (ed N. E. Miller and G. D. Miller), pp. 187–216. Elsevier, Amsterdam.

Moutafis, C. D. and Myant, N. B. (1976). The distribution of [^{14}C]cholesterol in muscle and skin of Rhesus monkeys after intravenous injection. *Clin. Sci. Mol. Med.* **50**, 307–310.

Reichl, D., Myant, N. B., Rudra, D. N. and Pflug, J. J. (1980). Evidence for the presence of tissue free cholesterol in low density lipoproteins of human peripheral lymph. *Atherosclerosis* **37**, 489–495.

Rhoads, G. G., Gulbrandsen, C. L. and Kagan, A. (1976). Serum lipoproteins and coronary heart disease in a population study of Hawaii Japanese men. *N. Engl. J. Med.* **294**, 293–298.

Sloop, C. H., Dory, L., Hamilton, R., Krause, B. R. and Roheim, P. S. (1983).

Characterization of dog peripheral lymph lipoproteins: the presence of a disc-shaped "nascent" high density lipoprotein. *J. Lipid Res.* **24**, 1429–1440.

Stein, O. and Stein, Y. (1973). The removal of cholesterol from Landschutz ascites cells by high-density apolipoprotein. *Biochim. Biophys. Acta* **326**, 232–244.

Stein, Y., Glangeaud, M. C., Fainaru, M. and Stein, O. (1975). The removal of cholesterol from aortic smooth muscle cells in culture and Landschutz ascites cells by fractions of human high-density apolipoprotein. *Biochim. Biophys. Acta* **380**, 106–118.

Thompson, G. R., Lowenthal, R. and Myant, N. B. (1975). Plasma exchange in the management of homozygous familial hypercholesterolaemia. *Lancet* **i**, 1208–1211.

Thompson, G. R., Myant, N. B., Kilpatrick, D., Oakley, C. M., Raphael, M. J. and Steiner, R. E. (1980). Assessment of long-term plasma exchange for familial hypercholesterolaemia. *Br. Heart J.* **43**, 680–688.

Thompson, G. R. (1981). Plasma exchange for hypercholesterolaemia. *Lancet* **i**, 1246–1248.

Warnick, G. R. and Albers, J. J. (1978). Heparin–Mn quantitation of high-density-lipoprotein cholesterol: an ultrafiltration procedure for lipemic samples. *Clin. Chem.* **25**, 596–604.

Wolinsky, H. and Daly, M. M. (1970). A method for the isolation of intima-media samples from arteries. *Proc. Exp. Biol. Med.* **135**, 265–275.

Yokoyama, S., Hayashi, R., Kikkawa, T., Tani, N., Takada, S., Hatanaka, K. and Yamamoto, A. (1984). Specific sorbent of apolipoprotein B-containing lipoproteins for plasmapheresis. Characterization and experimental use in hypercholesterolemic rabbits. *Arteriosclerosis* **4**, 276–282.

Yokoyama, S., Hayashi, R., Satani, M. and Yamamoto, A. (1985). Selective removal of low density lipoprotein by plasmapheresis in familial hypercholesterolemia. *Arteriosclerosis* **5**, 613–622.

8

Lipids, Coagulability and Ischaemic Heart Disease

T. W. MEADE

MRC Epidemiology and Medical Care Unit, Northwick Park Hospital, Harrow, UK

1 Introduction

Over thirty years ago, Morris, in two classical studies of the epidemiological pathology of ischaemic heart disease (IHD), showed that the clinical epidemic that had been growing since the 1920s could not be explained solely in terms of atheroma (Morris, 1951; Morris and Crawford, 1958). It was clear that some other process must be involved, and thrombogenesis was an obvious possibility. Despite these indications, however, it is only comparatively recently that much attention has been paid to the study of thrombogenesis and its contribution to IHD. There are several reasons. The first is the overwhelming predominance of hypotheses for IHD that centre round the dietary intake of fat and its influence on blood lipid levels and atherogenesis. A second reason has been that, although a thrombogenic contribution to IHD has always been recognized by some, the view has not been unanimous. It is not very long since many argued that thrombosis follows rather than causes infarction, and it is only comparatively recently that this particular controversy has been resolved (Chandler *et al.*, 1974). Over the last few years developments in angiography and imaging techniques have helped to clarify further the undoubted role of thrombosis in myocardial infarction. Even more controversial has been the place of thrombosis in sudden coronary death. Many previously thought of this manifestation as non-thrombotic in origin, though the careful pathological studies by Davies and Thomas (1984) now leave little doubt that thrombogenesis contributes to some extent to nearly all sudden deaths due to IHD. Thirdly, the technical difficulties of studying haemostatic mechanisms on an epidemiological scale have to be borne in mind.

HYPERLIPIDAEMIA AND ATHEROSCLEROSIS
ISBN 0.12.675645-7

Given that there is a strong case for investigating the thrombotic as well as lipid component of IHD, the main question for the epidemiologist is whether identifiable characteristics of the haemostatic system are associated with the subsequent risk of IHD. So far, it is the coagulation system rather than platelet function that has been more rewarding.

2 Coagulation system

Figure 1 is a highly simplified representation of the coagulation system. Its physiological function is to secure haemostasis after injury by the production of thrombin and thus the conversion of soluble fibrinogen to insoluble fibrin. Thrombin is also a potent platelet aggregating agent. The final common pathway can be activated through the intrinsic or the extrinsic system, the latter being so called because a constituent from outside the circulation—tissue factor—is needed. As Fig. 1 shows, factor VII can also be activated via the intrinsic or contact system. This pathway is probably of considerable relevance in considering the relationship between lipids, coagulability and IHD and will be referred to again later.

Since the epidemiological findings to be discussed point to the level of factor VII activity and to the plasma fibrinogen concentration as being of greatest interest, it is useful first to review their characteristics.

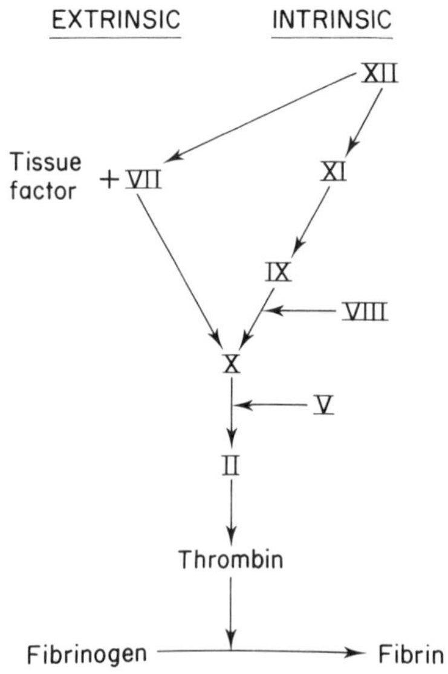

Fig. 1 A summary of the coagulation cascade.

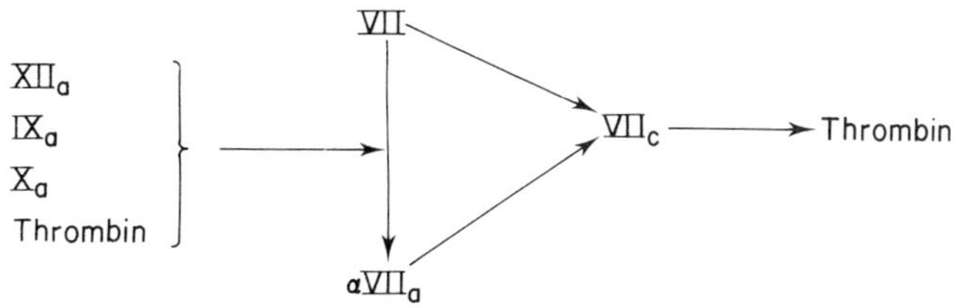

Fig. 2 Determinants and effect of factor VII coagulant activity, VII_c.

2.1 *Factor VII activity, VII_c*

Within the arterial circulation, it is not hard to imagine that the rupture of an atheromatous plaque might provide the tissue factor necessary to initiate extrinsic coagulation by complexing with factor VII. Figure 2 illustrates some of the determinants of factor VII coagulant activity. First, the factor VII zymogen is unusual in itself having some biological activity, and this will influence the result of a factor VII biological activity assay, i.e. VII_c. However, VII_c is largely an expression of the extent to which the native single-chain form, or zymogen, has been converted to the double-chain form, factor αVII_a, which is between 100 and 150 times more active. As Fig. 2 shows, the level of factor XII activity influences the extent to which factor VII is converted to factor αVII_a (already referred to) and so do factor X and, to some extent, thrombin itself. Secondly, factor VII activity is not inhibited, at any rate to any marked extent, by antithrombin III, for example. As a result, the level of factor VII coagulant activity is a useful general index of the level of "coagulability".

The level of VII_c can be considerably increased by the cold activation of plasma. When this is done there is, as Fig. 3 shows, a remarkably parallel increase in thrombin production, measured by fibrinopeptide A (Miller *et al.*, 1986a). When hirudin is used to inhibit thrombin production, it is clear that it is VII_c activation that precedes the increase in thrombin production, and not *vice versa*. This experiment strongly suggests that VII_c may be a determinant of thrombin production and there is further evidence to this effect (Meade, 1987).

2.2 *Fibrinogen*

Fibrinogen is an acute-phase protein. Plasma concentrations rise as a result of a wide range of stimuli, many of a somewhat non-specific nature. Examples are after surgery and in malignant disease. Atheroma has some of the characteristics of an inflammatory response, and this has led to the suggestion that the high levels associated with an increased risk of IHD (see later) may be no more

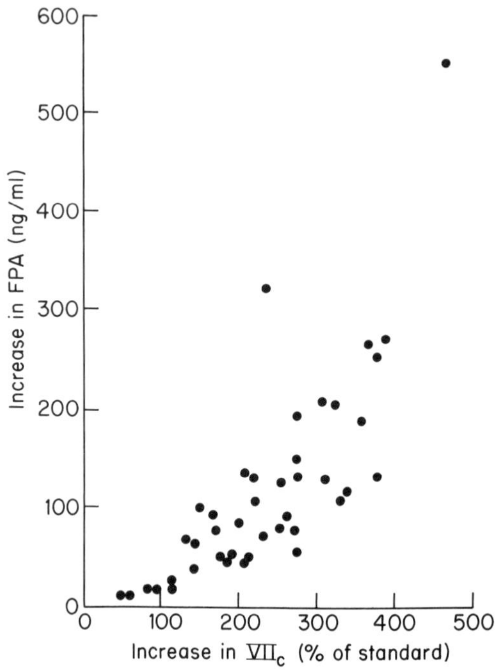

Fig. 3 Relationship between increase in VII$_c$ and increase in fibrinopeptide A (FPA) following surface/cold activation of plasma from 42 individuals. From Miller *et al.* (1986a); for details see reference.

than an index of the extent of atheroma. Even if this were the full and only explanation, the strong association of fibrinogen with IHD that has now been demonstrated would still be of considerable value. However, there are at least four ways in which high fibrinogen levels are likely to predispose to thrombosis, whatever the explanation for high levels in the first place. Thus fibrinogen and fibrin are important constituents of the atheromatous plaque itself (Smith, 1986). Secondly, the plasma fibrinogen concentration is a leading determinant of plasma and blood viscosity (Lowe, 1985). Thirdly, increasing levels of fibrinogen within the physiological range increase *in vitro* measures of platelet aggregability (Meade *et al.*, 1985a, b). Finally, work in experimental animals suggests that the amount of fibrin formed is determined by the initial concentration of fibrinogen (Gurewich *et al.*, 1976). There is no reason why the high fibrinogen levels that certainly are associated with an increased risk of IHD should not be partly due to "non-specific" influences, for example environmental causes such as cigarette smoking. Genetic contributions are

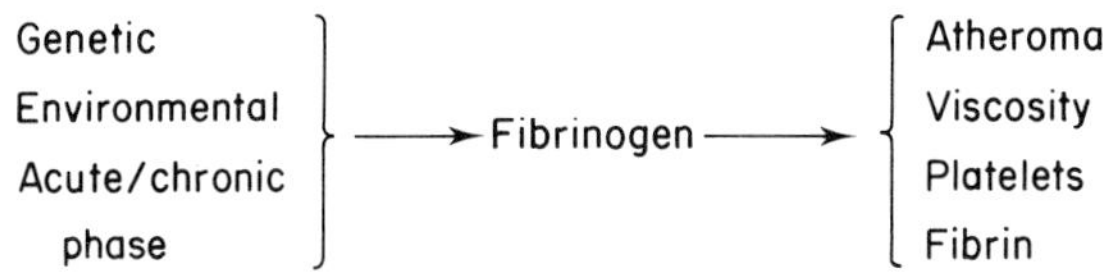

Fig. 4 Determinants and effects of fibrinogen.

also important, as has now been demonstrated (Humphries *et al.*, 1987). These points are summarized in Fig. 4. But whatever the explanation, there are clearly several pathogenetic pathways through which high levels of fibrinogen—however they are determined—may operate.

3 Prospective studies

In 1980 Meade *et al.* (1980) reported strong associations in the Northwick Park Heart Study of high levels of VII_c and plasma fibrinogen with mortality from cardiovascular disease, principally IHD. The main results of this study (Meade *et al.*, 1986a) are summarized in Fig. 5. They are based on data from

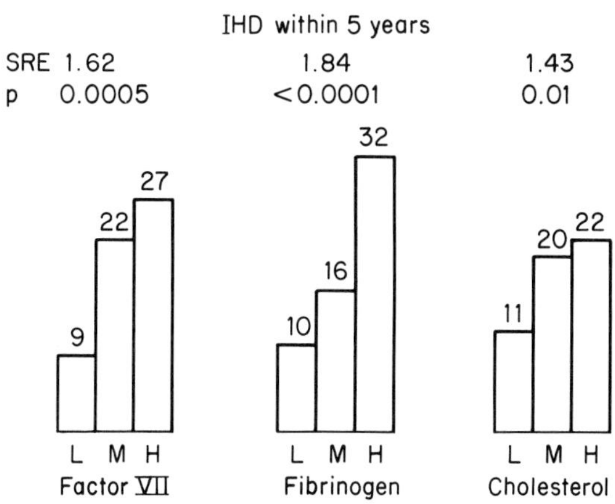

Fig. 5 Numbers of events of IHD (fatal and non-fatal) within 5 years of examination by low (L), middle (M) and high (H) thirds of distributions of factor VII activity, fibrinogen and cholesterol at entry to the Northwick Park Heart Study. SREs (standardized regression effects) show the increase in risk of an event for a standard deviation (SD) increase; for example, a 1 SD increase in factor VII activity increases the risk of an event within 5 years by 62%. (From Meade *et al.* (1986a); for further details see reference.)

Table 1 Mean fibrinogen levels (g/1) at entry to the Göteborg Study according to subsequent outcome.

Ischaemic heart disease ($n = 92$)	Stroke ($n = 37$)	Deaths from other causes ($n = 60$)	No event ($n = 608$)
3.56[a]	3.70[a]	3.37	3.30

[a]Significantly different from "No event" subjects; $p < 0.01$; n = number of subjects.

the 1511 white men aged between 40 and 64 when first recruited, who were then followed up six years later. The relationships of VII_c and fibrinogen with the incidence of IHD were, if anything, stronger than for cholesterol, though the latter relationship was also demonstrated.

In a study of 792 men born in 1913, Wilhelmsen *et al.* (1984) showed a relationship between high fibrinogen levels and the incidence of both IHD and stroke. Their findings are summarized in Table 1. There was an interaction between fibrinogen and systolic blood pressure in their effect on stroke. Men with high levels of both were at considerably greater risk than would have been expected from the sum of the two effects separately.

In 1985 Stone and Thorp reported an association between high fibrinogen levels and IHD incidence in a group of 297 men aged between 40 and 69. This relationship was stronger than in the case of cholesterol, blood pressure or smoking. In this study, too, there was an interaction between fibrinogen and blood pressure, this time in their association with IHD.

In 1987 Kannel *et al.* reported an association between high fibrinogen levels and the incidence of cardiovascular disease in both men and women.

The most recent report is the preliminary one from the Prospective Cardiovascular Münster Study confirming the finding in the Northwick Park Heart Study on VII_c as well as the results from this and other studies on fibrinogen (Balleisen *et al.*, 1987).

In summary, there is no real doubt as to the relationship between high fibrinogen levels and the risk of cardiovascular disease, both IHD and stroke. In fact, the fibrinogen level is almost certainly the strongest biochemical index of the risk of cardiovascular disease and probably, also, of IHD and stroke separately. Two studies have demonstrated a relationship between high VII_c levels and the risk of IHD. It may therefore be that the biochemical disturbance in IHD lies at least as much in the coagulation system as in the metabolism of lipids.

4 Hypercoagulability and IHD

Clearly, it is important to establish how far the association between high clotting-factor levels and IHD is of causal significance, since this will have a major bearing on approaches to primary prevention. Some of the additional evidence required has already been referred to, for example the mechanisms by which fibrinogen may predispose to thrombosis and the association between VII_c and thrombin production. Much of this evidence is summarized elsewhere (Meade, 1987). In the case of VII_c, the considerable benefits of oral anticoagulants on the incidence of thromboembolism after myocardial infarction should be borne in mind (Meade, 1984) since factor VII is the procoagulatory clotting factor most rapidly and extensively affected by these agents. The probable association between high VII_c levels and deep vein thrombosis (Boyer *et al.*, 1986) is of particular interest because it can with some confidence be attributed to characteristics of the blood rather than to vessel wall changes. The evidence that high VII_c levels are associated either with an increased incidence of IHD itself or with other high-risk situations is consistent, and much of it does suggest that the relationship with IHD is of causal significance.

5 Diet, lipids and coagulability

5.1 *Observational studies*

Table 2 summarizes the general epidemiological characteristics of VII_c and fibrinogen. Besides their general consistency with the results of prospective studies, they tend also to be paralleled by higher (or lower) levels of cholesterol. This is particularly true of VII_c. In the Northwick Park Heart Study the correlation between VII_c and cholesterol was 0.24. Higher values (unpublished) were found in several related studies. This phenomenon has been studied in detail by Miller *et al.* (1985). Scarabin *et al.* (1985) have reported a similar association. Most of the rest of this chapter is concentrated on the relationship between diet, lipids and VII_c. The correlation between fibrinogen and cholesterol in the Northwick Park Heart Study is 0.06. There is little if any evidence that diet affects fibrinogen levels, at any rate in the short term.

What is the explanation of the association between VII_c and cholesterol levels? In 1960 Merskey *et al.* included factor VII and fibrinogen in a study of African blacks and whites. The starting point was the clear dietary differences between the two groups, particularly in fat intake. Both cholesterol and VII_c were lower in the blacks. This finding has now been repeated in at least three

Table 2 General epidemiological characteristics of factor VII coagulant activity (VII_c) and fibrinogen levels in plasma.

VII_c		Fibrinogen
	Higher levels	
Increasing age		Increasing age
Obesity		Obesity
Use of oral contraceptives		Use of oral contraceptives
Menopause		Menopause
Diabetes		Diabetes
"Imprudent" diet		Smoking
		Low employment grade
	Lower levels	
Black ethnic group		Moderate alcohol intake
Vegetarians		

other studies (Meade *et al.*, 1978, 1986b; Miller *et al.*, 1988). One of these studies is summarized in Tables 3 and 4. As Table 3 shows, black Gambians, who experience little or no IHD, have low VII_c levels by comparison with whites, and these levels are contained within a relatively narrow range, as indicated by the standard deviations. In white groups in high IHD mortality countries (England and Czechoslovakia) levels are higher than in Gambians,

Table 3 Mean values of factor VII coagulant activity (VII_c) and fibrinogen levels in plasma from inhabitants of Gambia (no IHD), in Czechoslovakia and England (high IHD mortality) and in Scotland and Finland (very high IHD mortality).

	n	VII_c (%)	Fibrinogen (g/l)
Gambia			
Urban	54	71	2.90
Rural	36	70	3.86
Rural	67	67	4.19
Prague	101	87	3.48
London	26	86	2.82
Scotland			
Glasgow	81	94	3.00
Aberdeen	80	96	3.05
Finland			
South West	87	92	3.46
Central	51	88	3.32
East	45	92	3.62

SD in VII_c in Gambians = 11; SD in the other studies shown = 19.

Table 4 Mean factor VII biological coagulant activity (VII_c) and fibrinogen levels in plasma from black Gambians and white European expatriates in Gambia.

	n	VII_c (%)	Fibrinogen (g/l)
Blacks			
Rural	36	72	3.35
Rural	25	67	4.19
Urban (police)	52	72	2.90
Blood donors	23	71	2.69
Technical/nursing	10	102	3.45
Whites			
Expatriates	11	113	2.63

and they are highest of all in those with the highest IHD mortality rates (Scotland and Finland). The standard deviations are larger than in Gambians. An explanation of this latter observation might be the effect of some environmental stimulus tending to raise VII_c levels from an intrinsically lower level. Table 4 shows that among Gambians levels are highest in those who are economically most developed. It is also clear from Tables 3 and 4 that the highest fibrinogen levels (probably due to parasitic infection) are found in rural Gambians.

Merskey *et al.* (1960) had also found possibly higher fibrinogen levels in blacks than whites. If the high fibrinogen levels associated with IHD risk in endemic populations are of causal significance then the observation of high levels in groups where the disease is practically unrecorded suggests that high levels interact with some other characteristic to cause IHD. Attention has already been drawn to the interaction in two of the prospective studies between fibrinogen and blood pressure. By way of analogy, Japanese men are among the heaviest cigarette smokers in the world, yet they experience relatively little IHD. Few would seriously argue that this means that cigarette smoking is not involved in the onset of the disease. The probable explanation is that Japanese men also on average have low blood cholesterol levels (Keys, 1980) and are therefore not exposed to the degree of atheroma found in populations with higher cholesterol levels. Like cigarette smoking itself, therefore, the plasma fibrinogen level may only be of significance when the scene has been set by some other process—but when this process is fully established the effects may be very substantial. In passing, the likelihood that a major part of the effect of smoking on IHD is mediated through the plasma fibrinogen concentration (Meade *et al.*, 1987) should be emphasized. It is also worth noting that vegetarians have substantially lower levels of VII_c than non-vegetarians (Haines *et al.*, 1980).

The observational data therefore strongly suggest that diet may influence VII_c as well as cholesterol levels. A number of experimental studies and laboratory work also support this conclusion.

5.2 Experimental studies

Table 5 summarizes the results of a seven-week randomized cross-over trial of the effects of high- and low-fat diets on VII_c and fibrinogen (Miller *et al.*, 1986b). Healthy volunteers weighed all they ate over a six- or seven-week period during which the first two weeks were spent on normal diet and the remaining time on a high-fat and a low-fat diet, the order being randomly determined for each person. It was intended that the high- and low-fat diets should be isocaloric. In the event, energy intake was greater during the high-fat period. VII_c was significantly lower on the low-fat diet, and *vice versa*. This is illustrated for one individual in Fig. 6. There was no significant difference in fibrinogen levels. Three other experimental studies (Elkeles *et al.*, 1980; Simpson *et al.*, 1982; Simpson *et al.*, 1983) also indicate that dietary and/or drug modifications that lower blood cholesterol levels also lower VII_c levels. None of these studies, however, demonstrated a beneficial effect on plasma fibrinogen levels.

These observations in man are now being supplemented by animal studies (Mitropoulos *et al.*, 1987; Mitropoulos and Esnouf, 1987) which point to the same conclusion: dietary alterations leading to elevations in lipoproteins also increase VII_c. Which kinds of dietary fat are mainly responsible is currently under study.

The intrinsic coagulation system is contact-activated, depending on the exposure of blood to negative charges, for example on glass. Large lipoproteins such as chylomicrons and VLDL are also negatively charged. It may therefore be that these particles provide the physiological surface for the activation of factor XII, which in turn activates factor VII (see Fig. 1). Work on this possible explanation is currently in progress and suggests that it may be well

Table 5 Summary of results of seven-week randomized cross-over trial of effects of high- and low-fat diets on factor VII coagulant activity (VII_c) and fibrinogen levels in plasma of healthy volunteers.

	High-fat	Low-fat	*p*
VII_c (%)	98	82	0.001
Fibrinogen (g/l)	2.95	3.08	NS

NS: not significant.

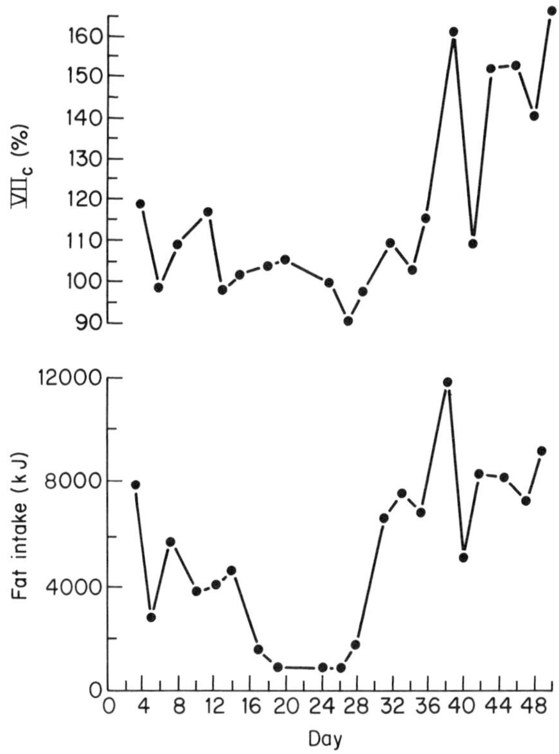

Fig. 6 VII_c activity and dietary fat intake in an individual over 50 days. (From Miller *et al.* (1986b); for details see reference.)

founded. If so, the relationship between dietary fat intake, lipids, VII_c and IHD may be along the lines set out in Fig. 7. Thus a high-fat intake causes hypercholesterolaemia, which in turn promotes atherogenesis and thus the risk of IHD. At the same time, the effect of diet on coagulability, reflected in higher VII_c, may predispose to thrombogenesis and thus to the acute complications of atheroma. (Hypercoagulability may also contribute to the thrombotic component of atheroma itself as indicated by the diagonal arrow in Fig. 7.)

There are several implications of a scheme of this kind. First, it is inappropriate that views about the pathogenesis of IHD should be polarized between lipid and thrombogenic hypothesis. It seems increasingly likely that diet influences both the chronic and acute pathways to IHD. Secondly, it is at least possible that measures designated to prevent IHD by lowering lipid levels may have done so partly and perhaps mainly by their effects on coagulability, bearing in mind the difficulty of achieving the regression of atheroma. Indeed,

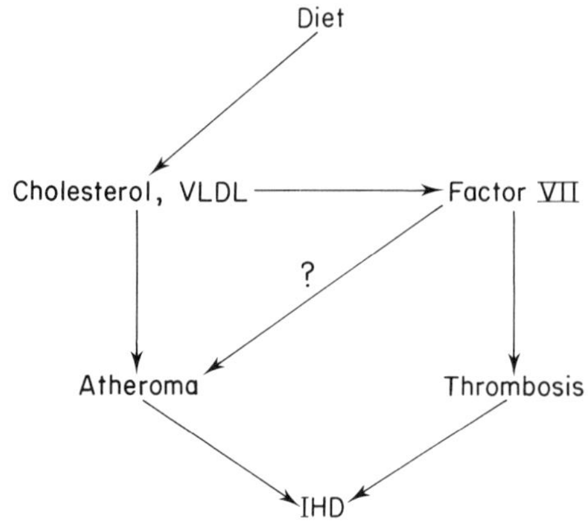

Fig. 7 Scheme of dietary contribution to pathogenesis of ischaemic heart disease (IHD). (Fibrin, partially due to coagulation initiated by extrinsic system, contributes to atheroma as well as thrombosis, as does fibrinogen.) (From Meade, T. W. (1987) *Blood Reviews* **1**, 2–8.)

the beneficial effects of gemfibrozil on the incidence of IHD in high-risk men (Frick *et al.*, 1987) may have been due not only to the effects of the drug on lipids, as well as on coagulability, but also to an effect on fibrinogen levels. Thirdly, the apparent resistance of the plasma fibrinogen level to dietary manipulation may place a limit on the extent to which primary prevention can be achieved by dietary means. Finally, to the extent that primary prevention cannot be achieved by attempting to reverse or slow the process of atherogenesis, for whatever reason, it may be necessary to give increasing attention to the prevention of thrombosis by pharmacological means. Besides the use of platelet-active agents, the possibility that gemfibrozil may be beneficial as a result of its fibrinogen-lowering properties has already been referred to. Consideration is also being given (Meade, 1987) to the possibility that lower doses of warfarin than those used in conventional anticoagulation may be effective, coupled as they almost certainly would be with a lower risk of bleeding.

References

Balleisen, L., Schulte, H., Assmann, G., Epping, P. H. and Van de Loo, J. (1987). Coagulation factors and the progress of coronary heart disease. *Lancet* **ii**, 461.

Boyer, C., Wolf, M., Rothschild, C. *et al.* (1986). An enzyme immunoassay ELISA for the quantitation of human factor VII. *Throm. Haemostasis* **56**, 250–255.

Chandler, A. B., Chapman, I., Erhardt, L. R., Roberts, W. C., Schwartz, C. J.,

Sinapius, D., Spain, D. M., Sherry, S., Ness, P. M. and Simon, T. L. (1974). Coronary thrombosis in myocardial infarction. Report of a workshop on the role of coronary thrombosis in the pathogenesis of acute myocardial infarction. *Am. J. Cardiol.* **34**, 823–833.

Davies, M. J. and Thomas, D. (1984). Thrombosis and acute coronary-artery lesions in sudden cardiac ischemic death. *N. Engl. J. Med.* **310**, 1137–1140.

Elkeles, R. S., Chakrabarti, R., Vickers, M., Stirling Y. and Meade, T. W. (1980). Effect of treatment of hyperlipidaemia on haemostatic variables. *Br. Med. J.* **281**, 973–974.

Frick, M. H., Elo, O. and Haapa K. *et al.* (1987). Helsinki Heart Study: Primary-prevention trial with gemfibrozil in middle-aged men with dyslipidemia. Safety of treatment, changes in risk factors, and incidence of coronary heart disease. *N. Engl. J. Med.* **317**, 1238–1245.

Gurewich, V., Lipinski, B. and Hyde, E. (1976). The effect of the fibrinogen concentration and the leukocyte count on intravascular fibrin deposition from soluble fibrin monomer complexes. *Thromb. Haemost.* **36**, 605–614.

Haines, A. P., Chakrabarti, R., Fisher, D., Meade, T. W., North, W. R. S. and Stirling, Y. (1980). Haemostatic variables in vegetarians and non-vegetarians. *Thromb. Res.* **19**, 139–148.

Humphries, S. E., Cook, M., Dubowitz, M., Sterling, Y. and Meade, T. W. (1987). Role of genetic variation at the fibrinogen locus in determination of plasma fibrinogen concentrations. *Lancet* **i**, 1452–1455.

Kannel, W. B., Wolf, P. A., Castelli, W. P. and D'Agostino, R. B. (1987). Fibrinogen and risk of cardiovascular disease. The Framingham Study. *J. Am. Med. Assoc.* **258**, 1183–1186.

Keys, A. (1980). *Seven Countries: A Multivariate Analysis of Death and Coronary Heart Disease.* Harvard University Press.

Lowe, G. D. (1985). Platelet volume subpopulations in acute myocardial infarction: an investigation of their homogeneity for smoking, infarct size and site. *Clin. Sci.* **68**, 419–425.

Meade, T. W., Brozovic , M., Chakrabarti, R., Haines, A. P., North, W. R. S. and Stirling, Y. (1978). Ethnic group comparisons of variables associated with ischaemic heart disease. *Br. Heart J.* **40**, 789–795.

Meade, T. W., North, W. R. S., Chakrabarti, R. *et al.* (1980). Haemostatic function and cardiovascular death: early results of a prospective study. *Lancet* **i**, 1050–1054.

Meade, T. W. (1984). In *Anticoagulants and Myocardial Infarction: A Reappraisal* (ed. T. W. Meade), pp. 91–111. Wiley, Chichester.

Meade, T. W., Vickers, M. V., Thompson, S. G., Stirling, Y., Haines, A. P. and Miller, G. J. (1985a). Epidemiological characteristics of platelet aggregability. *Br. Med. J.* **290**, 428–432.

Meade, T. W., Vickers, M. V., Thompson, S. G. and Seghatchian, M. J. (1985b). The effect of physiological levels of fibrinogen on platelet aggregation. *Thromb. Res.* **38**, 527–534.

Meade, T. W., Mellows, S. and Brozovic, M. *et al.* (1986a). Haemostatic function and ischaemic heart disease: principal results of the Northwick Park Heart Study. *Lancet,* **ii**, 533–537.

Meade, T. W., Stirling, Y., Thompson, S. G. *et al.* (1986b) An international and interregional comparison of haemostatic variables in the study of ischaemic heart disease. Report of a working group. *Intl J. Epidemiol.* **15**, 331–336.

Meade, T. W. (1987). In *Thrombosis and Haemostasis 1987* (ed. M. Verstraete, J. Vermylen, R. Lynen, J. Arnout), pp. 37–60. Leuven University Press.

Meade, T. W., Imeson, J. D. and Sterling, Y. (1987). Effects of changes in smoking and other characteristics on clotting factors and the risk of ischaemic heart disease. *Lancet* **ii**, 986–988.

Merskey, C., Gordon, H., Lackner, H. *et al.* (1960). Blood coagulation and fibrinolysis in relation to coronary heart disease. A comparative study of normal white men, white men with overt coronary heart disease, and normal Bantu men. *Br. Med. J.* **i**, 219–227.

Miller, G. J., Walter, S. J., Sterling, Y., Thompson, S. G., Esnouf, M. P. and Meade, T. W. (1985). Assay of factor VII activity by two techniques: evidence for increased conversion of VII to alpha VIIa in hyperlipidaemia, with possible implications for ischaemic heart disease. *Br. J. Haematol.* **59**, 249–258.

Miller, G. J., Seghatchian, M. J., Walter, S. J. *et al.*. (1986a). An association between the factor VII coagulant activity and thrombin activity induced by surface/cold exposure of normal human plasma. *Br. J. Haematol.* **62**, 379–384.

Miller, G. J., Martin, J. C., Webster, J. *et al.* (1986b). Association between dietary fat intake and plasma factor VII coagulant activity—a predictor of cardiovascular mortality. *Atherosclerosis* **60**, 269–277.

Miller, G. J., Kotecha, S., Wilkinson, W. H. *et al.* (1988). *Atherosclerosis* (in press).

Mitropoulos, K. A., Esnouf, M. P. and Meade, T. W. (1987). Increased factor VII coagulant activity in the rabbit following diet-induced hypercholesterolaemia. Evidence for increased conversion of VII to alpha VIIa and higher flux within the coagulation pathway. *Atherosclerosis* **63**, 43–52.

Mitropoulos, K. A. and Esnouf, M. P. (1987). Turnover of factor X and of prothrombin in rabbits fed on a standard or cholesterol-supplement diet. *Biochem. J.* **244**, 263–269.

Morris, J. N. (1951). Recent history of coronary disease. *Lancet* **i**, 1–7; 69–73.

Morris, J. N. and Crawford, M. D. (1958). Coronary heart disease and physical activity of work. Evidence of a national necroscopy survey. *Br. Med. J.* **4**, 1485–1496.

Scarabin, P. Y., Bara, L., Samama, M. and Orssaud, G. (1985). Further evidence that activated factor VII is related to plasma lipids. *Br. J. Haematol.* **61**, 186–187.

Simpson, H. C. R., Mann, J. L., Chakrabarti, R., Imeson, J. D., Stirling, Y., Tozer, M., Woolf, L. and Meade, T. W. (1982). Effect of high-fibre diet on haemostatic variables in diabetes. *Br. Med. J.* **284**, 1608.

Simpson, H. C. R., Mann, J. I., Meade, T. W., Chakrabarti, R., Stirling, Y. and Woolf, L. (1983). Hypertriglyceridaemia and hypercoagulability. *Lancet* **i**, 786–789.

Smith, E. B. (1986). Fibrinogen, fibrin and fibrin degradation products in relation to atherosclerosis. *Clinics in Haematology* **15**, 355–370.

Stone, M. C. and Thorp, J. M. (1985). Plasma fibrinogen—a major coronary risk. *J. R. Coll. Gen. Pract.* **35**, 565–569.

Wilhelmsen, L., Svardsudd, K., Korsan-Bengtsen, K., Larsson, B., Welin, L. and Tibblin, G. (1984). Fibrinogen as a risk factor for stroke and myocardial infarction. *N. Engl. J. Med.* **311**, 501–505.

9

Macrophages and Ceroid in Atherosclerosis

M. J. MITCHINSON, R. Y. BALL,
K. L. H. CARPENTER and D. V. PARUMS
University of Cambridge, Department of Pathology, Cambridge, UK

1 Introduction

1.1 Ceroid in atherosclerosis

Ceroid is the name given to insoluble material, thought to be composed of oxidized lipid and protein, that is found in a variety of circumstances in mammalian tissues (Wolman, 1975). It is especially abundant in animals deficient in the natural anti-oxidant vitamin E. Ceroid found in different circumstances is not of constant chemical structure. It can be produced artificially by the oxidation of a variety of lipids, in association with various proteins (Wolman, 1975). Ceroid is therefore defined only loosely as an autofluorescent material that is insoluble in lipid solvents and yet reacts with histological stains for lipid such as Oil Red O (Pearse, 1972).

It has been known for many years that ceroid occurs in human atherosclerotic plaques (Pappenheimer and Victor, 1946; Burt, 1952). Because of this, there have been occasional speculations about a role for lipid oxidation in the development of the lesions (Nishida and Kummerow, 1960; Porta and Hartroft, 1969).

1.2 Hypothesis

A more recent survey of ceroid distribution in human atherosclerosis showed that granules of ceroid were always present, not only in the necrotic base of

HYPERLIPIDAEMIA AND ATHEROSCLEROSIS
ISBN 0.12.675645-7

advanced lesions but also in at least some of the lipid-laden foam cells of the lesions, even very small fatty streaks in children (Mitchinson, 1982). These foam cells were thought to resemble macrophages. The presence of ceroid within them suggested a hypothetical role for lipid and protein oxidation in lesion development (Mitchinson, 1982, 1983):

(1) the human foam cells are macrophages, derived from blood monocytes;
(2) these macrophages oxidize some of their lipid burden, producing not only ceroid but also soluble oxidized lipids;
(3) the soluble oxidation products include some that are cytotoxic and others that influence plaque development by affecting the behaviour of nearby cells.

A similar view was put forward by Fowler (1983) as one of the possible contributions of macrophages to lesion development.

This hypothesis derived originally from the presence of ceroid in foam cells, but there were already a number of reports in the literature to provide support for one or other of the three components.

1.3 Existing support for the hypothesis

In 1982 the prevailing view was that most human arterial foam cells were derived from smooth muscle cells, but some electron microscopic and cell-marker studies in experimental animals were beginning to suggest that they might be monocyte-derived macrophages (Fowler *et al.*, 1979; Gaton and Wolman, 1977; Gerrity *et al.*, 1979; Gerrity, 1981a,b). Incidentally, this was by no means a new idea: a number of workers had held this opinion over the years (e.g. Anitschkow, 1933). Hard evidence as to the nature of human arterial foam cells was, however, lacking.

The oxidative free-radical-mediated microbicidal function of phagocytes was well established (Badwey and Karnovsky, 1980), and there were also existing reports that macrophages can cause lipid peroxidation (Mason *et al.*, 1972; Stossel *et al.*, 1974). Enzymatic oxidation of arachidonic acid with production of prostaglandins and leukotrienes was also, of course, well documented (Scott *et al.*, 1978).

There was some evidence that certain oxidized lipids were atherogenic when added to the diet of animals (e.g. Cook and MacDougal, 1968; Imai *et al.*, 1976) and were cytotoxic *in vitro* (e.g. Peng *et al.*, 1979; Baranowski *et al.*, 1982). Furthermore, various oxidized lipids had been detected in human atherosclerotic lesions (e.g. Glavind *et al.*, 1952; Smith and van Lier, 1970; Brooks *et al.*, 1971; Harland *et al.*, 1971, 1973). The hypothesis therefore appeared to be worth pursuing.

1.4 Remaining questions

Clearly the identity of the foam cells was of prime importance. The work of Goldstein and Brown and others had shown that lipid uptake by macrophages was very different from that of most other cells (Goldstein *et al.*, 1979; Fogelman *et al.*, 1980; Mahley *et al.*, 1979). Most cells take up low density lipoprotein (LDL) by means of a high-affinity LDL receptor, which is down-regulated when the cell's cholesterol content is adequate. However, chemically modified (e.g. acetylated) LDL is taken up by macrophages via different receptors, which are not down-regulated by increased cellular cholesterol content. These findings provided support for the attractive theory that foam cells were macrophages.

It was also clear that much more needed to be learned about the uptake and metabolism of lipids by macrophages, including whether or not they were capable of producing ceroid, and the soluble oxidized lipids known to be present in the arterial lesions. Above all, it was important to find out, if possible, whether such oxidation of lipids and proteins occurs in humans.

2 The identity of foam cells

Recent years have seen increasingly compelling ultrastructural evidence in experimental animals that monocytes adhere to endothelium and migrate into the intima to become macrophage foam cells (e.g. Joris *et al.*, 1983; Faggiotto *et al.*, 1984; Schwartz *et al.*, 1985). Evidence as to the nature of human foam cells was less abundant, until Stary (1983) produced particularly clear electron micrographs strongly suggesting that they were macrophages.

Morphology alone was not completely convincing, but studies detecting enzymes and other markers characteristic of macrophages in experimental arterial lesions added significantly to the accumulating evidence (e.g. Davis *et al.*, 1984; Adams and Bayliss 1976; Schaffner *et al.*, 1980; Fowler, 1983). Numano *et al.* (1983) introduced the use of monoclonal antibodies in immunocytochemical methods for the identification of the macrophages in experimental lesions.

In 1984, Vedeler and his associates, in a study of early human lesions, used a variety of cell-markers, and the results suggested that most foam cells in these early plaques were macrophages. Their methods also included the use of a monoclonal antibody to HLA-DR antigen.

We had begun to study human lesions with a panel of three monoclonal antibodies reacting with macrophages but not smooth muscle cells, and the findings suggested that all human arterial foam cells were macrophages (Aqel *et al.*, 1984). Similar results were obtained by Klurfeld (1985). At this stage we were fortunate to acquire also a monoclonal antibody to a component of smooth muscle cells. The use of these monoclonal antibodies against macrophages and smooth muscle cells produced a clear-cut differentiation between the cell-types (Aqel *et al.*, 1985). The "mirror-image" patterns of cell reactions resulting from this work are in our view particularly convincing, and have been confirmed by other groups using different monoclonals (Jonasson *et al.*, 1986; Gown *et al.*, 1986).

More recent studies, using monoclonal antibodies or scanning electron microscopy, continue to support the monocyte–macrophage origin of foam cells in experimental atherosclerosis (Watanabe *et al.*, 1985; Tsukada *et al.*, 1986; Taylor and Lewis, 1986).

It is important to emphasize that all these groups are using the term "foam cells" for cells whose cytoplasm is literally bulging with lipid droplets. Although smooth muscle cells in human atherosclerosis often contains some lipid droplets, they never become bloated with them as do macrophages. Therefore, after experience of monoclonal antibody studies, it becomes much easier to distinguish the two cell-types even in conventionally stained sections.

There can now be little doubt that the large, distended foam cells of both human and experimental atherosclerosis are indeed macrophages. This validates the first component of the hypothesis and indicates that the macrophage is of considerable importance in atherogenesis.

Some have chosen to interpret the identification of foam cells as macrophages to mean that their presence is beneficial, like their scavenger role in a healing wound. However, their role as scavengers in a wound depends on their ability, when loaded, to depart the scene via the lymphatics, but this is not possible from the arterial intima. There are suggestions that macrophage foam cells might leave the intima by migrating back through the endothelium into the blood (e.g. Gerrity, 1981b; Faggiotto *et al.*, 1984). This would be an attractive explanation of the regression of some early lesions, but must be regarded as not yet proved.

However, in human advanced lesions, macrophages appear to be dying to give rise to the necrotic gruel in the base of the plaque (Schaefer, 1981; Stary, 1983; Aqel *et al.*, 1985). This can scarcely be regarded as beneficial. Indeed, our own interpretation of the histological appearances of lesions is that in plaques that are progressing, macrophage foam cells are abundant and adding to the bulk of the necrotic base. Spillage of contents of living or dead macrophages may therefore be enlarging the lesion; the ingrowth of smooth muscle cells seems to us to be secondary and essentially reparative, like fibroblasts in a healing wound. Lesions are sometimes seen consisting mainly or only of smooth muscle cells. These do not protrude much into the lumen, and in our view are healed and virtually never cause complications. There are many chronic inflammatory conditions in which macrophage spillage or death seems to perpetuate the lesion, such as the pneumoconioses. We believe that atherosclerosis is in the same category.

To judge from our studies with monoclonal antibodies, only macrophages contain ceroid, in the form of granules or "ring" forms; endothelial cells and smooth muscle cells do not (Aqel *et al.*, 1985; Mitchinson *et al.*, 1985).

3 Accumulation of ceroid by macrophages *in vitro*

The second component of the hypothesis was tested by a series of experiments on macrophages in culture. Early experiments showed that mouse peritoneal macrophages cultured in medium containing 33% foetal calf serum rapidly accumulated membrane-bound lipid droplets, which within a day contained a peripheral skin of ceroid (Ball *et al.*, 1984). The "ring" structures produced were very similar to those often seen in human arterial foam cells, by light and electron microscopy (Ball *et al.*, 1984; Mitchinson *et al.*, 1985). The appearances supported the idea that oxidation was occurring at the periphery of the membrane-bound droplets. Similar lipid droplets surrounded by a ceroid skin are present in the necrotic base of advanced plaques, presumably having been spilled from dead macrophages (Mitchinson *et al.*, 1985). This raises the possibility that these insoluble ceroid skins are preventing dispersal of the soluble lipid droplets within them.

Mouse peritoneal macrophages were then cultured with native human LDL and various forms of artificially modified LDL in medium containing lipoprotein-deficient serum. All the cultures showed accumulation of lipid droplets, but granules of ceroid accumulated only in the cells exposed to partially preoxidized LDL and not in those given native, acetylated or dextran-sulphate-modified LDL (Ball *et al.*, 1986). This raises the question whether, in order to produce ceroid, macrophages need to take up lipoprotein that has already been oxidized to some degree, the macrophage itself perhaps merely completing the process of oxidation to ceroid.

These early experiments on ceroid accumulation in macrophages told us very little about the chemistry of the process, except that the artificial oxidation of LDL was accompanied by depletion of linoleic (18:2) and arachidonic (2:4) acids. Experiments were therefore conducted in which mouse peritoneal macrophages were exposed to artificial emulsions of bovine serum albumin with particular cholesteryl esters or acylglycerols (Ball *et al.*, 1987a, b). All the emulsions were avidly taken up to produce multiple droplets within the cell. Ceroid accumulation occurred within all the cells in 12 hours, when the emulsion had contained cholesteryl linoleate, cholesteryl arachidonate, trilinolein or 1,3-dilinolein. However, no ceroid appeared in cells exposed to emulsions containing cholesterol, cholesteryl oleate or triolein (Ball *et al.*, 1987a,b). Thus it appeared that the more easily oxidized lipids, with one or more bisallylic carbon atoms, led to ceroid production.

An unexpected finding was that the ceroid morphology depended on the lipid species in the emulsion. Cholesteryl arachidonate was associated with intracellular granules of ceroid, cholesteryl linoleate with "rings" and di- or trilinolein with granules and coarse lumps of ceroid. Incorporation of the free-radical scavengers butylated hydroxytoluene (BHT) or butylated hydroxyanisole (BHA) into the emulsions did not seem to affect the production of ceroid from arachidonate, but greatly diminished that from linoleate and altered its morphology, with no ring forms visible (Ball *et al.*, 1987a,b). The ultrastructural appearance of the ceroid was once again analogous to the range of appearances seen in human foam cells (Ball *et al.*, 1987b). Thus the range of appearances of ceroid seen in the human plaque might result partly from the oxidation of different lipid species.

4 Depletion of linoleate and arachidonate

As previously mentioned, artificial oxidation of LDL, in our method using cupric ions as a catalyst, leads to depletion of linoleic (18:2) and arachidonic (20:4) acids relative to oleic (18:1) (Ball *et al.*, 1986). Similar changes have been noted as a result of other forms of oxidation such as bubbling oxygen through LDL solutions (Esterbauer *et al.*, 1987). The chemical composition of ceroid is difficult to study, but hydrolysates of the ceroid-rich insoluble fraction of human atheroma show similar depletion of linoleate and arachidonate (Ball *et al.*, 1987c).

In experiments using a mixture of cholesteryl oleate-BSA and cholesteryl linoleate-BSA emulsions, mouse peritoneal macrophages also produced linoleate depletion relative to oleate (Carpenter *et al.*, 1987).

The interest of these observations lies in comparing them with the chemistry of lipids of the human arterial wall. Lipoproteins containing apolipoprotein B extracted from human aorta have been reported to show linoleate depletion (Hoff and Gaubatz, 1982), and Smith and her colleagues showed long ago that there was relative depletion of both cholesteryl linoleate and arachidonate in the foam-cell-rich lesions of human aorta when compared with LDL or to fibrous lesions (Smith *et al.*, 1967). These findings are therefore compatible with the view that LDL oxidation occurs in the arterial wall, perhaps especially in foam-cell-rich areas.

5 Oxidized lipids

Oxidized lipids have been found in human serum and plasma, aortic tissue (including human atherosclerotic plaques and atherosclerotic aorta from

Watanabe Hereditable Hyperlipodaemic (WHHL) rabbits) and in mouse peritoneal macrophages cultured with polyunsaturated lipids *in vitro*. These findings are summarized in Table 1. In addition, there are numerous reports of prostaglandin and leukotriene production from arachidonic acid by macrophages of various types (e.g. Aderem *et al.*, 1986 and references therein; MacDermot *et al.*, 1984). The data are obviously incomplete, but it is interesting that the best documented oxidized lipids are oxidation products of cholesterol, linoleic acid and arachidonic acid. However, many other lipid oxidation products may be present, such as lipid peroxides (e.g. Glavind *et al.*, 1952).

The significance of these compounds in development of atherosclerosis is not yet clear. Some oxidation products of cholesterol and of linoleic acid have been shown to induce arterial lesions in dietary experiments in rabbits (Imai *et al.*, 1976; Cutler and Schneider, 1974) and to be cytotoxic *in vivo* (Imai *et al.*, 1980) and *in vitro* (Baranowski *et al.*, 1982). This might be a contributing factor to the necrosis seen in more advanced plaques. 12-L-Hydroxy-5,8,10,14-eicosatetraenoic acid, the main hydroxyeicosatetraenoic acid produced by mouse peritoneal macrophages from arachidonic acid, is chemokinetic for

Table 1 Some oxidized lipids of possible relevance in atherosclerosis.

(Extracted from)	Serum/plasma	Aorta	Macrophages *in vitro*
Cholesterol epoxides	a		
Cholest-5-en-3β-ol-7-one	a, b		
Cholest-5-en-3β, 26-diol	a, b	b, c	
Cholest-5-en-3β, 25-diol	b	b	
Cholest-5-en-3β, 24-diol	b	b, c	
Cholest-5-en-3β, 7-diols	b	b, c	d
Hydroxyoctadecadienoic acids (HODES)	g	c, f	d, e
Hydroxyeicosatetraenoic acids (HETES)	g		d, e, i
Cholesterol linoleate hydroperoxides		h	

Sources

a. Brooks *et al.* (1983)	Lipoproteins from type II hypercholesterolaemic serum.
b. Smith *et al.* (1982)	Human plasma—and human aorta (intima + media).
c. Brooks *et al.* (1971)	Human atherosclerotic plaques.
d. Carpenter *et al.* (1988)	Cellular lipids of mouse peritoneal macrophages incubated with cholesteryl linoleate/BSA or cholesteryl arachidonate/BSA.
e. Rabinovitch *et al.* (1981)	Incubation products of mouse peritoneal macrophages with linoleic acid or arachidonic acid.
f. Mowri *et al.* (1986)	Atherosclerotic aorta of WHHL rabbit.
g. Aisen *et al.* (1985)	Human familial Mediterranean fever serum.
h. Harland *et al.* (1973)	Advanced human atherosclerosis.
i. Pawlowski *et al.* (1983)	Human monocytes in culture with arachidonic acid.

smooth muscle cells (Nakao *et al.*, 1983), and might cause smooth muscle cell recruitment.

A number of short-chain breakdown products of polyunsaturated fatty acids have been found, for example during artificial oxidation of LDL (Esterbauer *et al.*, 1987). These compounds identified by HPLC include 4-hydroxynonenal, malondialdehyde and other aldehydes. The above two compounds are able to modify LDL *in vitro*, enabling it to be taken up by the scavenger receptor of macrophages (Esterbauer *et al.*, 1987). However, these compounds are volatile and very reactive, making their analysis in aorta and serum difficult. The time-honoured technique of malondialdehyde assay, the thiobarbituric acid test, on which much of the available data relies, is non-specific (Esterbauer *et al.*, 1987) and only gives nominal "malondialdehyde equivalent" values.

Oxidized LDL is reported to be cytotoxic (e.g. Hessler *et al.*, 1983; Cathcart *et al.*, 1985) and to be chemotactic for monocytes (Quinn *et al.*, 1987).

6 Similarities between ceroid and oxidized LDL

In view of the likely role of modified LDL in atherosclerosis and the possibility that oxidized LDL may be one form of modified LDL that occurs *in vivo*, it is interesting to consider whether ceroid might be an end-product of LDL oxidation.

Artificially oxidized LDL was found to contain tiny floccules, amounting to 10% of the total weight. Ultrastructurally, these floccules showed a focal multilamellar appearance similar to that seen in human foam cells and in the macrophages in the experiments described previously (Ball *et al.*, 1986, 1987b). Oxidized LDL and human ceroid also show similar autofluorescence (Ball *et al.*, 1986).

There are also some serological data that suggest ceroid is at least partly composed of oxidized LDL. To explain these, it is necessary to digress briefly.

The chronic inflammatory response seen in the media and adventitia of many advanced atherosclerotic plaques, especially those with attenuated or breached media, has been interpreted as suggesting an autoimmune reaction to a component of the plaque (Mitchinson, 1970, 1986). IgG is found in such plaques, attached to the ceroid in the necrotic base (Parums *et al.*, 1986). An enzyme-linked immunosorbent assay (ELISA) technique was therefore devised in which ceroid extracted from human atheroma was used as the antigen, to try to detect circulating antibodies to ceroid. This was attempted in the hope of providing a diagnostic test for the most severe form of this atherosclerosis-induced inflammation, which is called chronic periaortitis (Mitchinson, 1986). However, in view of the possibility that ceroid is partly oxidized LDL, in each assay four antigens were used: native human LDL;

LDL oxidized for 24 hours using cupric ions as a catalyst; LDL similarly oxidized for 72 hours; and ceroid from human atheroma. In essence the results showed that all of 20 patients with clinically evident chronic periaortitis had detectable circulating antibodies to ceroid and to oxidize LDL. Such antibodies were also present in 16 out of 20 necropsy subjects with histological, but not clinical, evidence of chronic periaortitis (i.e. a less severe form), in 10 out of 20 patients with clinical ischaemic heart disease, and in 10 out of 20 elderly control subjects. Twenty young healthy adults had no detectable antibodies (Parums, 1987; Parums and Mitchinson, 1987; Parums *et al.*, 1987).

These findings suggest that there probably is some correlation between this form of inflammation and the presence of such antibodies, but they are not entirely conclusive. Two other findings in the study, however, are of considerable interest. The first is that none of these 100 subjects had antibodies to native LDL, when careful precautions were taken to prevent auto-oxidation during rapid preparation of the ELISA plates. Claims from a number of groups (e.g. Szondy *et al.*, 1983) that a proportion of ischaemic heart disease patients have anti-LDL antibodies are therefore now highly suspect. This is particularly so because when their slower method of preparation of native LDL-coated walls was used in our assay, with serum known to contain anti-oxidized LDL antibodies, the negative result with native LDL became positive. Therefore we believe at least some of the reported anti-LDL antibodies were in fact anti-oxidized LDL.

The most significant finding, however, is that pre-absorption of the positive human sera with LDL oxidized for 24 or 72 hours inhibited by 64% and 67% respectively the reaction with ceroid. Furthermore, 11 out of the 20 sera samples from patients with chronic periaortitis showed positive immunoblots on some of the various low-molecular-weight polypeptides (80–190 KD), found on Western electrophoresis of oxidized apo B (Parums *et al.*, 1986; Parums *et al.*, 1987). We regard this as the best evidence so far of the similarity of ceroid in human atherosclerosis to oxidized LDL.

7 Factors diminishing experimental atherosclerosis

The view that in atherosclerosis the macrophage is doing harm to the arterial wall is supported by inhibition of experimental atherosclerosis by various anti-inflammatory drugs (e.g. Gordon *et al.*, 1954; Bailey and Butler, 1985).

The role of oxidation of lipid derives support from human epidemiological studies linking vitamin E or selenium deficiency with enhanced risk of complications of atherosclerosis (e.g. Ellis *et al.*, 1984). A number of reports have suggested a beneficial effect of anti-oxidants in experimental atherosclerosis. The most striking to date is the effect of probucol, which inhibits cupric-ion-catalysed LDL oxidation (Parthasarathy *et al.*, 1986a) and greatly decreases the atherosclerosis developing in WHHL rabbits (Kita *et al.*, 1987).

It is even possible that the widely canvassed anti-atherogenic effects of the fatty acids of fish oils may be related to their reported inhibition of the oxidative inflammatory activity of phagocytes (Lee *et al.*, 1985, Leslie *et al.*, 1985; Fisher *et al.*, 1986).

One natural anti-oxidant, vitamin E, is carried in LDL and taken up by cells in the LDL particle. It is therefore interesting to note that, in one study of artificial oxidation of LDL, vitamin E content was noted to be exhausted before the lipid oxidation ensued (Esterbauer *et al.*, 1987).

8 Possible sites of lipid or lipoprotein oxidation

If lipid oxidation is important in atherogenesis, intervention in the process to prevent the disease progressing should be aimed at the sites where most of the oxidation occurs. Our own work has been centred on the macrophage foam cell as the culprit, but there are many other candidates (Fig. 1).

First, some foods, such as finely divided, dehydrated milk or eggs are susceptible to oxidation on the shelf or during cooking (Taylor *et al.*, 1979) and some of the oxidation products can probably be absorbed from the gut (Fornas *et al.*, 1984). Oxidation might also occur in the blood (Harman, 1957; Schuh *et al.*, 1978; and see Table 1), where lipid peroxides are said to be more concentrated in atherosclerotic and hyperlipidaemic human patients (Goto, 1982; Szczeklik *et al.*, 1985). There is very little oxidized LDL in the blood (Szczeklik *et al.*, 1981), but this might conceivably be due to rapid clearance by the acetyl-LDL receptors of endothelial cells (Stein and Stein, 1980; Pitas *et al.*, 1985).

The circulating monocyte might theoretically take up and oxidize LDL, but blood monocytes contain very few lipid droplets indeed and no ceroid (Mitchinson, unpublished observation); and Montgomery and his colleagues (1986) were unable to demonstrate LDL oxidation in freshly isolated human blood monocytes.

The major contributions of Steinberg and his colleagues to this field include the finding that endothelial cells modify LDL *in vitro* (Henriksen *et al.*, 1981) by oxidizing it (Steinbrecher *et al.*, 1984). This oxidation seems to be mediated by free radicals (Morel *et al.*, 1984). Endothelial cell-mediated LDL oxidation *in vivo* could therefore explain the fact that intimal LDL is found to be modified (Hoff and Gaubatz, 1982) and would certainly help to explain enhanced LDL uptake by foam cells. This is because LDL oxidized either artificially or by endothelial cells *in vitro*, like other forms of modified LDL, is taken up by the macrophage more avidly than native LDL (Henriksen *et al.*, 1981; Prescott *et al.*, 1984; Parthasarathy *et al.*, 1987).

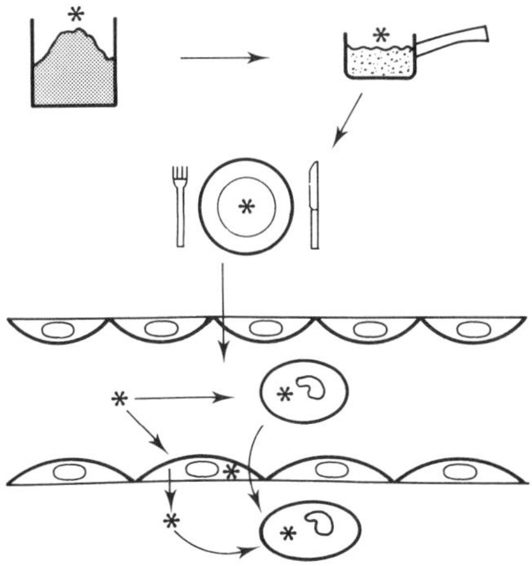

Fig. 1 Possible sites of lipid or lipoprotein oxidation, marked by asterisks (see text).

Oxidation of LDL might also occur theoretically extracellularly in the intima. If so, it is unlikely to be essential to have high intimal oxygen concentrations for the accumulation of oxidized LDL in macrophages, because ceroid is no less common in the foam cells of pulmonary artery atherosclerosis than in systemic arteries (Mitchinson, unpublished observations).

Finally, as discussed above, the macrophage itself is a likely site for LDL oxidation *in vivo*. Human monocyte-derived macrophages can oxidize LDL *in vitro* (Parthasarathy *et al.*, 1986b), resulting in cytotoxicity (Cathcart *et al.*, 1985).

The findings, mentioned above, that young healthy adults do not have antibodies to oxidized LDL, whereas many older patients with advanced atherosclerosis do, suggests that in earlier stages of development of atherosclerosis oxidized LDL is a sequestered antigen. This allows the tentative opinion that oxidation of LDL sufficient to render it antigenic must occur within the intima and not in the blood.

The relative contributions of all these possible sites and oxidative mechanisms *in vivo* is, however, at present unknown.

9 Conclusions

The hypothesis that we set out to test has now been supported by the identification of human arterial foam cells as macrophages and by the ability of macrophages *in vitro* to accumulate ceroid, probably by oxidizing lipoprotein. Such chemical evidence as has emerged so far suggests that cytotoxic and biologically active oxidized lipids can be produced by macrophages *in vitro* and are present in human lesions. Clearly this is a long way from establishing that these events do occur in human atherosclerosis, and more investigation will be needed. However, the serological similarity of ceroid to oxidized LDL is strongly suggestive that LDL oxidation does indeed occur *in vivo*.

The macrophage probably contributes in many other ways to the development of the lesions, and these too will require detailed study (Mitchinson and Ball, 1987). The most pressing need is for more non-invasive studies of human subjects and human tissue.

Eventually, of course, the significance of lipid or lipoprotein oxidation in atherogenesis can only be assessed by intervening in the process, in the most susceptible human patients, such as those with familial hypercholesterolaemia, coronary by-pass grafts, or accelerated atherosclerosis in heart transplants. If the experimental evidence continues to accumulate as it has in the last five years or so, the time for such studies may not be far off.

Acknowledgements

Dr Ball was supported by the Wellcome Trust, Dr Carpenter by the John Lucas Walker Fund of Cambridge University and Dr Parums by the British Heart Foundation. Additional support was provided by the East Anglian Regional Health Authority and the British Heart Foundation. We are very grateful to Drs D. E. Bowyer and E. Gherardi for advice, to Jacqui Enright for technical assistance and Helen Wilson for secretarial assistance.

References

Adams, C. W. M. and Bayliss, O. B. (1976). Detection of macrophages in atherosclerotic lesions with cytrochrome oxidase. *Br. J. Exp. Path.* **57**, 30–36.

Aderem, A. A., Cohen, D. S., Wright, S. D. and Cohn, Z. A. (1986). Bacterial lipopolysaccharides prime macrophages for enhanced release of arachidonic acid metabolites. *J. Exp. Med.* **164**, 165–179.

Aisen, P. S., Haines, K. A., Given, W., Abramson, S. B., Pras, M., Serhan, C., Hamberg, M., Samuelsson, B. and Weissman, G. (1985). Circulating hydroxy fatty acids in familial Mediterranean fever. *Proc. Natl Acad. Sci. USA* **82**, 1232–1236.

Anitschkow, N. (1933). Experimental arteriosclerosis in animals. *Arteriosclerosis: A Survey of the Problem* (ed. E. V. Cowdry), pp. 271–322. Macmillan, New York.

Aqel, N., Ball, R. Y., Waldmann, H. and Mitchinson, M. J. (1984). Monocytic origin of foam cells in human atherosclerotic plaques. *Atherosclerosis* **53**, 265–271.

Aqel, N., Ball, R. Y., Waldmann, H. and Mitchinson, M. J. (1985). Identification of macrophages and smooth muscle cells in human atherosclerosis using monoclonal antibodies. *J. Path.* **146**, 197–204.

Badwey, J. A. B. and Karnovsky, M. L. (1980). Active oxygen species and the functions of phagocytic leucocytes. *Ann. Rev. Biochem.* **49**, 695–726.

Bailey, J. M. and Butler, J. (1985). Anti-inflammatory drugs in experimental atherosclerosis. Part 6 (combination therapy with steroid and non-steroid agents). *Atherosclerosis* **54**, 205–212.

Ball, R. Y., Brodley, H., Brooks, P. N. and Mitchinson, M. J. (1984). The production of ceroid by mouse peritoneal macrophages *in vitro*. *Br. J. Exp. Path.* **65**, 719–724.

Ball, R. Y., Bindman, J. P., Carpenter, K. L. H. and Mitchinson, M. J. (1986). Oxidized low density lipoprotein induces ceroid accumulation by murine peritoneal macrophages *in vitro*. *Atherosclerosis* **60**, 173–181.

Ball, R. Y., Carpenter, K. L. H., Enright, J. H., Hartley, S. L. and Mitchinson, M. J. (1987a). Ceroid accumulation by murine peritoneal macrophages exposed to artificial lipoproteins. *Br. J. Exp. Path.* **68**, 427–438.

Ball, R. Y., Carpenter, K. L. H. and Mitchinson, M. J. (1987b). Ceroid accumulation by murine peritoneal macrophages exposed to artificial lipoproteins: ultrastructural observations. *Br. J. Exp. Path.* (in press).

Ball, R. Y., Carpenter, K. L. H. and Mitchinson, M. J. (1987c). What is the significance of ceroid in human atherosclerosis? *Arch. Path.* (in press).

Baranowski, A., Adams, C. W. M., Bayliss High, O. B. and Bower, D. E. (1982). Connective tissue responses to oxysterols. *Atherosclerosis* **41**, 255–266.

Brooks, C. J. W., Steel, G., Gilbert, J. D. and Harland, W. A. (1971). Polar sterol esters in human atherosclerotic plaques. *Atherosclerosis* **13**, 223–237.

Brooks, C. J. W., McKenna, R. M., Cole, W. J., MacLachlan, J. and Veitchlaurie, T. D. (1983). "Profile" analysis of oxygenated sterols in plasma and serum. *Biochem. Soc. Trans.* **11**, 700–701.

Burt, R. C. (1952). The incidence of acid-fast pigment (ceroid) in aortic atherosclerosis. *Am. J. Clin. Path.* **22**, 135–139.

Carpenter, K. L. H., Ballantine, J. A., Ball, R. Y. and Mitchinson, M. J. (1987). Lipid uptake and oxidation by murine peritoneal macrophages *in vitro*. *J. Path.* **151**, 32A.

Carpenter, K. L. H., Ball, R. Y. Ardeshna, K. M., Bindman, J. P., Enright, J. H., Hartley, S. L., Nicholson, S. and Mitchinson, M. J. (1988). Production of ceroid and oxidised lipids by macrophages *in vitro*. *Lipofuscin 1987—State of the Art* (ed. I.Z.s.-Nagy), pp. 245–268. Elsevier, Amsterdam.

Cathcart, M. K., Morel, D. W. and Chisolm, G. M. (1985). Monocytes and neutrophils oxidize low density lipoprotein making it cytotoxic. *J. Leukocyte Biol.* **38**, 341–350.

Cook, R. P. and MacDougal, J. D. B. (1968). Experimental atherosclerosis in rabbits after feeding cholestanetriol. *Br. J. Exp. Path.* **49**, 265–271.

Cutler, M. G. and Schneider, R. (1974). Linoleate oxidation products and cardiovascular lesions. *Atherosclerosis* **20**, 383–394.

Davis, H. R., Vesselinovitch, D. and Wissler, R. W. (1984). Histochemical detection and quantification of macrophages in rhesus and cynomolgus monkey atherosclerotic lesions. *J. Histochem. Cytochem.* **32**, 1319–1327.

Esterbauer, H., Jurgens, G., Quehenberger, O. and Koller, E. (1987). Autoxidation of human low density lipoprotein: loss of polyunsaturated fatty acids and vitamin E and generation of aldehydes. *J. Lipid. Res.* **28**, 495–509.

Ellis, N. I. A., Lloyd, B., Lloyd, R. S. and Clayton, B. E. (1984). Selenium and vitamin E in relation to risk factors for coronary heart disease. *J. Clin. Path.* **37**, 220–260.

Faggiotto, A., Ross, R. and Harker, L. (1984). Studies of hypercholesterolemia in the non human primate. I. Changes that lead to fatty streak formation. *Arteriosclerosis* **4**, 323–340.

Fisher, M., Upchurch, K. S., Levine, P. H., Johnson, M. H., Vaudreuil, C. H., Natale, A. and Hoogasian, J. J. (1986). Effects of dietary fish oil supplementation on polymorphonuclear leukocyte inflammatory potential. *Inflammation* **10**, 387–392.

Fogelman, A. M., Schechter, I., Seager, J., Hokom, M. and Child, J. S. (1980). Malondialdehyde alteration of low density lipoproteins leads to cholesteryl ester accumulation in human monocyte-macrophages. *Proc. Natl Acad. Sci. USA* **77**, 2214–2218.

Fornas, E., Martinez-Sales, V., Camanas, A. and Bagnena, J. (1984). Intestinal absorption of cholesterol autoxidation products in the rat. *Arch. Pharmacol. Toxicol.* **10**, 175–182.

Fowler, S. D. (1983). Role of macrophage foam cells in arterial lesions. *Atherosclerosis VI* (ed. G. Schettler *et al.*), pp. 452–456. Springer-Verlag, New York.

Fowler, S., Shio, H. and Haley, N. J. (1979). Characterization of lipid-laden aortic cells from cholesterol-fed rabbits. IV. Investigation of macrophage-like properties of aortic cell populations. *Lab. Invest.* **41**, 372–378.

Gaton, E. and Wolman, M. (1977). The role of smooth muscle cells and hematogenous macrophages in atheroma. *J. Path.* **123**, 123–128.

Gerrity, R. G., Naito, H. K., Richardson, M. and Schwartz, C. J. (1979). Dietary-induced atherosclerosis in swine: morphology of the intima in prelesion stages. *Am. J. Path.* **95**, 775–786.

Gerrity, R. G. (1981a). The role of the monocyte in atherogenesis. I. Transition of blood-borne monocytes into foam cells in fatty lesions. *Am. J. Path.* **103**, 181–190.

Gerrity, R. G. (1981b). The role of the monocyte in atherogenesis. II. Migration of foam cells from atherosclerotic lesions. *Am. J. Path.* **103**, 191–200.

Glavind, J., Hartmann, S., Clemmesen, J., Jessen, K. E. and Dam, H. (1952). Studies on the role of lipoperoxides in human pathology. II. The presence of peroxidised lipids in the atherosclerotic aorta. *Acta Path. Microbiol. Scand.* **30**, 1–6.

Goldstein, J. L., Ho, Y. K., Basu, S. K. and Brown, M. S. (1979). Binding site on macrophages that mediates uptake and degradation of acetylated LDL, producing massive cholesterol deposition. *Proc. Natl Acad. Sci. USA.* **76**, 333–337.

Gordon, D., Kobernick, S. D., McMillan, G. C. and Duff, G. L. (1954). The effect of cortisone on the serum lipids and on the development of experimental cholesterol atherosclerosis in the rabbit. *J. Exp. Med.* **99**, 371–376.

Goto, Y. (1982). Lipid peroxides as a cause of vascular diseases. *Lipid Peroxides in Biology and Medicine* (ed. K. Yagi), pp. 295–303. Academic Press, New York.

Gown, A. M., Tsukada, T. and Ross, R. (1986). Human atherosclerosis: II. Immunocytochemical analysis of the cellular composition of human atherosclerotic lesions. *Am. J. Path.* **125**, 191–207.

Harland, W. A., Gilbert, J. D., Steel, G. and Brooks, C. J. W. (1971). Lipids of human atheroma. Part 5—The occurrence of a new group of polar sterol esters in various stages of human atherosclerosis. *Atherosclerosis* **13**, 239–246.

Harland, W. A., Gilbert, J. D. and Brooks, C. J. W. (1973). Lipids of human atheroma VIII. Oxidised derivatives of cholesteryl linoleate. *Biochim. Biophys. Acta* **316**, 378–385.

Harman, D. (1957). Atherosclerosis: a hypothesis concerning the initiating steps in pathogenesis. *J. Gerontol.* **12**, 199–202.

Henriksen, T., Mahoney, E. M. and Steinberg, D. (1981). Enhanced macrophage degradation of LDL previously incubated with cultured endothelial cells: recognition by receptors for acetylated LDL's. *Proc. Natl Acad. Sci. USA* **78**, 6499–6503.

Hessler, J. R., Morel, D. W., Lewis, L. J. and Chisolm, G. M. (1983). Lipoprotein oxidation and lipoprotein-induced cytotoxicity. *Arteriosclerosis* **3**, 215–222.

Hoff, H. F. and Gaubatz, J. W. (1982). Isolation, purification and characterization of a lipoprotein containing apo B from the human aorta. *Atherosclerosis* **42**, 273–279.

Imai, H., Werthessen, N. T., Taylor, C. B. and Lee, K.-T. (1976). Angio-toxicity and arteriosclerosis due to contaminants of USP-grade cholesterol. *Arch. Path.* **100**, 565–572.

Imai, H., Werthessen, N. T., Subramanyam, V., LeQuesne, P. W., Soloway, A. H. and Kanisawa, M. (1980). Angiotoxicity of oxygenated sterols and possible precursors. *Science* **207**, 651–653.

Jonasson, L., Holm, J., Skalli, O., Bondjers, G. and Hansson, G. K. (1986). Regional accumulations of T cells, macrophages and smooth muscle cells in the human atherosclerotic plaque. *Arteriosclerosis* **6**, 131–138.

Joris, I., Zand, T., Nunnari, J. J., Krolikowski, F. J. and Majno, G. (1983). Studies on the pathogenesis of atherosclerosis. I. Adhesion and emigration of mononuclear cells in the aorta of hypercholesterolemic rats. *Am. J. Path.* **113**, 341–358.

Kita, T., Nagano, Y., Yokode, M., Ishii, K., Kume, N., Ooshima, A., Yoshida, H. and Kawai, C. (1987). Probucol prevents the progression of atherosclerosis in Watanabe heritable hyperlipidemic rabbit, an animal model for familial hypercholesterolemia. *Proc. Natl Acad. Sci. USA* **84**, 5928–5931.

Klurfeld, D. M. (1985). Identification of foam cells in human atherosclerotic lesions as macrophages using monoclonal antibodies. *Arch. Path.* **109**, 445–449.

Lee, T. H., Hoover, R. L., Williams, J. D., Sperling, R. I., Ravalese, J., Spur, B. W., Robinson, D. R., Corey, E. J., Lewis, R. A. and Austen, K. F. (1985). Effect of dietary enrichment with eicosapentaenoic and docosahexaenoic acids on *in vitro* neutrophil and monocyte leukotriene generation and neutrophil function. *N. Engl. J. Med.* **312**, 1217–1224.

Leslie, C. A., Gonnermann, W. A., Ullman, M. D., Hayes, K. C., Franzblau, C. and Cathcart, E. S. (1985). Dietary fish oil modulates macrophage fatty acids and decreases arthritis susceptibility in mice. *J. Exp. Med.* **162**, 1336–1349.

MacDermot, J., Kelsey, C. R., Waddell, K. A., Richmond, R., Knight, R. K., Cole, P. J., Dollery, C. T., Landen, D. N. and Blair, I. A. (1984). Synthesis of leukotriene B4 and prostanoids by human alveolar macrophages: analysis by gas chromatography/ mass spectrometry. *Prostaglandins* **27**, 163–179.

Mahley, R. W., Innerarity, T. L., Weisgraber, K. H. and Oh, S. Y. (1979). Altered metabolism (*in vivo* and *in vitro*) of plasma lipoproteins after selective chemical modification of lysine residues of the apo proteins. *J. Clin. Invest.* **64**, 743–750.

Mason, R. J., Stossel, T. P. and Vaughan, M. (1972). Lipids of alveolar macrophages, polymorphonuclear neutrophil leukocytes and their phagocytic vesicles .*J. Clin. Invest.* **51**, 2399–2407.

Mitchinson, M. J. (1970). The pathology of idiopathic retroperitoneal fibrosis. *J. Clin. Path.* **23**, 681–689.

Mitchinson, M. J. (1982). Insoluble lipids in human atherosclerotic plaques. *Atherosclerosis* **45**, 11–15.

Mitchinson, M. J. (1983). Macrophages, oxidised lipids and atherosclerosis. *Med. Hypotheses* **12**, 171–178.

Mitchinson, M. J., Hothersall, D. C., Brooks, P. N. and de Burbure, C. Y. (1985). The distribution of ceroid in human atherosclerosis. *J. Path.* **145**, 177–183.

Mitchinson, M. J. (1986). Retroperitoneal fibrosis revisited. *Arch. Path.* **110**, 784–786.

Mitchinson, M. J. and Ball, R. Y. (1987). Macrophages and atherogenesis—a new opportunity. *Lancet* **ii**, 146–149.

Montgomery, R. R., Nathan, C. F. and Cohn, Z. A. (1986). Effects of reagent and cell-generated hydrogen peroxide on the properties of low density lipoprotein. *Proc. Natl Acad. Sci. USA* **83**, 6631–6635.

Morel, D. W., DiCorleto, P. E. and Chisolm, G. M. (1984). Endothelial and smooth muscle cells alter low density lipoprotein *in vitro* by free radical oxidation. *Arteriosclerosis* **4**, 357–364.

Mowri, H., Chinen, K., Ohkuma, S. and Takano, T. (1986). Peroxidised lipids isolated by HPLC from atherosclerotic aorta. *Biochem. Int.* **12**, 347–352.

Nakao, J., Ito, H., Ooyama, T., Chang, W.-C. and Murota, S. (1983). Calcium dependency of aortic smooth muscle cell migration induced by 12-L-hydroxy-5,8,10,14-eicosatetraenoic acid. Effects of A23187, nicardipine and trifluoperazine. *Atherosclerosis* **46**, 309–319.

Nishida, T. and Kummerow, F. A. (1960). Interaction of serum lipoproteins with the hydroperoxide of methyl linoleate. *J. Lipid. Res.* **1**, 450–458.

Numano, F., Tsukada, T., Kishi, Y., Nishiyama, K., Yajima, M. and Adachi, K. (1983). Identification of macrophages in atherosclerotic lesions by hybridmonoclonal antibody. *Arteriosclerosis* **3**, 470a.

Pappenheimer, A. M. and Victor, J. (1946). Ceroid pigment in human tissues. *Am. J. Path.* **22**, 395–413.

Parthasarathy, S., Young, S. G., Witztum, J. L., Pittman, R. C. and Steinberg, D. (1986a). Probucol inhibits oxidative modification of LDL. *J. Clin. Invest.* **77**, 641–644.

Parthasarathy, S., Printz, D. J., Boyd, D., Joy, L. and Steinberg, D. (1986b). Macrophage oxidation of LDL generates a modified form recognized by the scavenger receptor. *Arteriosclerosis* **6**, 505–510.

Parthasarathy, S., Fong, L. G., Otero, D. and Steinberg, D. (1987). Recognition of solubilized apoproteins from delipidated, oxidized low density lipoprotein (LDL) by the acetyl-LDL receptor. *Proc. Natl Acad. Sci. USA* **84**, 537–540.

Parums, D. V. (1987). Studies on inflammation in atherosclerosis. Ph.D. Dissertation, University of Cambridge.

Parums, D. V., Chadwick, D. R. and Mitchinson, M. J. (1986). The localisation of immunoglobulin G in chronic periaortitis. *Atherosclerosis* **61**, 117–123.

Parums, D. V., Mitchinson, M. J. and Brown, D. L. (1987). Serum antibodies to oxidised LDL and ceroid in chronic periaortitis. Submitted for publication.

Parums, D. V. and Mitchinson, M. J. (1987). Serum antibodies to oxidised LDL and ceroid in chronic periaortitis. *J. Path.* **151**, 57A.

Pawlowski, N. A., Kaplan, G., Hamill, A. L., Cohn, Z. A. and Scott, W. A. (1983). Arachidonic acid metabolism by human monocytes. *J. Exp. Med.* **158**, 393–412.

Pearse, A. G. E. (1972). The lipid pigments. *Histochemistry*, 3rd edn, pp. 1076–1089. Churchill Livingstone, Edinburgh.

Peng, S., Tham, P., Taylor, C. B. and Mikkelson, B. (1979). Cytotoxicity of oxidation derivatives of cholesterol on cultured aortic smooth muscle cells and their effect on cholesterol biosynthesis. *Am. J. Clin. Nutr.* **32**, 1033–1042.

Pitas, R. E., Boyles, J., Mahley, R. W. and Bissell, D. M. (1985). Uptake of chemically modified low density lipoproteins *in vivo* is mediated by specific endothelial cells. *J. Cell. Biol.* **100**, 103–117.

Porta, E. A. and Hartroft, W. S. (1969). Lipid pigments in relation to aging and dietary factors. *Pigments in Pathology* (ed. M. Wolman), pp. 191–235. Academic Press, New York.

Prescott, M. F., Muller, K. R., Flammer, R. and Feige, U. (1984). The effect of LDL and modified LDL on macrophage secretion products. *Agents and Actions Suppl.* **16**, 163–170.

Quinn, M. T., Parthasarathy, S., Fong, L. G. and Steinberg, D. (1987). Oxidatively-modified LDL's: a potential role in recruitment and retention of monocyte-macrophages during atherogenesis. *Proc. Natl Acad. Sci. USA* **84**, 2995–2998.

Rabinovitch, H., Durand, J., Gualde, N. and Rigaud, M. (1981). Metabolism of polyunsaturated fatty acids by mouse peritoneal macrophages: the lipoxygenase metabolic pathway. *Agents and Actions* **11**, 580–583.

Schaefer, H.-E. (1981). The role of macrophages in atherosclerosis. *Disorders of the Monocyte Macrophage System* (ed. F. Schmalzl, D. Huhn and H.-E. Schaefer), pp. 137–142. Springer-Verlag, Berlin.

Schaffner, T., Taylor, K., Bartucci, E. J., Fischer-Dzoga, K., Beeson, J. H., Glagov, S. and Wissler, R. W. (1980). Arterial foam cells with distinctive immunomorphological and histochemical features of macrophages. *Am. J. Path.* **100**, 57–80.

Schuh, J., Fairclough, G. F. Jr. and Haschemeyer, R. H. (1978). Oxygen mediated heterogeneity of apo-low density lipoprotein. *Proc. Natl Acad. Sci. USA* **75**, 3173–3177.

Schwartz, C. J., Sprague, E. A., Kelley, J. L., Valente, A. J. and Suenram, C. A. (1985). Aortic intimal monocyte recruitment in the normo and hypercholesterolemic baboon (*Papio cynocephalus*). *Virch. Arch. Path. Anat.* **405**, 175–191.

Scott, W. A., Zrike, J. M., Hamill, A. L., Kempe, J. and Cohn, Z. A. (1978). Regulation of arachidonic acid metabolites in macrophages. *J. Exp. Med.* **152**, 324–335.

Smith, E. B., Evans, P. H. and Downham, M. D. (1967). Lipids in the aortic intima. The correlation of morphological and chemical characteristics. *J. Atherosclerosis Res.* **7**, 171–186.

Smith, L. L. and van Lier, J. E. (1970). Sterol metabolism: Part 9. 26-hydroxycholesterol levels in the human aorta. *Atherosclerosis* **12**, 1–14.

Smith, L. L., Teng, J. I., Lin, Y. Y., Seitz, P. K. and McGhee, M. F. (1982). Lipid peroxides of cholesterol. *Lipid Peroxides in Biology and Medicine* (ed. K. Yagi), pp. 89–105. Academic Press, New York.

Stary, H. C. (1983). Macrophages in coronary artery and aortic intima and in atherosclerotic lesions of children and young adults up to age 29. *Atherosclerosis VI* (ed. G. Schettler *et al.*), pp. 462–466. Springer-Verlag, New York.

Stein, O. and Stein, Y. (1980). Bovine aortic endothelial cells display macrophage-like properties toward acetylated ^{125}I-labelled LDL. *Biochim. Biophys. Acta* **620**, 631–635.

Steinbrecher, U. P., Parthasarathy, S., Leake, D. S., Witztum, J. L. and Steinberg, D. (1984). Modification of low density lipoprotein by endothelial cells involves lipid peroxidation and degradation of low density lipoprotein phospholipids. *Proc. Natl Acad. Sci. USA* **81**, 3883–3887.

Stossel, T. P., Mason, R. J. and Smith, A. L. (1974). Lipid peroxidation by human blood phagocytes. *J. Clin. Invest.* **54**, 638–645.

Szczeklik, A., Gryglewski, R. J., Domagala, B., Zmuda, A., Hartwich, J., Wozny, E., Grzywacz, M., Madej, J. and Gryglewska, T. (1981). Serum lipoproteins, lipid peroxides and prostacyclin synthesis in patients with coronary heart disease. *Prostaglandins* **22**, 795–807.

Szczeklik, A., Gryglewski, R. J., Domagala, B., Dworski, R. and Basista, M. (1985). Dietary supplementation with vitamin E in hyperlipoproteinaemias: effects on plasma lipid peroxides, antioxidant activity, prostacyclin generation and platelet aggregability. *Thromb. Haemost.* **54**, 425–430.

Taylor, C. B., Peng, S.-K., Werthessen, N. T., Tham, P. and Lee, K.-T. (1979). Spontaneously occurring angiotoxic derivatives of cholesterol. *Am. J. Clin. Nutr.* **32**, 40–57.

Taylor, R. G. and Lewis, J. C. (1986). Endothelial cell proliferation and monocyte adhesion to atherosclerotic lesions of white Carneau pigeons. *Am. J. Path.* **125**, 152–160.

Tsukada, T., Rosenfeld, M., Ross, R. and Gown, A. M. (1986). Immunocytochemical analysis of cellular components in atherosclerotic lesions. Use of monoclonal antibodies with the Watanabe and fat-fed rabbit. *Arteriosclerosis* **6**, 601–613.

Vedeler, C. A., Nyland, H. and Matre, R. (1984). *In situ* characterisation of the foam cells in early human atherosclerotic lesions. *Acta Path. Microbiol. Immunol. Scand.* **C92**, 133–137.

Watanabe, T., Hirata, M., Yoshikiwa, Y., Nagafuchi, Y., Toyoshima, H. and Watanabe, T. (1985). Role of macrophages in atherosclerosis: sequential observations of cholesterol-induced rabbit aortic lesions by the immunoperoxidase technique using monoclonal antimacrophage antibody. *Lab. Invest* **53**, 80–90.

Wolman, M. (1975). *Biological Peroxidation of Lipids and Membranes* Supplement to *Isr. J. Med. Sci.* **11**.

10

Low Density Lipoprotein Interaction with Arterial Proteoglycans: Effects on Lipoprotein Interaction with Arterial Cells

G. BONDJERS, O. WIKLUND, S.-O. OLOFSSON, G. FAGER, E. HURT and G. CAMEJO

Arterial Biology Group, Wallenberg Laboratory for Cardiovascular Research, University of Göteborg, Sahlgren's Hospital, Göteborg, Sweden

1 Introduction

In this discussion we shall try to summarize recent observations in our laboratories about the interactions between low density lipoproteins (LDL) and the arterial tissue. The basis for our interest in this subject is the well-established relationship between LDL and atherosclerosis as demonstrated both in clinical studies and in experimental studies. Our ability to penetrate the molecular basis for the interaction between LDL and arterial tissue has increased to a new level during the last two to three years, after the cloning of the cDNA for apoB and the subsequent unravelling of the primary amino acid structure of apoB (Knott *et al.*, 1986; Yang *et al.*, 1986; Olofsson *et al.*, 1987). We have chosen to describe the interaction between LDL and the arterial tissue as a drama, with LDL as the main character. The minor characters involved in the drama as we see it in this particular representation are the cells of the atherosclerotic lesion—endothelial cells, smooth muscle cells, macrophages and lymphocytes, and the various extracellular structures found in the arterial tissue.

HYPERLIPIDAEMIA AND ATHEROSCLEROSIS
ISBN 0.12.675645-7

2 The cellular constituents of the atherosclerotic lesion

Until recently, almost exclusive attention was given to one of the minor constituents, the arterial smooth muscle cell (Ross and Glomset, 1976; Schwartz *et al.*, 1981). We now know much about the control of arterial smooth muscle cell growth, with the platelet-derived growth factor (PDGF) as a major growth promotor, possibly together with other growth factors of the epidermal growth factor and insulin growth factor family (Ross, 1986), and with heparin-like substances as potential growth inhibitors (Castelot *et al.*, 1981). Growth-promoting substances are released in endothelial injury, at the same time as growth-inhibitor levels may be decreased by the loss of endothelial cells. This may explain why endothelial injury gives rise to cell-rich and atherosclerosis-like intimal thickenings (Ross and Glomset, 1976; Björkerud and Bondjers, 1976). The arterial reactions to injury are now well described, and involve not only the formation of a lipid-rich intimal thickening but also with time the complete regression of such intimal thickenings. We have suggested that failure to achieve repair after injury may be a key process in the development of clinical complications to atherosclerosis (Bondjers *et al.*, 1981). Others have suggested that such failure may be due to repeated or chronic injury (Ross, 1981, 1986). The cholesterol balance of the smooth muscle cell is subject to several control mechanisms, involving the expression of the LDL receptor, of HMG-CoA reductase, and of a cholesteryl ester synthetase activity (Goldstein and Brown, 1984). In spite of these intricate control mechanisms, which should counteract accumulation of lipids in the cell, the presence of smooth muscle foam cells in atherosclerotic lesions has been reported, both in rabbits that are hypercholesterolaemic due to LDL receptor deficiency and to dietary factors (Rosenfeld *et al.*, 1987a,b). The mechanisms that lead to lipid deposition in the smooth muscle cells are currently unknown.

During the last few years, a new supporting actor has attracted interest. The monocyte-derived macrophage actually may be a major cell type in the atherosclerotic lesion, as demonstrated both in man (Jonasson *et al.*, 1986; Tsukada *et al.*, 1987) and in various animal models (Haley *et al.*, 1977; Fowler *et al.*, 1979, 1980; Rosenfeld *et al.*, 1987a,b; Seddon *et al.*, 1987). In addition, these cells appear to be recruited to the arterial tissue as an effect of endothelial injury (Hansson *et al.*, 1981; Ross, 1986). The macrophage may be an ominous guest in the arterial tissue, as it may release a number of proteases and protease inhibitors (for a review with references see Adams and Hamilton, 1984), which may affect normal functions in the arterial tissue. We know that in the macrophage, control of the cholesterol balance is different from that in most other cells. Thus, in addition to the benevolent and well-controlled LDL receptor, the macrophage expresses a lipoprotein receptor that is not subject to feedback control. This receptor interacts with modified LDL (for a review with references see Brown *et al.*, 1980a). However, we do not know yet how or even if LDL may be modified outside the laboratory, although oxidative modification recently has been suggested as a potential mechanism (Parthasarathy *et al.*, 1986).* On the other hand, we do know that macrophages in the atherosclerotic tissue accumulate lipids and transform into lipid-rich foam cells. In view of the uncertainties about how LDL may be modified, the mechanisms involved in this transformation are another unsolved mystery. In addition, accepting that macrophage foam cells do exist, another mystery is why it would be harmful to harbour them in the arterial tissue. In other tissues lipid-rich cells do not appear to present a major problem apart from aesthetic ones.

Two minor cell types that have not attracted much interest, but still may be of major significance in the broader context of the mechanisms involved in atherogenesis, are the endothelial cell and the T lymphocyte. Injury to the endothelial cell may in fact be the initial event in atherogenesis (Reidy, 1985), even if recent observations question the significance of the endothelial cell layer as a barrier to lipoproteins (Wiklund *et al.*, 1987). The T lymphocyte has been noticed as an inhabitant in the atherosclerotic lesion only quite recently (Jonasson *et al.*, 1986; Tsukada *et al.*, 1986) and we do not yet know its significance.

3 Low density lipoprotein interaction with arterial proteoglycans

We have now set the stage for the role of LDL, and we shall try to evaluate what happens once it has entered the arterial wall. The endothelial cell layer was once regarded as a major barrier for lipoprotein penetration into the arterial tissue (for a review see Bondjers, 1975). This conclusion was based on observations on cholesterol transfer into arterial tissue, following experimental injury or spontaneously occurring injury (Bondjers and Björkerud, 1973a,b). However, it was later pointed out that, in spite of faster transfer of lipoproteins into areas without endothelium, retention of the lipoproteins might be the major factor involved in lipid deposition during arterial injury (Minick *et al.*, 1981). Therefore both increased levels of labelled lipoproteins and increased lipid levels in areas of injury may rather be due to secondary changes induced by injury in the subendothelial tissue than due to the endothelial injury itself. This conclusion is supported by recent observations in an *in vitro* perfusion system, which is more easily controlled than the *in vivo* system (Wiklund *et al.*, 1987). The obstacles raised by the endothelial cell layer will not be considered

*This topic is discussed further in Chapter 9 by Mitchinson *et al.*

further in this chapter. Once through the endothelium, the lipoprotein encounters the extracellular space of the arterial tissue, containing a number of substances unknown to the lipoprotein in serum. It is important to emphasize that the effects of the extracellular matrix on the LDL particle will affect the significance of all the data gathered in the past about lipoprotein–cell interactions in tissue culture experiments. We shall now try to review which of the previously described effects may be of significance.

There is much evidence to suggest that, in particular, the proteoglycans of the arterial tissue have profound effects on the lipoprotein (for a review see Camejo, 1982). Thus in intimal thickenings induced by injury, there is a co-localization of lipoproteins and acid glycosaminoglycans (Minick *et al.*, 1981). A similar association has been observed in lesion-prone areas of cholesterol-fed pigs and monkeys (Hoff and Bond, 1983; Hoff and Wagner, 1986). Finally, complexes of proteoglycans and lipoproteins may be isolated from the atherosclerotic intima in man (Camejo *et al.*, 1985). In view of the recent establishment of the primary amino acid structure of apolipoprotein B, we wanted to clarify the molecular basis for the interaction between LDL and arterial proteoglycans. Using frontal affinity chromatography, we observed that a sequence of 20 amino acids in the vicinity of the border between the T_2 and T_3 fragments (thrombin cleavage products of apoB) of apoB (residues 3359–3377) bound with high affinity to human aortic proteoglycans (Camejo *et al.*, 1987). The ligand for the arterial proteoglycan would be within the putative ligand for the LDL receptor (Yang *et al.*, 1986), and therefore we considered it quite possible that binding of LDL to the proteoglycan might affect the interaction between LDL and the cellular LDL receptor, a possibility that will be discussed later in this chapter. The affinity of LDL for the arterial proteoglycan varied considerably between individuals, and when myocardial infarction patients were compared with controls, significantly higher binding was found in the patients (Lindén *et al.*, 1987a). Actually, the affinity of LDL for arterial proteoglycan discriminated infarction patients from controls better than any of the conventional risk factors. Whether the variation may be correlated to differences in the primary amino acid structure is presently unknown, but this is an exciting possibility. However, within a given individual, the LDL-proteoglycan affinity might also be altered by external factors. Thus beta-blockers, suggested as exerting an anti-atherogenic effect (for a review with references see Kaplan *et al.*, 1987), decrease binding of LDL to proteoglycans (Lindén *et al.*, 1987b). These effects, though, were far smaller than the differences between the myocardial infarction patients and the controls. Thus there is evidence to suggest that binding of LDL to the arterial proteoglycans might be of significance for the development of cardiovascular disease. We must now consider whether this is a direct effect, or if it also could be due to secondary effects induced by the reaction of LDL with proteoglycans on the interaction between the lipoproteins and the cells of the atherosclerotic tissue.

4 The effects of proteoglycan treatment on the interaction of LDL with arterial smooth muscle cells

As discussed above, the arterial smooth muscle cell expresses a high-affinity receptor for native LDL. The putative ligand for this receptor is in the same region as the amino acid sequence binding to the arterial proteoglycans. Therefore it appeared reasonable to hypothesize that the interaction between the lipoprotein and the arterial smooth muscle cell might be blocked by the interaction between the lipoprotein and the proteoglycan. This hypothesis was tested experimentally, and, as is so often the case with beautiful hypothesis, it turned out to be incorrect. In short, lipoprotein uptake actually was stimulated if LDL first was exposed to arterial proteoglycans and then to arterial smooth muscle cells (Fig. 1). The increase in lipoprotein uptake was partly mediated by the receptor for native LDL and could be competed for by an excess of native, unlabelled LDL. Why previous exposure to proteoglycans would have such an effect is entirely unclear at present, but it might be related to changes in the tertiary structure of LDL that have been observed (Camejo, 1982). However, some of the increase in LDL uptake could also be accounted for by low-affinity binding and uptake of LDL. Thus even in LDL receptor-deficient cells a stimulation of lipoprotein uptake by previous exposure of the LDL to proteoglycans was observed. As this type of uptake is not subject to feedback control such as that regulating the uptake via the specific LDL receptor, it may eventually lead to cholesterol deposition in the smooth muscle cells. This mechanism might explain why Rosenfeld *et al.* (1987a,b) observed smooth muscle foam cells in the LDL receptor-deficient rabbit, an otherwise perplexing observation. So the proteoglycan-altered lipoprotein may enter the smooth muscle cell either via conventional routes, but more efficiently than the LDL that comes directly from plasma, or it might sneak into the cell via unspecific pathways, routes normally not much used but perhaps deleterious to the cells as they are not subject to control in relation to cellular cholesterol levels. What happens to the arterial smooth muscle cell once it has become a foam cell is unclear, but will be speculated on later in this chapter.

5 The effects of proteoglycan treatment on the interaction of LDL with arterial macrophages

If the lipoprotein, following its meeting with a proteoglycan, does not encounter a smooth muscle cell, it may instead come across a macrophage.

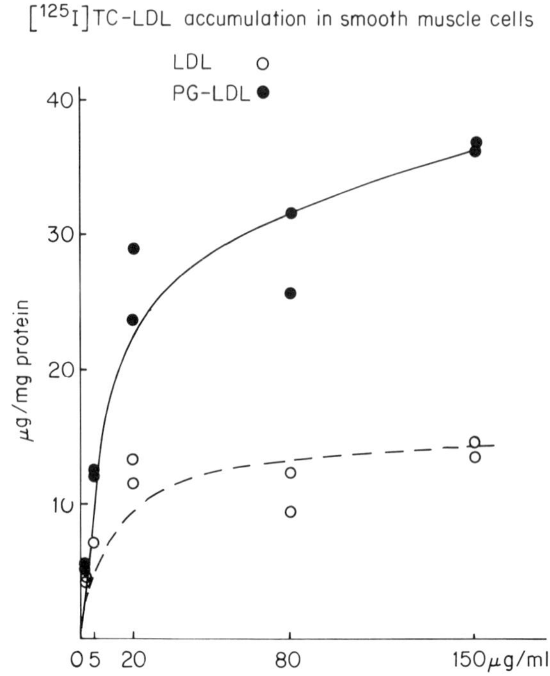

Fig. 1 Uptake of native and proteoglycan-treated LDL in arterial smooth muscle cells. Human arterial smooth muscle cell cultures were established from the intima of human uterine arteries and grown in Waymouth's medium with 10% human serum and 10% foetal calf serum. The cultures were split once a week at a ratio of 1 : 4–1 : 6. These particular experiments were performed at the fifth passage of the cells. The medium was substituted to Eagle's Minimum Essential Medium with 10% lipoprotein-deficient, apoB-free medium for 24 hours. Then the cells were exposed to Eagle's medium with various concentration of [^{125}I]tyramine cellobiose labelled LDL, which in some cases had been pre-treated with human arterial proteoglycans. In short such treatment involved exposure of labelled LDL to the proteoglycan under conditions of low ionic strength in the solution, formation of an LDL-proteoglycan precipitate, and resolubilization of the LDL at physiological ionic strength. The smooth muscle cells were exposed to the lipoproteins for 6 hours, washed with a physiological solution three times and then trypsinized off the petri dishes. Radioactivity in the supernate, representing surface association of lipoproteins, and in a cell pellet at 1000*g*, representing internalized lipoproteins, were calculated. Radioactivity was normalized against cellular protein levels.

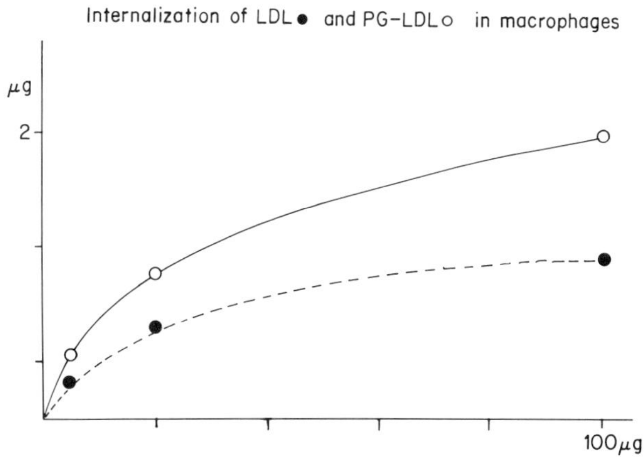

Fig. 2 Uptake of native and proteoglycan treated LDL in human monocyte-derived macrophages. Human monocytes were derived from the buffy-coat of blood-bank blood, from healthy volunteers. The cells were isolated from other blood cells through centrifugation with Ficoll–Paque, and left to adhere to plastic petri dishes, in Waymouth's medium with 10% foetal calf serum. Non-adherent cells were washed away with repeated washes with a balanced salt solution. Twenty-four hours before the experiment, the medium was substituted to Eagle's medium with 10% lipoprotein-deficient, apoB-free medium as described in the legend for Fig. 1. Further treatment was identical to that for smooth muscle cells (see Fig. 1).

This cell expresses both a receptor for native LDL and one for modified LDL. How is the interaction with these receptors affected by the previous interaction between the lipoprotein and the proteoglycan? It seemed a reasonable possibility to us that pre-treatment with proteoglycan might lead to a recognition of the LDL by the receptor for modified LDL. However, we were not able to demonstrate any interaction between proteoglycan-LDL and the receptor for modified LDL (Hurt, Camejo and Bondjers, work in progress). On the other hand, in these cells too, we observed a potentiation of the uptake via the native-LDL receptor by pre-treatment of the lipoprotein by arterial proteoglycans (Fig. 2). In addition, low-affinity uptake of LDL was increased several-fold when the lipoprotein had been exposed to proteoglycans. In fact, the increased uptake of LDL, induced by the pre-treatment with the proteoglycan, leads to lipid accumulation in the cells, to the formation of the hallmark cells of atherosclerosis—the foam cells (Hurt and Camejo, 1987).

This takes us to another unresolved mystery. Why would it be deleterious for the arterial tissue to have foam cells in it? One possible deleterious effect of the formation of foam cells has been suggested by Brown *et al.* (1980b). They proposed that in its effort to control the free cholesterol levels in cells, the combination of free cholesterol esterification and cholesteryl ester hydrolysis might form an energy-consuming metabolic futile cycle in foam cells. If this were significantly the case, we would be able to show changes in the energy consumption in isolated foam cells from arterial tissue, and, in fact, at least oxygen consumption was observed to be increased in such cells (Björnheden and Bondjers, 1987). These observations may explain why an increased oxygen consumption accompanies the development of atherosclerotic lesions (see Björnheden and Bondjers, 1987). In the arterial tissue an increased oxygen consumption might create particular problems, as the distance for diffusion of oxygen and nutrients is particularly large. Apart from cartilage, no other tissue in the body is so far from its supply of nutrients as the arterial tissue. In central regions of advanced atherosclerosis lesions, zero levels of oxygen have been observed (Jurrus and Weiss, 1977). The decrease in tissue oxygen levels may induce a number of changes in the metabolism of arterial smooth muscle cells, including an altered pattern of synthesis of proteoglycans. Thus when fibroblasts are exposed to decreased oxygen levels in the cell culture condition, synthesis of acid glycosaminoglycans is stimulated at the expense of other types of glycosaminoglycans (Kittlietz, 1986). If these observations are relevant also for smooth muscle cells, they may close a vicious circle leading to even more lipoprotein retention, cellular lipid deposition, further decrease in oxygen levels, and so on (Fig. 3). The increased oxygen consumption and increased metabolic strain may be one reason why cell death is such a typical phenomenon in the necrotic core of atherosclerotic lesions. Death of macrophage foam cells, with release of a number of proteases, may in itself lead to continuous irritation of the cells, and transfer the acute reactions to injury into a chronic phase (as discussed above as the turning-point in atherogenesis). We propose that cell death and its consequences, induced by lipid accumulation, may be the link connecting hyperlipidaemia with chronic inflammatory changes in arterial tissue. However, it is possible that the particular problems induced by the interactions of proteoglycan with LDL are part of a more physiological mechanism, devoted to an efficient removal of lipoproteins from the arterial intima that goes out of control only if too much LDL is deposited.

6 Conclusions

In this chapter we have tried to describe a scenario where the lipoprotein, in itself a harmless particle, through its interaction with the arterial tissue (Fig. 3a) undergoes a metamorphosis. The cellular uptake of the lipoprotein is increased, and part of the uptake now occurs via mechanisms not subject to control. This may lead to transformation, both of smooth muscle cells and of

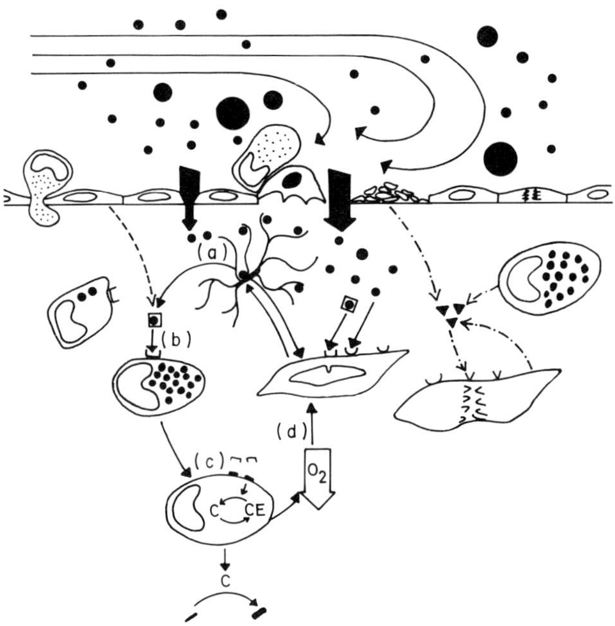

Fig. 3 Schematic and hypothetical representation of lipoprotein interaction with arterial cells, and the vicious circle promoting lipoprotein uptake, and increased metabolic demands in atherosclerosis. (a) LDL interacts with chondroitin-6-sulphate-rich proteoglycans, leading to an increased uptake of LDL both in smooth muscle cells and in macrophages. (b) Following the increased uptake of LDL, both macrophages and smooth muscle cells transform into foam cells. (c) The increased cellular cholesterol levels leads to increased energy consumption in the cells. (d) Decreased oxygen tensions in the tissue stimulate smooth muscle cells to synthesize more chondroitin-6-sulphate-rich proteoglycans, which leads to even further increases in LDL retention and uptake in the cells.

macrophages to foam cells (Fig. 3b). At least in the macrophages, one effect of the transformation is an increased energy consumption (Fig. 3c). We do not yet know whether such an increased energy consumption is found in smooth muscle cells even though this seems to be a reasonable assumption. Decreased oxygen tensions in the arterial tissue may stimulate smooth muscle cells to form more LDL-binding proteoglycans (Fig. 3d), and even further stimulate lipoprotein binding and uptake. It is as yet unclear how this sequence of events may be interrupted. However, one obvious point of intervention may be to take measures to decrease serum lipid levels. A second point of intervention may be to decrease the LDL affinity for proteoglycans, as may be done by beta-blockers and in the future possibly also by other more specific drugs. A third point of intervention may be to try to inhibit the cycle of cholesterol esterification and cholesteryl ester hydrolysis. The cholesteryl ester hydrolases may be equivalent to the hormone-sensitive lipase, which we know is subject to hormonal regulation (Belfrage *et al.*, 1984).* The relevance of these proposed points of interventions should be tested in the future, in experimental models as well as in the clinic.

So, in the final act of our drama, it appears that the key figure, the low density lipoprotein, has changed considerably since the first act. Following its rendezvous with the arterial proteoglycan, the properties of the lipoprotein have changed so that arterial cells have difficulties controlling its uptake. The low density lipoprotein may induce lipid deposition and foam cell transformation, both in the macrophages and in the smooth muscle cell. In the macrophage, and perhaps also in the smooth muscle cell, the increased cellular cholesterol levels may lead to an increased energy consumption, with tissue oxygen levels incompatible with further cell life. When the macrophage dies, it may release toxic products leading to cell death in surrounding smooth muscle cells as well. Thus the encounter between the lipoprotein, the arterial proteoglycans and the cells of the arterial intima may lead to the repeated trauma that has been speculated upon as the critical event in atherogenesis.

* *Editors' note:* There is evidence for hormonal regulation of cholesteryl ester hydrolase in macrophages, smooth muscle cells and steroid hormone-producing tissue.

Acknowledgements

These investigations were supported by grants from the Swedish Medical Research Council (Projects No. 4531 and 7142), the Swedish National Association against Heart and Lung Diseases, King Gustaf V's and Queen Victoria's Foundation, the Medical Society of Göteborg and the Medical Faculty at the University of Göteborg. The secretarial assistance of A. Ladström and E. Landegren is gratefully acknowledged.

References

Adams, D. O. and Hamilton, T. A. (1984). The cell biology of macrophage activation. *Ann. Rev. Immunol.* **2**, 283–322.

Belfrage, P., Fredrikson, G., Strålfors, P. and Tornqvist, H. (1984). In *Lipases* (ed. P. Borgström and H. L. Brockman), pp. 365–416. Elsevier/North Holland, Amsterdam.

Björkerud, S. and Bondjers, G. (1976). Repair responses and tissue lipid after experimental injury to the artery. *Ann. NY Acad. Sci.* **275**, 180–198.

Björnheden, T. and Bondjers, G. (1987). Oxygen consumption in aortic tissue from rabbits with diet-induced atherosclerosis. *Arteriosclerosis* **7**, 238–247.
Bondjers, G. (1975). In *Blood and Arterial Wall in Atherosclerosis and Arterial Thrombosis* (ed. J. G. A. J. Hautvast, R. J. J. Hermus and F. Van der Haar), pp. 55–67. E. J. Brill, Leiden.
Bondjers, G. and Björkerud, S. (1973a). Cholesterol accumulation and content in regions with defined endothelial integrity in the normal rabbit aorta. *Atherosclerosis* **17**, 71–83.
Bondjers, G. and Björkerud, S. (1973b). Arterial repair and atherosclerosis after mechanical injury. 3. Cholesterol accumulation and removal in morphologically defined regions of aortic atherosclerosis lesions in the rabbit. *Atherosclerosis* **17**, 85–94.
Bondjers, G., Wiklund, O., Olofsson, S.-O., Gustafson, A. and Björkerud, S. (1981). In *High-Density Lipoproteins*, (ed. C. E. Day), pp. 463–503. Marcel Dekker, New York.
Brown, M. S., Basu, S. K., Falck, J. R., Ho, Y. K. and Goldstein, J. L. (1980a). The scavenger cell pathway for lipoprotein degradation: specificity of the binding site that mediates the uptake of negatively-charged LDL by macrophages. *J. Supramol. Structure* **13**, 67–81.
Brown, M. S., Ho, Y. K. and Goldstein, J. L. (1980b). The cholesteryl ester cycle in macrophage foam cells. Continual hydrolysis and re-esterification of cytoplasmic cholesteryl esters. *J. Biol. Chem.* **255**, 9344–9352.
Camejo, G. (1982). The interaction of lipids and lipoproteins with the intercellular matrix of arterial tissue: its possible role in atherogenesis. *Adv. Lipid Res.* **19**, 1–51.
Camejo, G., Hurt, E. and Romano, M. (1985). Properties of lipoprotein complexes isolated by affinity chromatography from human aorta. *Biomed. Biophys. Acta* **44**, 389–396.
Camejo, G., Olofsson, S.-O., Lopez, F., Carlsson, P. and Bondjers, G. (1987). *Arteriosclerosis* (in press).
Castelot, I. J., Addonizio, M. L., Rosenberg, E., Karnovsky, K. S. (1981). Cultured endothelial cells produce a heparinlike inhibitor of smooth muscle cell growth. *J. Cell Biol.* **90**, 372–379.
Fowler, S., Shio, H. and Haley, N. J. (1979). Characterization of lipid-laden aortic cells from cholesterol-fed rabbits. IV. Investigation of macrophage-like properties of aortic cell populations. *Lab. Invest.* **41**, 372–378.
Fowler, S., Berberian, P. A., Shio, H., Goldfischer, S. and Wolinsky, H. (1980). Characterization of cell populations isolated from aortas of rhesus monkeys with experimental atherosclerosis. *Circ. Res.* **46**, 520–530.
Goldstein, J. L. and Brown, M. J. (1984). Progress in understanding the LDL receptor and HMG-GoA reductase, two membrane proteins that regulate the plasma cholesterol. *J. Lipid Res* **25**, 1450–1461.
Haley, N. J., Shio, H. and Fowler, S. (1977). Characterization of lipid-laden aortic cells from cholesterol-fed rabbits. I. Resolution of aortic cell populations by metrizamide density gradient centrifugation. *Lab. Invest.* **37**, 287–296.
Hansson, G. K., Bjornheden, T., Bylock, A. and Bondjers, G. (1981). Fc-dependent binding of monocytes to areas with endothelial injury in the rabbit aorta. *Exp. Molec. Path.* **34**, 264–280.
Hoff, H. F. and Bond, G. M. (1983). Apolipoprotein B localization in coronary atherosclerotic plaques from cynomolgus monkeys. *Artery* **12**, 104–117.
Hoff, H. F. and Wagner, W. D. (1986). Plasma low density lipoprotein accumulation in aortas of hypercholesterolemic swine correlates with modifications in aortic glycosaminoglycan composition. *Atherosclerosis* **61**, 231–236.

Hurt, E. and Camejo, G. (1987). Effect of arterial proteoglycans on the interactions of LDL with human monocyte-derived macrophages. *Atherosclerosis* **67**, 115–126

Jonasson, L., Holm, J., Bondjers, G., Skalli, O. and Hansson, G. K. (1986). Regional accumulations of T cells, macrophages, and smooth muscle cells in the human atherosclerotic plaque. *Arteriosclerosis* **6**, 131–138.

Jurrus, E. R. and Weiss, H. S. (1977). *In vitro* tissue oxygen tensions in the rabbit aortic arch. *Atherosclerosis* **28**, 223–232.

Kaplan, J. R., Manuck, S. B., Adams, M. R. and Clarkson, T. B. (1987). The effect of beta-adrenergic blocking agents on atherosclerosis and its complications. *Eur. Heart J.* **87**, 928–944.

Kittlietz, P. D. (1986). Inflammation, glycolytic metabolism, and glycosaminoglycans. *Exp. Path.* **30**, 1–19.

Knott, T. J., Pease, R. J., Powell, L. M., Wallis, S. C., Innerarity, T. L., Blackhart, B., Taylor, W. H., Marcel, Y., Milne, R., Johnson, D., Fuller, M., Lusis, A. J., McCarthy, B. J., Mahley, R. W., Levy-Wilson, B. and Scott, J. (1986). Complete protein sequence and identification of structural domains of human apolipoprotein B. *Nature* **323**, 734–738.

Lindén, T., Bondjers, G., Camejo, G. and Wiklund, O. (1987a). Submitted for publication.

Lindén, T., Wiklund, O., Camejo, G. and Bondjers, G. (1987b). Submitted for publication.

Minick, C. R., Hajjar, D. P., Falcone, D. J., Fowler, S., Eldor, A. and Weksler, B. B. (1981). Arterial injury alters metabolism of the arterial wall. *Thromb. Haemost.* **46**, 781–788.

Olofsson, S.-O., Bjursell, G., Boström, K., Carlsson, P., Elovson, J., Protter, A. A., Reuben, M. A. and Bondjers, G. (1987). Apolipoprotein B: structure, biosynthesis and role in the lipoprotein assembly process. *Atherosclerosis* **68**, 1–17.

Parthasarathy, S., Printz, D. J., Boyd, D., Joy, L. and Steinberg, D. (1986). Macrophage oxidation of low density lipoprotein generates a modified form recognised by the scavenger receptor. *Arteriosclerosis* **6**, 505–510.

Reidy, M. A. (1985). A reassessment of endothelial injury and arterial lesion formation. *Lab. Invest.* **53**, 513–520.

Rosenfeld, M. E., Tsukada, T., Chait, A., Bierman, E. L., Gown, A. M. and Ross, R. (1987a). Fatty streak expansion and maturation in Watanabe Heritable Hyperlipemic and comparably hypercholesterolemic fat-fed rabbits. *Arteriosclerosis* **7**, 24–34.

Rosenfeld, M. E., Tsukada, T., Gown, A. M. and Ross, R. (1987b). Fatty streak initiation in Watanabe Heritable Hyperlipemic and comparably hypercholesterolemic fat-fed rabbits. *Arteriosclerosis* **7**, 9–23.

Ross, R. (1981). Arteriosclerosis: A problem of the biology of arterial cell walls and their interactions with blood components. *Arteriosclerosis* **1**, 293–311.

Ross, R. (1986). The pathogenesis of atherosclerosis—an update. *N. Engl. J. Med.* **314**, 488–500.

Ross, R. and Glomset, J. A. (1976). The pathogenesis of atherosclerosis. *N. Engl. J. Med.* **295**, 369–377; 420–425.

Schwartz, S. M., Gajdusek, C. M. and Selden, S. C. (1981). Vascular wall growth control: the role of the endothelium. *Arteriosclerosis* **1**, 107–121.

Seddon, A. M., Woolf, N., La Ville, A., Pittilo, R. M., Rowles, P. M., Turner, P. R. and Lewis, B. (1987). Hereditary hyperlipidemia and atherosclerosis in the rabbit due to overproduction of lipoproteins. II. Preliminary report of arterial pathology. *Arteriosclerosis* **7**, 113–124.

Tsukada, T., Rosenfeld, M., Ross, R. and Gown, A. M. (1986). Immunocytochemical analysis of cellular components in atherosclerotic lesions. Use of monoclonal antibodies with the Watanabe and fat-fed rabbit. *Arteriosclerosis* **6**, 601–613.

Wiklund, O., Björnheden, T., Olofsson, S.-O. and Bondjers, G. (1987). *Arteriosclerosis* (in press).

Yang, C. Y., Chen, S.-H., Gianturco, S. H., Bradley, W. A., Sparrow, J. T., Tanimura, M., Li, W.-H., Sparrow, D. A., DeLoof, H., Rosseneu, M., Lee, F.-S., Gu, Z.-W., Gott, A. M. Jr. and Chan, L. (1986). Sequence, structure, receptor-binding domains and internal repeats of human apolipoprotein B-100. *Nature* **323**, 738–742.

11

Proliferation of Vascular Smooth Muscle Cells *In Vivo*

MICHAEL A. REIDY, JÜRGEN FINGERLE and MARK W. MAJESKY

Department of Pathology, University of Washington, Seattle, Washington, USA

1 Introduction

It is now well established that vascular smooth muscle cells play a major role in the development of atherosclerotic lesions, and considerable effort has been spent to understand what factors cause proliferation of these cells. Despite intensive work on this issue, it is surprising that there is still only limited information regarding what factors are important for the stimulation of these cells *in vivo*. Moreover, data obtained from *in vivo* studies are often at odds with data obtained *in vitro*. In this chapter we shall review some potential mechanism for the stimulation of smooth muscle cells *in vivo*.

The reaction to injury theory proposed by Ross and Glomset (1976) suggested that platelet interaction with the vessel wall could stimulate smooth muscle cell growth. This process was thought to be mediated by the release of platelet-derived growth factor (PDGF), which *in vitro* has been shown to be mitogenic for smooth muscle cells (Heldin *et al.*, 1979; Ross *et al.*, 1974, 1977; Rutherford and Ross, 1976). In part, major support for the existence of this pathway has been derived from studies in which the endothelium is removed from intact vessels. These studies have shown that endothelial loss is immediately followed by platelet adherence, and within a few days these injuries cause a very significant increase in smooth muscle cell proliferation with a subsequent intimal thickening (Bjorkerud and Bondjers, 1971; Fishman *et al.*, 1975; Haudenschild and Schwartz, 1979; Stemerman *et al.*, 1972). A major problem with these studies has been that the devices used to denude the

HYPERLIPIDAEMIA AND ATHEROSCLEROSIS
ISBN 0.12.675645-7

endothelium often create such widespread injury to the entire vessel that it is difficult to attribute the resultant changes to simply endothelial denudation. For example, we have used a Fogarty balloon catheter to denude arteries in rat and have found that a loss of up to 25% of the vessel wall DNA occurs within the first 24 hours (Clowes *et al.*, 1983a). Since only a small percentage of this DNA can be attributed to loss of endothelium, we are left with the conclusion that the balloon catheter technique damages a significant percentage of the medial smooth muscle cells. Therefore it is somewhat presumptive to interpret the results of these *in vivo* experiments as evidence of the resultant effects of endothelial injury.

For several years a major thrust of our work was to remove vascular endothelial cells without inflicting injury to the subendothelium and to examine the consequences of this action. We developed a procedure using a fine flexible nylon filament that would remove endothelium in a highly reproducible manner, and that did not distend the artery or cause any detectable perturbation to the underlying medial cells (Reidy and Schwartz, 1981). This procedure was also designed so that only a limited region of endothelium was removed from the artery in order to mimic more realistically endothelial denudation *in vivo*. The results of this study showed that when arteries were denuded with this catheter a similar platelet response as with the balloon catheter was observed, but, somewhat surprisingly, no intimal proliferation could be observed and no change was observed in the proliferation rate of the underlying smooth muscle cells. This experiment has been repeated in different species (Prescott and Muller, 1983; Ramsay *et al.*, 1982) and with a larger catheter so as to remove a larger zone of endothelium (Reidy and Silver, 1985), and the result has always been that endothelial loss caused in this fashion did not precipitate intimal thickening (Table 1). These data prompted us to suggest that *in vivo* loss of endothelium in the absence of medial injury was not sufficient to cause proliferation of smooth muscle cells and that other

Table 1 Effect of injury to rat aorta using a nylon filament.

Size of wound[b]	Time of closure	Intimal thickening[a]	Intimal replication[a]
3–5	48 h	No	No
10–15	90 h	No	No
90–120	180 h	No	No
Total denudation with balloon catheter	>6 months	Yes	Yes

[a]Intimal thickening and replication were assessed from five sections cut from each segment of aorta ($n = 9$).

[b]Width of wound measured by number of cells removed.

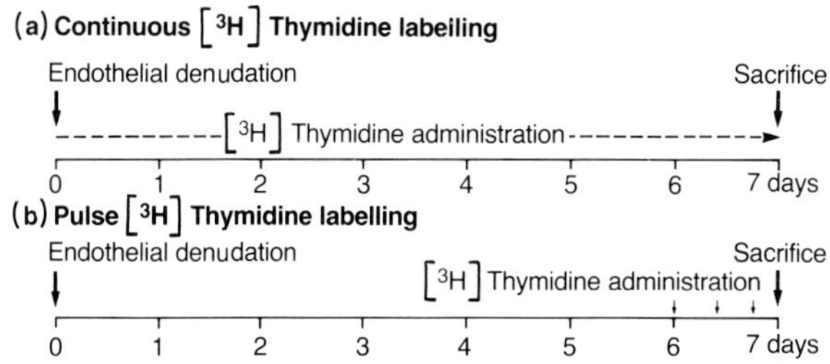

Fig. 1 Schematic diagram illustrating protocols for administration of [^{3}H]thymidine to experimental animals. (a) The implanted osmotic pump continuously infuses [^{3}H]thymidine for the entire experimental period of 7 days. (b) [^{3}H]Thymidine is administered during the last 24 hours of the experiment by three bolus injections.

factors, as yet undetermined, must play a controlling role in stimulating these cells. This conclusion, as discussed below, turned out to be only partially correct, but the above data stimulated us to propose other mechanisms by which smooth muscle cells can undergo replication; these pathways will be discussed later in this chapter.

Our conclusion that endothelial loss and platelet interaction with damaged vessel wall led to no increase in smooth muscle proliferation was based on studies where [^{3}H]thymidine was administered to animals and smooth muscle cell proliferation assessed from cross-sections of the injured arteries using conventional autoradiography. Each animal received [^{3}H]thymidine (50 μCi/100 g body weight) at 1, 9 and 17 hours prior to sacrifice (Schwartz and Benditt, 1973). These times were chosen because the S-phase of endothelial cell cycle has been estimated to be approximately 8 hours and therefore by following this protocol we should have captured all cell division over a 24 hour period (Fig. 1). Recently we have administered [^{3}H]thymidine continuously for periods of up to 1 week by means of an indwelling osmotic pump and have found this procedure to be more sensitive for detecting cell replication than the protocol used above (Clowes and Schwartz, 1985; Tada and Reidy, 1987). The advantages of such a procedure are that it eliminates any concern regarding the length of the S-phase and that it allows us to obtain the cumulative rate of cell replication that occurred throughout the experimental period. We have recently repeated the studies that examined the effect of limited endothelial denudation on smooth muscle cell proliferation and used an indwelling osmotic pump to administer [^{3}H]thymidine (10 μCi/h) continuously for 7 days (Tada and Reidy, 1987). The results of this study (Table 2) showed that there was a slight but significant increase in smooth muscle cell replication in those aortas with endothelial denudation as compared with sham operated controls. As previously reported, this limited denudation did not lead to any

Table 2 Smooth muscle cell replication in rat aortas after limited denudation with continuous thymidine labelling for 7 days.

	Denuding injury	Sham operation	Control
Thymidine index[a]	1.02 ± 0.44[b]	0.19 ± 0.13	0.15 ± 0.12

[a]The cumulative thymidine index is the number of replicating cells/total number of cells counted ×100 (see text for details).
[b]Mean ± standard deviation (SD) (n = 5 for each group). p <0.005.

intimal thickening (Reidy and Schwartz, 1981). We consider these new data to be important since they show that a small relatively non-traumatic injury to the vessel wall does indeed elicit a response by the underlying smooth muscle cells. If the cell replication had been triggered by the platelet then we should have been able to localize this replication only to those zones subjected to endothelial denudation. Somewhat surprisingly, there was a poor correlation between the sites of denudation visualized by the presence of replicating endothelial cells and smooth muscle cell proliferation (Table 3). However, this lack of any clear association may be due to the fact that endothelial repair can occur without cell division (Reidy and Schwartz, 1981). Of great interest to us was the finding that smooth muscle cell proliferation was not followed by migration of cells into the intima. These data are in striking contrast with the results obtained with vessels subjected to a balloon catheter injury, where smooth muscle cells were observed in the intima within 4 days and a very substantial intimal thickening observed after 7 days (Clowes *et al.*, 1983a,b).

Table 3 Location of replicating smooth muscle cells at sites of endothelial replication.

	Number of replicating smooth muscle cells[a] (%)
Adjacent to endothelial replication[b]	34.5 ± 26.7
Distant to endothelial replication	65.5 ± 26.7

[a]Data expressed as a percentage of total labelled smooth muscle cells ± SD.
[b]Includes those smooth muscle cells that were directly covered by replicating endothelial cells or lay within one cell length of a replicating endothelial cell.

At the present time there are no firm data to explain the differences elicited by these denuding injuries, but one possibility relates to the speed of endothelial regrowth. After injury with the nylon filament, total endothelial regrowth occurred within approximately 3 days, but after balloon catheter denudation, endothelial regrowth was very slow and at certain sites was never complete. *In vitro* endothelial cells have been shown to inhibit the growth of smooth muscle cells, possibly by the action of a secreted heparin-like molecule (Castellot *et al.*, 1982). Thus the presence of endothelial cells over the proliferating smooth muscle cells may be an important controlling factor in intimal lesion development. Some support for this concept can be found in the study of Haudenschild and Schwartz (1979), where it was observed that after aortic denudation the dorsal wall of the aorta, which was rapidly repopulated with endothelium, showed little or no intimal thickening. The ventral wall, however, showed a significant intimal thickening. We have started to reexamine the role of endothelium in injured arteries and have chosen the rat common carotid artery as our model. This has the advantage that endothelial regrowth occurs in a well-defined manner with new endothelial cells arising from the bifurcation with the aorta and with the internal carotid artery. After balloon catheter injury to this vessel, the regrowth of endothelium over this injured artery caused a marked decrease in the proliferation rate of the smooth muscle cells (Table 4) at all the times studied (Clowes *et al.*, 1983a). Perhaps more surprising was that in a similar study in which total endothelial denudation of the carotid artery was achieved with a new less abrasive catheter, intimal thickening was not observed in those areas of the artery that were not rehealed by endothelium within approximately 7 days (see Fig. 2). It should be noted that this was despite the fact that immediately after denudation medial smooth

Table 4 Replication rate of smooth muscle cells in balloon injured rat carotid arteries.

	Areas not covered by endothelium	Areas covered by endothelium[a]
4 Weeks		
Intima	1.2 ± 0.6[b]	0.36 ± 0.05
Media	0.8 ± 0.06	0.3 ± 0.2
8 Weeks		
Intima	0.03 ± 0.1	0.04 ± 0.02
Media	0.1 ± 0.08	0.1 ± 0.2

[a]Vessels were completely denuded of endothelium and endothelial regrowth occurred from both ends of the carotid artery.
[b]Mean thymidine index (%) of smooth muscle cells in balloon injured rat common carotid artery.

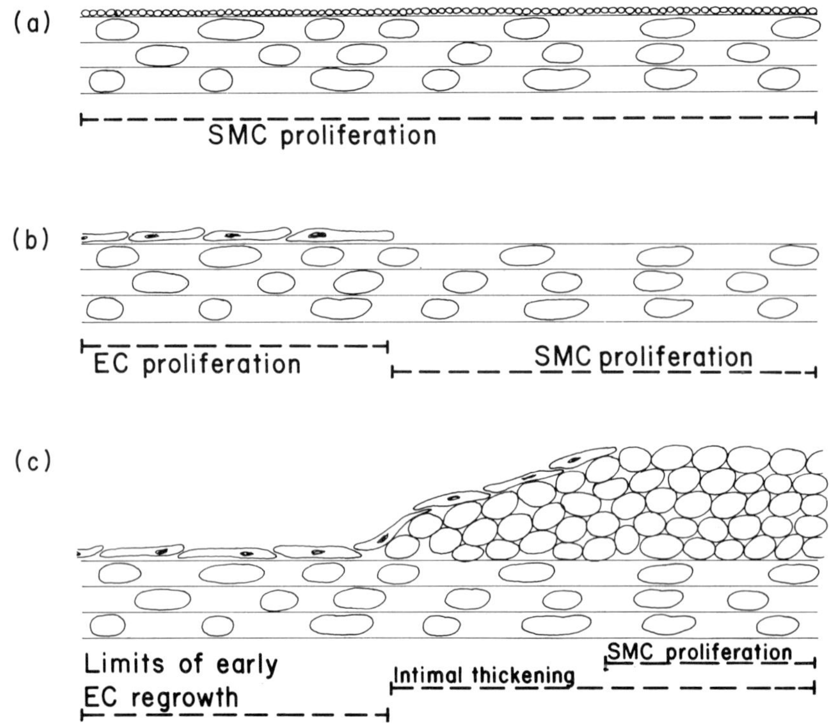

Fig. 2 Growth of rat carotid smooth muscle after total endothelial denudation. (a) Immediately after endothelial loss, there is a significant increase in smooth muscle cell replication throughout the entire carotid which continues for several days. (b) Regrowth of endothelium starts immediately after denudation, and those zones rapidly recovered by endothelium show a marked reduction in smooth muscle cell proliferation as compared with adjacent denuded areas. (c) Rapid endothelial regrowth (i.e. by approximately 7 days) retards the migration of smooth muscle cells into the intima. Those areas not repopulated by endothelium at this time develop a thickened intima and continue to have an increase in smooth muscle cell replication.

muscle cell proliferation was significantly elevated throughout the entire vessel and was maintained at this high rate for several days. It would therefore appear that smooth muscle proliferation and smooth muscle migration are separate events and that regrowth of endothelium plays an important modulating role in intimal lesion formation. The presence of endothelial cells not only inhibits smooth muscle cell replication but also appears to block the migration of smooth muscle cells into the intima (see Fig. 2). This finding has direct relevance to initiation of early atherosclerotic lesions where in experimental animals only very small zones of endothelial denudation have ever been observed. If we assume the regenerative properties of the endothelial cells are not impaired, then the denuded zones should be rapidly covered by new endothelium and thereby prevent the migration of smooth muscle cells into the intima. It is worth remembering, however, that in at least three species of animals, endothelial regrowth can be extremely slow, and in some instances total endothelial regrowth is never achieved (Reidy *et al.*, 1982, 1983, 1986). In these circumstances, therefore, this lack of rapid endothelial repair may significantly contribute to the formation of atherosclerotic lesions both by continuing to allow platelets to adhere to the exposed subendothelium and by allowing smooth muscle cells to migrate from the media to the intima. Thus, as was suggested by Ross as early as 1976, the endothelium plays a major pivotal role in atherogenesis.

2 Smooth muscle proliferation in vascular lesions

So far our discussion has focused on proliferation of smooth muscle cells in deliberately injured arteries where the endothelium is known to be absent. If platelet-PDGF is important for the initiation of diet-induced lesions then we should be able to detect endothelial cell denudation prior to lesion formation. Early studies by Bowyer and co-workers in Cambridge showed an intact endothelium was found over developing lesions in rabbits receiving a cholesterol-rich diet (Fig. 3) (Davies *et al.*, 1976; Goode *et al.*, 1977; Reidy and

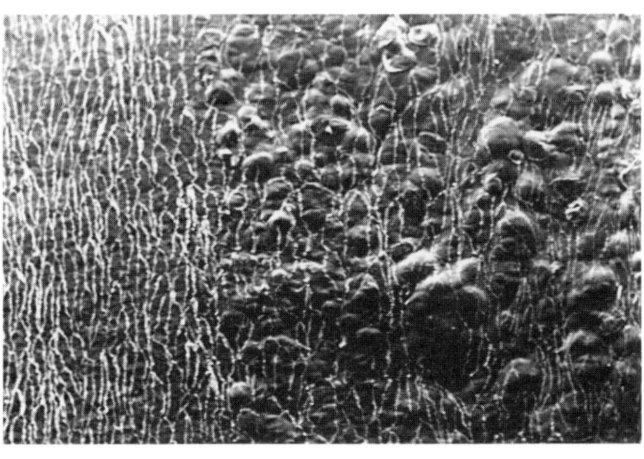

Fig. 3 Aortic endothelium of a rabbit fed a cholesterol diet viewed with scanning electron microscopy. On the right side of the micrograph there is a developing raised intimal lesion and endothelial cells can clearly be visualized over this area. Cells were stained with silver nitrate (0.25%) to highlight their boundaries.

Table 5 Labelling index of aortic smooth muscle cells in cholesterol-fed rabbits.

Time on diet (weeks)	Intimal index (±SD)	Media index (±SD)
0	0.0 (±0.0)	0.016 (±0.024)
4	0.0 (±0.0)	0.032 (±0.051)
6	0.025 (±0.137)	0.024 (±0.044)
10	0.0 (±0.0)	0.010 (±0.057)
20	0.885 (±1.611)[a]	0.073 (±0.136)[b]

[a] $p < 0.005$.
[b] $p < 0.05$.

Bowyer, 1978). These data have been confirmed by many laboratories and in several different species (Gerrity, 1981; Faggiotto and Ross, 1984; Joris *et al.*, 1983; Scott *et al.*, 1986), although endothelial injury has been found in animals with significant lesion involvement after approximately 4–5 months of dietary cholesterol feeding. An important issue raised by these studies is that presumably smooth muscle cell growth occurred in these lesions despite the presence of an intact endothelium and therefore in the absence of PDGF. Kim and co-workers provided the first definite evidence of increased thymidine labelling in pig intimal cell cushions induced by hyperlipidaemia (Kim *et al.*, 1985), and work from this laboratory in conjunction with David Bowyer (Walker *et al.*, 1986a) showed that after 20 weeks of feeding a 0.1% cholesterol diet the proliferation rate of both intimal and medial smooth muscle cells was significantly elevated (Table 5). Furthermore, both studies confirmed the presence of an intact endothelium over these lesions. In light of the absence of any platelets, these data have important implications because they suggest that cells other than platelets may play a role in stimulating smooth muscle cell growth.

3 Mitogen production by vascular smooth muscle cells

In recent years it has been shown that many cells can produce PDGF-like activity, for example, *in vitro* endothelial cells will readily synthesize PDGF and there is some evidence that this occurs *in vivo* (Barrett *et al.*, 1984; Collins *et al.*, 1985, 1987). Furthermore, recent work has shown that macrophages that are known to be present in diet-induced lesions can also synthesize and secrete a PDGF-like molecule (Shimokado *et al.*, 1985). Finally, as will be discussed below, it has been shown that smooth muscle cells can also secrete a PDGF-like mitogen (Seifert *et al.*, 1984; Walker *et al.*, 1986b).

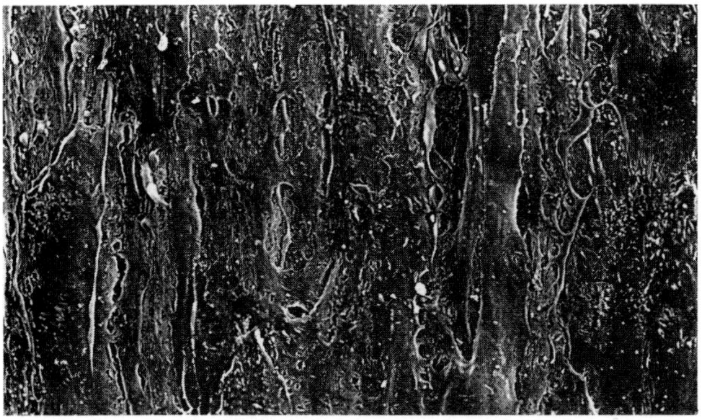

Fig. 4 Luminal surface of rat carotid artery 12 weeks after endothelial cell denudation with a balloon catheter. These cells are non-thrombogenic and smooth muscle cells that have migrated from the media to form a pseudo-endothelium.

In an artery injured by a balloon catheter, vascular smooth muscle cells start to proliferate within 24 hours, which is a time when platelet interaction with the vessel wall is high (Clowes *et al.*, 1983a). At later times the denuded areas, now covered by smooth muscle cells, are almost non-thrombogenic (Fig. 4) (Reidy *et al.*, 1983) and yet those intimal smooth muscle cells continue to replicate (Clowes *et al.*, 1983a). A question raised by these observations is, if PDGF is the controlling mitogen then what is the source of the mitogen in these vessels? To try to answer this question, we again used our injured rat carotid artery model, which was subjected to balloon catheter injury as before. We have shown that after two weeks this injury induced a pronounced intima, and by using microdissection we were able to separate these cells from the media and grow them in culture. It was immediately apparent that the intimal smooth muscle cells were phenotypically different from medial cells *in vitro*. The intimal cells grew as a monolayer and morphologically strongly resembled cultured endothelial cells (Fig. 5). These cells, however, stained positive with an antibody against smooth muscle cell actin, did not express acetyl-LDL receptors and were negative when stained with an anti-von Willebrand factor antibody (Walker *et al.*, 1986b). Thus, by all these criteria, they were smooth muscle cells. The medial cells grew in the typical "hills and valleys" fashion and stained positive with the smooth muscle cell actin antibody. Conditioned media were collected from both sets of cells and assayed for secreted PDGF-like activity using a competitive-binding assay. Intimal smooth muscle cells secreted three to four times as much PDGF-like activity as did medial cells from the same animal (Table 6), and this activity was neutralized by addition

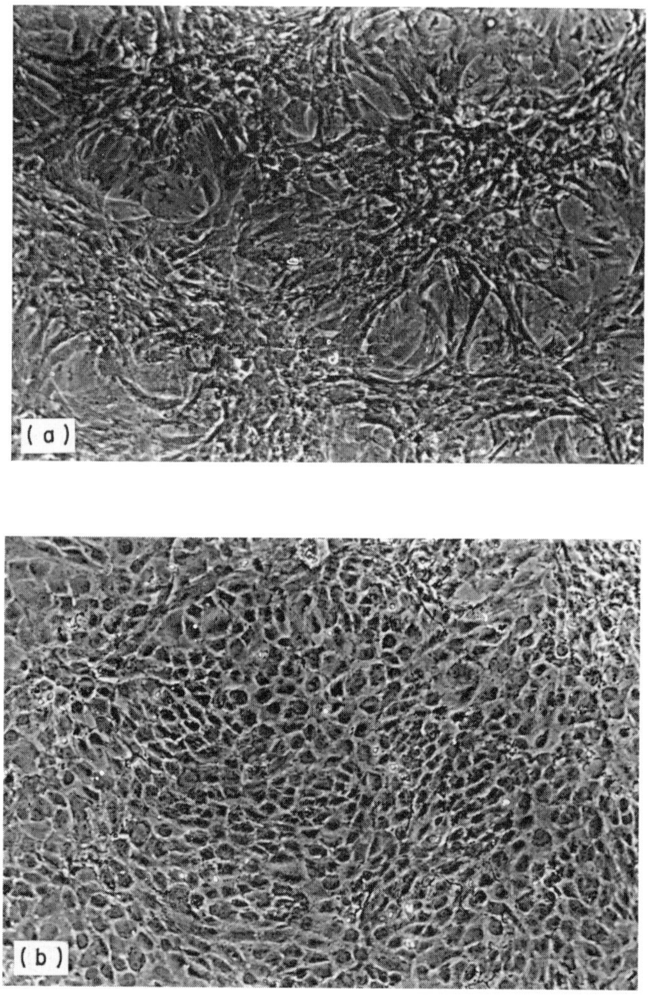

Fig. 5 *In vitro* cultures of rat smooth muscle cells. (a) Cells were derived from media and grown in the typical "hills and valleys" fashion. (b) Intimal smooth muscle cells that grow as monolayers and closely resemble endothelium. These cells do stain positive with antibody to smooth muscle cell actin, do not have acetyl-LDL receptors, and do not stain with an antibody to von Willebrand factor.

Table 6 Rate of production of PDGF-like activity by medial and intimal smooth muscle cells.

Culture no.	PDGF-like activity (ng per 10^6 cells) Medial smooth muscle cells	Intimal smooth muscle cells	Ratio, intimal/medial
1	0.63	1.01	1.60
2	0.11	0.46	4.18
3	0.09	0.56	6.20
4	0.06	0.48	8.00
5	0.20	0.63	3.15
6	0.04	0.59	14.80
7	0.44	0.90	2.05
8	0.23	0.41	1.78
9	0.08	0.43	5.38
10	—	1.33	—
11	0.38	0.25	0.66
12	0.06	0.34	5.70
Mean ± SD	0.21 ± 0.19	0.62 ± 0.31[a]	4.86 ± 4.00

Conditioned (48 h) medium collected from primary-passage intimal and medial smooth muscle cells was assayed for PDGF-like activity by competitive binding in a radioreceptor assay. In all cases, except culture no. 12, which was a pool of tissue from five animals, cultures were derived from individual animals.

[a] $p = 0.0014$.

of PDGF antibody (Fig. 6). These intimal cells were also found to grow well in low serum concentrations and did respond to exogenously added PDGF. Furthermore, these cells expressed fewer unoccupied receptors for PDGF than did the medial cells as assessed by quantitating specific binding of ^{125}I-labelled PDGF. This would suggest that PDGF receptors in the intimal cells were occupied by endogenous PDGF. Taken together, these data indicate that after vessel wall injury the underlying smooth muscle cells undergo a phenotypic change that leads to a different morphology and importantly to the secretion of a PDGF-like molecule. These data could therefore explain why *in vivo* the smooth muscle cells continued to replicate in the absence of an exogenous source of PDGF.

One concern about the above data is that they were derived from cells *in vitro* and it has been shown that culture conditions may very markedly change gene expression for PDGF. This was shown by the work of Barrett *et al.* (1984), who

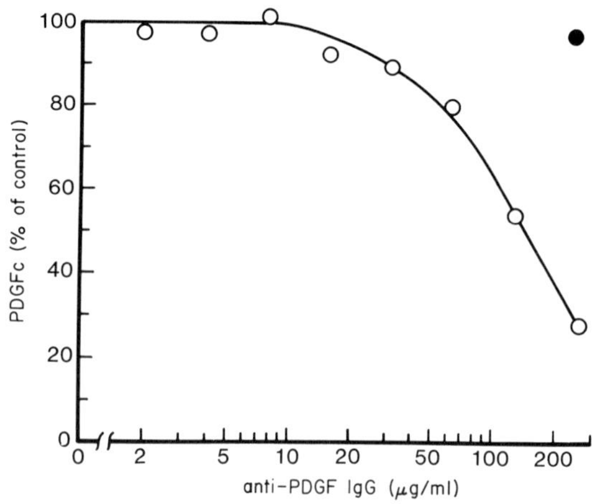

Fig. 6 Neutralization of PDGF-like activity in conditioned medium from rat intimal smooth muscle cells by antibodies to PDGF. Conditioned medium from cells was incubated with various concentrations of goat anti-human PDGF IgG (○) or non-immune goat IgG (●). Residual PDGF-like activity in the conditioned medium was then determined by radioreceptor assay and expressed as a percentage of activity determined in the absence of IgG.

conducted an experiment in which the expression of B-chain transcripts of PDGF were compared in endothelial cells immediately removed from the normal umbilical vein and in endothelial cells grown in culture. They showed that the cells *in vivo* expressed little message for the B-chain of PDGF, but after culturing these cells there was a 1000-fold increase in the transcripts for the same gene. Should smooth muscle cells behave in a similar fashion to *in vitro* conditions, then it might be difficult to relate our findings to the replication of these intimal smooth muscle cells *in vivo*. We have approached this problem using cDNA probes to both chains of PDGF, which were hybridized to the extracted mRNA from rat carotid arteries at various times after injury. An example of these Northern hybridizations is shown in Fig. 7. Our results showed that few or no transcripts from the B-chain of PDGF were seen in the uninjured controls nor in arteries subjected to injury. This was true for up to several weeks after injury. In contrast, increases in message levels for the A-chain of PDGF were detected in the injured arteries within six hours (Majesky *et al.*, 1987).

These data therefore support our original observation of secreted PDGF activity by intimal smooth muscle cells in culture and reinforce our notion that

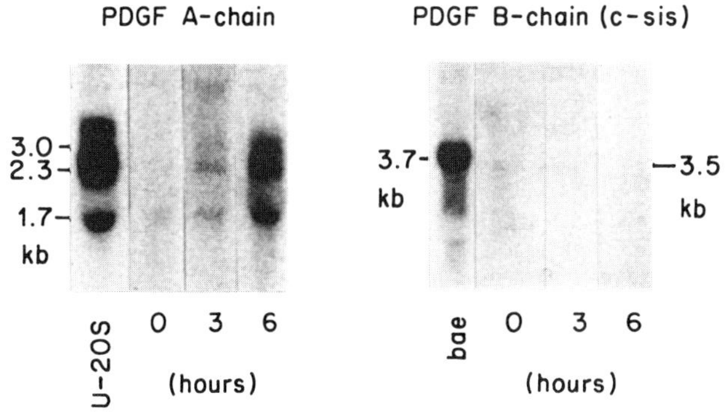

Fig. 7 Northern assay of mRNA extracted from rat carotid artery at various times after balloon catheter injury. A significant increase in A-chain transcripts was observed within 3 hours. The cells showed no change in the B-chain transcript.

smooth muscle cells can influence their own replication by the synthesis and secretion of PDGF activity. These studies raise many questions, but one that interests us is whether all smooth muscle cells can respond to injury in the manner described above. One hypothesis is that injury activates a subpopulation of cells that has maintained the properties of immature "blast" cells (Schwartz *et al.*, 1985). Normal young rat cells have also been shown to secrete PDGF activity, and one possibility is that, owing to their advantage in proliferative activity, these cells participate in intimal lesion formation. This form of selective proliferation of a subset of cells is consistent with the data of Clowes and Schwartz (1985), who found that only 50% of cells that migrate into the intima go on to divide actively. A proliferative response by a subset of cells could also account for the monoclonal phenotype of certain human atherosclerotic lesions. We shall however, need to know far more about the replicative properties of smooth muscle cells and the lineage of smooth muscle cells in lesions before this idea can be confirmed.

Acknowledgements

This work was supported by National Institutes of Health Grants HL-30203 and HL-03174. Dr Reidy is an Established Investigator for the American Heart Association and is supported in part from funds contributed by the Washington affiliate.

References

Barrett, T. B., Gajdusek, C. M., Schwartz, S. M., McDougall, J. K. and Benditt, E. P. (1984). Expression of the sis gene by endothelial cells in culture and *in vivo*. *Proc. Natl Acad. Sci. USA* **81**, 6772–6774.

Bjorkerud, S. and Bondjers, G. (1971). Arterial repair and atherosclerosis after mechanical injury. 2. Tissue response after induction of a total local necrosis deep longitudinal injury. *Atherosclerosis* **14**, 259–276.

Castellot, J. J., Favreau, L. V., Karnovsky, M. J. and Rosenberg, R. D. (1982). Inhibition of vascular smooth muscle cell growth by endothelial cell-derived heparin. Possible role of a platelet endoglycosidase. *J. Biol. Chem.* **257**, 11256–11260.

Clowes, A. W. and Schwartz, S. M. (1985). Significance of quiescent smooth muscle migration in the injured rat carotid artery. *Circ. Res.* **56**, 139–145.

Clowes, A. W., Reidy, M. A. and Clowes, M. M. (1983a). Kinetics of cellular proliferation after arterial injury. I. Smooth muscle growth in the absence of endothelium. *Lab. Invest.* **49**, 327–333.

Clowes, A. W., Reidy, M. A. and Clowes, M. M. (1983b). Mechanisms of stenosis after arterial injury. *Lab. Invest.* **49**, 208–215.

Collins, T., Ginsburg, D., Boss, J. M., Orkin, S. H. and Pober, J. S. (1985). Cultured human endothelial cells express platelet-derived growth factor B chain: cDNA cloning and structural analysis. *Nature* **316**, 748–750.

Collins, T., Pober, J., Gimbrone, M. A., Hammacher, A., Betscholtz, C., Westermark, B. and Heldin, C. H. (1987). Cultured human endothelial cells express platelet-derived growth factor A chain. *Am. J. Path.* **126**, 7–12.

Davies, P. F., Reidy, M. A., Goode, T. B. and Bowyer, D. E. (1976). Scanning electron microscopy in the evaluation of endothelial integrity of the fatty lesion in atherosclerosis. *Atherosclerosis* **25**, 125–130.

Faggiotto, A. and Ross, R. (1984). Studies of hypercholesterolemia in the non-human primate. II. Fatty streak conversion to fibrous plaque. *Arteriosclerosis* **4**, 341–356.

Fishman, J. A., Ryan, G. B. and Karnovsky, M. J. (1975). Endothelial regeneration in the rat carotid artery and the significance of endothelial denudation in the pathogenesis of myointimal thickening. *Lab. Invest.* **32**, 339–351.

Gerrity, R. G. (1981). The role of the monocyte in atherogenesis: I. Transmission of blood-borne monocytes into foam cells in fatty lesions. *Am. J. Path.* **103**, 181.

Goode, T. B., Davies, P. F., Reidy, M. A. and Bowyer, D. E. (1977). Aortic endothelial cell morphology observed *in situ* by scanning electron microscopy during atherogenesis in the rabbit. *Atherosclerosis* **27**, 235–251.

Haudenschild, C. C. and Schwartz, S. (1979). Endothelial regeneration. II. Restitution of endothelial continuity. *Lab. Invest.* **41**, 407–418.

Heldin, C.-H., Westermark, B. and Wasteson, A. (1979). Platelet-derived growth factor: purification and partial characterization. *Proc. Natl Acad. Sci. USA* **76**, 3722–3726.

Joris, I., Zand, T., Nunnari, J. J., Krolikowski, F. J. and Majno, G. (1983). Studies on the pathogenesis of atherosclerosis. I. Adhesion and emigration of mononuclear cells in the aorta of hypercholesterolemic rats. *Am. J. Path.* **113**, 341–358.

Kim, D. N., Imai, H., Schmee, J., Lee, K. T. and Thomas, W. A. (1985). Intimal cell mass-derived atherosclerotic lesions in the abdominal aorta of hyperlipidemic swine. Part 1. Cell of origin, cell divisions and cell losses in first 90 days on diet. *Atherosclerosis* **56**, 169–188.

Majesky, M., Reidy, M., Benditt, E. and Schwartz, S. M. (1987). Expression of platelet-derived growth factor (PDGF) A- and B-chain genes in smooth muscle during repair of arterial injury. *J. Mol. Cell Cardiol.* **19** (Suppl. 4), 58.

Prescott, M. F. and Muller, K. R. (1983). Endothelial regeneration in hypertensive and genetically hypercholesterolemic rats. *Arteriosclerosis* **3**, 206–214.

Ramsay, M. M., Walker, L. N. and Bowyer, D. E. (1982). Narrow superficial injury to rabbit aortic endothelium. The healing process as observed by scanning electron microscopy. *Atherosclerosis* **43**, 233–243.

Reidy, M. A. and Bowyer, D. E. (1978). Scanning electron microscope studies of rabbit aortic endothelium in areas of haemodynamic stress during induction of fatty streaks. *Virch. Arch. Path. Anat.* **377**, 237–248.

Reidy, M. A. and Schwartz, S. M. (1981). Endothelial regeneration. III. Time course of intimal changes after small defined injury to rat aortic endothelium. *Lab. Invest.* **44**, 301–308.

Reidy, M. A. and Silver, M. (1985). Endothelial regeneration. VII. Lack of intimal proliferation after defined injury to rat aorta. *Am. J. Path* **118**, 173–177.

Reidy, M. A., Standaert, D. and Schwartz, S. M. (1982). Inhibition of endothelial cell regrowth. Cessation of aortic endothelial cell replication after balloon catheter denudation. *Arteriosclerosis* **2**, 216–220.

Reidy, M. A., Clowes, A. W. and Schwartz, S. M. (1983). Endothelial regeneration. V. Inhibition of endothelial regrowth in arteries of rat and rabbit. *Lab. Invest.* **49**, 569–575.

Reidy, M. A., Chao, S. S., Kirkman, T. R. and Clowes, A. W. (1986). Endothelial regeneration. VI. Chronic nondenuding injury in baboon vascular grafts. *Am. J. Path.* **123**, 432–439.

Ross, R. and Glomset, J. (1976). The pathogenesis of atherosclerosis. *N. Engl. J. Med.* **295**, 369–377.

Ross, R., Glomset, J., Kariya, B. and Harker, L. (1974). A platelet-dependent serum factor that stimulates the proliferation of arterial smooth muscle cells *in vitro*. *Proc. Natl Acad. Sci. USA* **71**, 1207–1210.

Ross, R., Glomset, J. and Harker, L. (1977). Response to injury and atherogenesis. *Am. J. Path.* **86**, 675–684.

Rutherford, R. B. and Ross, R. (1976). Platelet factors stimulate fibroblasts and smooth muscle cells quiescent in plasma serum to proliferate. *J. Cell. Biol.* **69**, 196–203.

Schwartz, S. M. and Benditt, E. P. (1973). Cell replication in the aortic endothelium; a new method for study of the problem. *Lab. Invest.* **28**, 699–707.

Schwartz, S. M., Reidy, M. A. and Clowes, A. W. (1985). Kinetics of atherosclerosis: a stem cell model. *Ann. NY Acad. Sci.* **454**, 292–304.

Scott, R. F., Reidy, M. A., Kim, D. N., Schmee, J. and Thomas, W. A. (1986). Intimal cell mass-derived atherosclerotic lesions in the abdominal aorta of hyperlipidemic swine. Part 2. Investigation of endothelial cell changes and leukocyte adherence associated with early smooth muscle cell proliferative activity. *Atherosclerosis* **62**, 27–38.

Seifert, R. A., Schwartz, S. M. and Bowen-Pope, D. F. (1984). Developmentally regulated production of platelet-derived growth factor-like molecules. *Nature* **311**, 669–671.

Shimokado, K., Raines, E. W., Madtes, D. K., Barrett, T. B., Benditt, E. P. and Ross, R. (1985). A significant part of macrophage-derived growth factor consists of at least two forms of PGDF. *Cell* **43**, 277–286.

Stemerman, M. B., Spaet, T. H., Pitlick, F., Clinton, J., Lejneks, I. and Tiell, M. L. (1972). Intimal healing. The pattern of re-endothelialization and intimal thickening. *Am. J. Path.* **87**, 125.

Tada, T. and Reidy, M. A. (1987). Endothelial regeneration: IX. Arterial injury followed by rapid endothelial repair induces smooth muscle cell proliferation but not intimal thickening. *Am. J. Path.* **129**, 429–433.

Walker, L. N., Reidy, M. A. and Bowyer, D. E. (1986a). Morphology and cell kinetics of fatty streak lesion formation in the hypercholesterolemic rabbit. *Am. J. Path.* **125**, 450–459.

Walker, L. N., Bowen-Pope, D. F., Ross, R. and Reidy, M. A. (1986b). Production of platelet-derived growth factor-like molecules by cultured arterial smooth muscle cells accompanies proliferation after arterial injury. *Proc. Natl Acad. Sci. USA* **83**, 7311–7315.

12

Molecular Mechanism of Action of Newer Thrombolytic Agents

D. COLLEN

Centre for Thrombosis and Vascular Research, University of Leuven, Belgium

1 The fibrinolytic system

1.1 Components of the fibrinolytic system

The fibrinolytic system, schematically represented in Fig. 1, contains a proenzyme, plasminogen, which can be converted to the active enzyme plasmin by the action of several different types of plasminogen activators. Plasmin is a serine protease that digests fibrin to soluble degradation products.

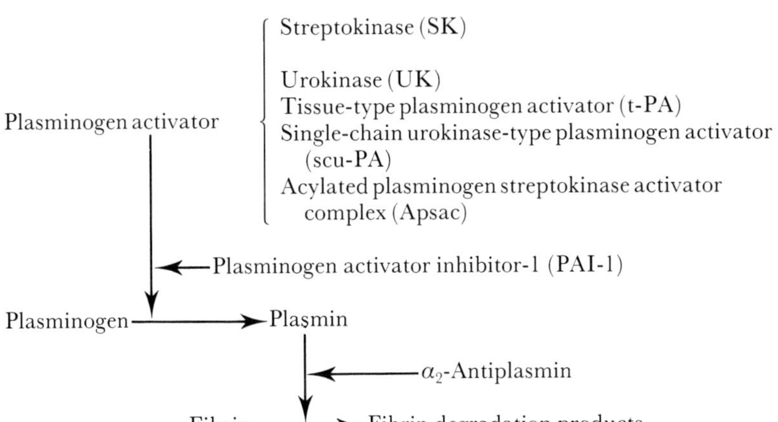

Fig. 1 Schematic representation of the fibrinolytic system.

HYPERLIPIDAEMIA AND ATHEROSCLEROSIS
ISBN 0.12.675645-7

Natural inhibition of the fibrinolytic system occurs both at the level of the plasminogen activator and also at the level of plasmin (Collen and Lijnen, 1986; Bachmann, 1987; Collen, 1987a).

Plasminogen

Plasminogen is a single-chain glycoprotein, consisting of 790 amino acids, which is converted to plasmin by cleavage of the Arg^{560}-Val^{561} peptide bond. The plasminogen molecule contains structures called lysine-binding sites that mediate its binding to fibrin and accelerate the interaction between plasmin and its physiological inhibitor α_2-antiplasmin. The lysine binding sites play a crucial role in the regulation of fibrinolysis (Wiman and Collen, 1978a; Collen, 1980).

Plasminogen activators

Plasminogen activators are serine proteases with a high specificity for plasminogen, which hydrolyse the Arg^{560}-Val^{561} peptide bond, yielding the active enzyme plasmin.

Streptokinase is a non-enzyme protein with molecular weight of 47 000, produced by beta-haemolytic streptococci, that activates the fibrinolytic system indirectly. Streptokinase forms a 1 : 1 stoichiometric complex with plasminogen that then undergoes a transition exposing an active site in the modified plasminogen moiety, whereby the complex becomes a potent plasminogen activator (Kosow, 1975).

Urokinase is a trypsin-like serine protease composed of two polypeptide chains, connected by a disulphide bridge, that activates plasminogen directly to plasmin (White *et al.*, 1966). Single-chain urokinase-type plasminogen activator (scu-PA) or pro-urokinase is a single-chain glycoprotein containing 411 amino acids that is converted to urokinase by hydrolysis of the Lys^{158}-Ile^{159} peptide bond (Holmes *et al.*, 1985). Scu-PA has very little activity towards low-molecular-weight substrates but has intrinsic plasminogen activating potential, with a catalytic efficiency about 5% of that of urokinase (Lijnen *et al.*, 1986a).

Tissue-type plasminogen activator (t-PA) is a trypsin-like serine protease composed of 527 amino acids (Pennica *et al.*, 1983). It occurs either as a single-chain glycoprotein or as a two-chain proteolytic derivative, but both forms have comparable enzymatic properties. t-PA is a poor plasminogen activator in the absence of fibrin, but it binds specifically to fibrin and activates plasminogen at the fibrin surface several hundred-fold more efficiently than in the circulation (Hoylaerts *et al.*, 1982).

α_2-Antiplasmin

α_2-Antiplasmin is a glycoprotein of the serine protease inhibitor (serpin) superfamily, composed of 452 amino acids with Arg^{364}-Met^{365} as the reactive site (Holmes *et al.*, 1987). α_2-Antiplasmin reacts very rapidly with plasmin, first to form a reversible but inactive complex, which is then slowly converted into an irreversible complex. The first step of the reaction is dependent on the presence of free lysine binding sites and a free active centre in the plasmin molecule (Wiman and Collen, 1978b).

Plasminogen activator inhibitor-1

Plasminogen activator inhibitor-1 (PAI-1) is a fast-acting inhibitor of t-PA and urokinase (Kruithof *et al.*, 1984) occurring at very low concentration in the blood, but which may be significantly increased in several disease states including venous thromboembolism and ischaemic heart disease. It is a serpin, composed of 379 amino acids with Arg^{364}-Met^{347} as the reactive site (Bachmann, 1987).

1.2 Mechanism of fibrin-specific thrombolysis

Plasmin, the proteolytic enzyme of the fibrinolytic system has a low substrate specificity. In purified systems it will degrade fibrinogen almost as well as fibrin, and, when circulating freely in the blood, it will degrade a number of plasma proteins including fibrinogen and the blood coagulation factors V and VIII. Plasmin generated in blood will, however, be rapidly neutralized by α_2-antiplasmin via interaction with both its lysine-binding sites and its active centre. Extensive systemic activation of the fibrinolytic system will result in α_2-antiplasmin consumption, excess free plasmin generation and secondary haemostatic breakdown. In contrast, plasmin that is generated at the fibrin surface has both its lysine-binding sites and active centre occupied and thus is only very slowly inactivated by α_2-antiplasmin (Collen, 1980).

Clot-specific thrombolysis will, in view of these interactions, require plasminogen activation at or in the vicinity of the fibrin clot. The two physiological plasminogen activators, t-PA and scu-PA, exert clot-specificity in a plasma environment; however, this is via entirely different molecular mechanisms (Collen, 1987a). t-PA is relatively, but not totally, inactive in the absence of fibrin. It binds specifically to fibrin, thereafter acquiring a high affinity for plasminogen, resulting in preferential plasminogen activation on the fibrin clot.

In a plasma milieu, relatively fibrin-specific clot lysis can be obtained within a rather narrow concentration range with scu-PA. In the absence of fibrin, no significant plasminogen activation occurs. Apparently, plasma exerts a competitive inhibitory effect, which is reversed by fibrin (Collen, 1987a). In addition, fibrin-bound plasminogen may be more sensitive to activation by scu-PA.

2 Clinical experience with thrombolytic agents

Thrombotic complications of cardiovascular diseases are a main cause of death and disability, and consequently one might assume that thrombolysis could favourably influence the outcome of such life-threatening diseases as myocardial infarction, cerebrovascular thrombosis and venous thromboembolism. The agents used for thrombolytic therapy in man can be classified in two main categories: (i) the "classical" thrombolytic agents, streptokinase and urokinase and (ii) the "second generation" thrombolytic agents presently under clinical investigation, now including t-PA, scu-PA and acylated plasminogen-streptokinase activator complex (Apsac).

Although streptokinase was first administered to man over 30 years ago, it is not yet widely used, mainly as a result of uncertainty about the optimum dose, fear of bleeding complications and a poor correlation between the results of laboratory parameters and the incidence of either therapeutic success or of bleeding complications. Interest in thrombolytic therapy has been renewed by the demonstration that acute myocardial infarction is most frequently caused by thrombotic occlusion of an atherosclerotic coronary artery and that the early administration of streptokinase significantly reduces mortality. The efficacy of streptokinase is, however, limited and rapidly decreases with time after the onset of coronary artery thrombosis. In addition, it has no fibrin-selectivity and its use is associated with extensive breakdown of the haemostatic system; yet the occurrence of life-threatening bleeding in association with high-dose short-duration therapy is consistently less than 1%.

A better understanding of the molecular mechanisms that regulate fibrinolysis *in vivo*, the identification of the physiological activators t-PA and scu-PA with higher degrees of fibrin-selectivity, and the development of recombinant DNA technology that allows large-scale production of these proteins, have fuelled the hope that newer and better thrombolytic drugs might become available. One of these new generation thrombolytic agents, t-PA, has now been studied in over 4000 patients. These studies have indicated that it is more efficacious, more fibrin-specific, and when used in adequate dose, at least as safe as streptokinase. Important issues such as its impact on morbidity and mortality and its cost–benefit ratio remain to be resolved. The physiological plasminogen activators t-PA and scu-PA, however, still suffer shortcomings, including the need for large doses to be therapeutically efficient, a limited fibrin-specificity and residual toxicity in terms of bleeding complications. Consequently, research into the development of still further improved therapeutic regimes or thrombolytic agents is intensifying. Recent progress in this area will be reviewed below.

3 New trends in research on thrombolytic therapy

Present research in this area is carried out along several lines. In addition to the studies described below, several groups have reported *in vitro* data on synergism of thrombolytic agents, mutants of t-PA or scu-PA, and hybrids of t-PA and scu-PA at the recent Congress of the International Society on Thrombosis and Haemostasis, Brussels, Belgium, 6–10 July 1987, with abstracts published in *Thrombosis and Haemostasis*, Vol. 58, No. 1 (1987).

3.1 Synergism between thrombolytic agents

Because the mechanisms that regulate the fibrin-specificity of t-PA and scu-PA are different, combined infusions of both agents might act synergistically, to produce enhanced efficacy with reduced side-effects on the haemostatic system. In an *in vitro* system, composed of a [^{125}I]fibrin-labelled plasma clot, immersed in citrated plasma, t-PA, scu-PA and urokinase in molar ratios between 4 : 1 and 1 : 4, do not display significant synergism (Collen *et al.*, 1986a; Lijnen *et al.*, 1986b; Gurewich and Pannell, 1987). *In vivo*, however, in a jugular vein thrombosis model in the rabbit, significant synergism between t-PA and scu-PA and between t-PA and urokinase for thrombolysis was observed (Collen *et al.*, 1986b). When t-PA and scu-PA were infused in a molar ratio of approximately 1 : 3, the specific thrombolytic activity of the mixture was approximately three times higher than was anticipated on the basis of additive effects of both agents. The synergistic effect of t-PA and urokinase was only of borderline significance. A synergistic effect of at least a factor of 2 between t-PA and scu-PA was also found on coronary arterial thrombolysis in dogs (Ziskind *et al.*, 1987).

Preliminary results in patients with acute myocardial infarction (Collen *et al.*, 1986c; Collen and Van de Werf, 1987) suggest that t-PA and scu-PA and t-PA and urokinase also act synergistically in man. Indeed, combination of t-PA and scu-PA at approximately one-fifth of their individual thrombolytic doses produced coronary artery reperfusion in patients with acute myocardial infarction without associated systemic fibrinogen breakdown. Although these results are still preliminary and need to be confirmed in larger studies, they are potentially of significant clinical importance. The synergistic effect of t-PA and urokinase on coronary reperfusion has, however, not been confirmed in a large-scale study, although the use of the combination was associated with a significant reduction of the frequency of reocclusion (Topol *et al.*, 1987).

3.2 Mutants of tissue-type plasminogen activator

Mutants of t-PA, which have a higher fibrin-affinity, a longer *in vivo* half-life or an improved fibrin-specificity may constitute potentially useful thrombolytic agents. Deletion mutants of t-PA with a more than five-fold prolonged half-life in rats have recently been described (Larsen *et al.*, 1987). The thrombolytic and pharmacokinetic properties of one of these variants were studied in a canine model of coronary artery thrombosis. The deletion mutant had a markedly slower clearance rate from plasma than intact t-PA, which rendered it more potent than natural t-PA after bolus injection (Cambier *et al.*, 1987).

3.3 Mutants of single-chain urokinase-type plasminogen activator

Scu-PA differs markedly from urokinase with respect to fibrin-specific thrombolytic properties, and site-directed mutagenesis of scu-PA at the cleavage site might therefore yield a more stable molecule. Recently, mutants of scu-PA were constructed and characterized in which Lys^{158} was substituted with Gly or with Glu (Nelles *et al.*, 1987a). Although these non-convertible mutants still activate plasminogen, the specific thrombolytic effect of the Gly mutant *in vivo* is approximately 10 times lower than that of natural scu-PA (Collen, 1987b). A low-molecular-weight form of scu-PA with Leu^{144} in the amino terminal position was found to be functionally indistinguishable from intact scu-PA (Stump *et al.*, 1986, 1987). This scu-PA may therefore be preferable to intact scu-PA for large-scale production by recombinant DNA technology.

3.4 Hybrid plasminogen activators

On the basis of the hypothesis that the fibrin-selectivities of t-PA and scu-PA are localized in different structural domains, a hybrid or chimeric molecule was recently produced, consisting of amino acids Ser^{1} through Thr^{263} of t-PA fused to amino acids Leu^{144} through Leu^{411} of scu-PA (Nelles *et al.*, 1987b). This hybrid has both the fibrin-affinity of t-PA and the enzymatic properties of scu-PA. In preliminary studies in animal models of thrombosis, it proved to be comparable but not superior to scu-PA (Collen, 1987b). Whether other chimeras developed on the basis of these concepts may constitute improved thrombolytic agents remains to be determined.

3.5 Antibody-targeted thrombolytic therapy

Several alternatives for targetting the action of thrombolytic agents towards the thrombus with the use of fibrin-specific antibodies are presently being investigated. These include chemical conjugates of fibrin-specific antibodies with streptokinase (Ito *et al.*, 1985), urokinase (Bode *et al.*, 1985) or t-PA (Runge *et al.*, 1986), or recombinant fusion proteins comprising a fibrin-specific antibody site and the B-chain of t-PA (Schnee *et al.*, 1987). Alternatively, chemical conjugates between a fibrin-specific and a t-PA-specific antibody (Bode *et al.*, 1987), and biosynthetically produced heteroduplex antibodies that are both fibrin- and t-PA-specific (Haber *et al.*, 1987), could bind to fibrin and localize endogenous or exogenous t-PA. These conjugates display significantly enhanced clot-specific lysis *in vitro* and, in an animal model, *in vivo* (Runge *et al.*, 1987).

4 Conclusions

Thrombolytic therapy, despite a 30 year period of relatively slow development, will probably become routine therapy for early acute myocardial infarction and possibly for other thrombotic cardiovascular diseases. Further improvements of thrombolytic agents to maximize efficacy, minimize side effects and optimize cost–benefit ratios are needed. It is anticipated that such improvements will emerge from several of the new lines of ongoing preclinical and clinical research.

References

Bachmann, F. (1987). In *Thrombosis and Haemostasis 1987* (ed M. Verstraete, J. Vermylen, R. Lijnen and J. Arnout), pp. 227–265. Leuven University Press, Leuven, Belgium.

Bode, C., Matsueda, G., Hui, K. and Haber, E. (1985). Antibody-directed urokinase: a specific fibrinolytic agent. *Science* **229**, 765–767.

Bode, C., Runge, M. S., Matsueda, G. R., Gold, H. K. and Haber, E. (1987). Can intrinsic tissue type plasminogen activator be concentrated at the site of a thrombus? *J. Am. Coll. Cardiol.* **9**, 81A.

Cambier, P., Van de Werf, F., Larsen, G. R. and Collen, D. (1987). *J. Cardiovasc. Pharmacol.* (in press).

Collen, D. (1980). On the regulation and control of thrombolysis. Edward Kowalski Memorial Lecture. *Thromb. Haemost.* **43**, 77–89.

Collen, D. (1987a). Molecular mechanisms of fibrinolysins and their application to fibrin-specific thrombolytic therapy. *J. Cell. Biochem.* **33**, 77–94.

Collen, D. (1987b). Synergism, mutants and hybrids of tissue-type plasminogen activator (t-PA) and single chain urokinase-type plasminogen activator (scu-PA): potential for thrombolytic therapy. *Thromb. Haemost.* **58**, 254 (Abstract 926).

Collen, D. and Lijnen, H. R. (1986). The fibrinolytic system in man. *CRC Crit. Rev. Hemat. Oncol.* **4**, 249–301.

Collen, D. and Van de Werf, F. (1987). Coronary artery thrombolysis with low-dose synergistic combinations of recombinant tissue-type plasminogen activator (rt-PA) and recombinant single-chain urokinase-type plasminogen activator (rscu-PA) for acute myocardial infarction. *Am. J. Cardiol.* **60**, 431–434.

Collen, D., De Cock, F., Demarsin, E., Lijnen, H. R. and Stump, D. C. (1986a). Absence of synergism between tissue-type plasminogen activator (t-PA), single-chain urokinase-type plasminogen activator (scu-PA) and urokinase on clot lysis in a plasma milieu *in vitro*. *Thromb. Haemost.* **56**, 35–39.

Collen, D., Stassen, J. M., Stump, D. C. and Verstraete, M. (1986b). Synergism of thrombolytic agents *in vivo*. *Circulation* **74**, 838–842.

Collen, D., Stump, D. C. and Van de Werf, F. (1986c). Coronary thrombolysis in patients with acute myocardial infarction by intravenous infusion of synergic thrombolytic agents. *Am. Heart J.* **112**, 1083–1084.

Gurewich, V. and Pannell, R. (1987). Synergism of tissue-type plasminogen activator (t-PA) and single-chain urokinase-type plasminogen activator (scu-PA) on clot lysis *in vitro* and a mechanism for this effect (letter). *Thromb. Haemost.* **57**, 372.

Haber, E., Runge, M., Bode, C., Branscomb, B., Schnee, J., Quertermous, T. and Matsueda, G. (1987). Antibody targetted fibrinolysis. *Thromb. Haemost.* **57**, 253.

Holmes, W. E., Pennica, D., Blaber, M., Rey, M. W., Guenzler, W. A., Steffens, G. J. and Heyneker, H. L. (1985). Cloning and expression of the gene for pro-urokinase in *E. coli*. *Biotechnology* **3**, 923–929.

Holmes, W. E., Nelles, L., Lijnen, H. R. and Collen, D. (1987). Primary structure of human α_2-antiplasmin, a serine protease inhibitor (serpin). *J. Biol. Chem.* **262**, 1659–1664.

Hoylaerts, M., Rijken, D. C., Lijnen, H. R. and Collen, D. (1982). Kinetics of the activation of plasminogen by human tissue plasminogen activator. Role of fibrin. *J. Biol. Chem.* **257**, 2912–2919.

Ito, R. K., David, G. L., Howanish, A. and Yunes, E. J. (1985). Development of a thrombolytic agent using a human fibrin-specific monoclonal antibody as a conjugate-carrier for streptokinase. *Circulation* **72**, 111–192.

Kosow, D. P. (1975). Kinetic mechanism of the activation of human plasminogen by streptokinase. *Biochemistry* **14**, 4459–4465.

Kruithof, E. K. O., Tran-Thang, C., Ransijn, A. and Bachmann, F. (1984). Demonstration of a fast-acting inhibitor of plasminogen activator in human plasma. *Blood* **64**, 907–913.

Larsen, G. R., Metzger, M., Blue, Y. and Henderson, K. (1987). Pharmacokinetics of genetically modified t-PA in rat. *Thromb. Haemost.* **57**, 491 (Abstract 1815).

Lijnen, H. R., Van Hoef, B. and Collen, D. (1986a). Comparative kinetic analysis of the activation of human plasminogen by natural and recombinant-single-chain urokinase-type plasminogen activator. *Biochim. Biophys. Acta* **884**, 402–408.

Lijnen, H. R., Zamarron, C., Blaber, M., Winkler, M. E. and Collen, D. (1986b). Activation of plasminogen by pro-urokinase I. Mechanism. *J. Biol. Chem.* **261**, 1253–1258.

Nelles, L., Lijnen, H. R., Collen, D. and Holmes, W. E. (1987a). Characterization of a fusion protein consisting of amino acids 1 to 263 of tissue-type plasminogen activator and amino acids 144 to 411 of urokinase-type plasminogen activator. *J. Biol. Chem.* **262**, 5682–5689.

Nelles, L., Lijnen, H. R., Collen, D. and Holmes, W. E. (1987b). Characterization of recombinant human single chain urokinase-type plasminogen activator mutants produced by site-specific mutagenesis of lysine 158. *J. Biol. Chem.* **262**, 10855–10862.

Pennica, D., Holmes, W. E., Kohr, W. J., Harkins, R. N., Vehar, G. A., Ward, C. A., Bennett, W. F., Yelverton, E., Seeburg, P. H., Heyneker, H. L., Goeddel, D. V. and Collen, D. (1983). Cloning and expression of human tissue-type plasminogen activator cDNA in *E. coli*. *Nature* **301**, 214–221.

Runge, M. S., Bode, C., Matsueda, G. R. and Haber, E. (1986). Tissue-type plasminogen activator-antifibrin monoclonal antibody conjugate enhances clot lysis in plasma. *Circulation* **74**, II-246.

Runge, M. S., Bode, C., Matsueda, G. R. and Haber, E. (1987). *Proc. Natl Acad. Sci. USA* (in press).

Schnee, J., Runge, M., Matsueda, G., Hudson, N., Seidman, J., Haber, E. and Quertermous, T. (1987). *Proc. Natl Acad. Sci. USA* (in press).

Stump, D. C., Lijnen, H. R. and Collen, D. (1986). Purification and characterization of a novel low molecular weight form of single-chain urokinase-type plasminogen activator. *J. Biol. Chem.* **261**, 17120–17126.

Stump, D. C., Stassen, J. M., Demarsin, E. and Collen, D. (1987). Comparative thrombolytic properties of single-chain forms of urokinase-type plasminogen activator. *Blood* **69**, 592–596.

Topol, E. J., Califf, R. M., O'Neill, W. W., George, B. S., Kereiakis, D. J., Pinkerton, C. A., Candela, R. J., Abbottsmith, C. W., Rothbaum, D. and Stack, R. S. (1987). Synergism of tissue-type and urokinase plasminogen activators for acute myocardial infarction: results of the multicenter TAMI-2 Trial. *Circulation* **76**, IV-307 (Abstract 1219).

White, W. F., Barlow, G. H. and Mozen, M. M. (1966). The isolation and characterization of plasminogen activators (urokinase) from human urine. *Biochemistry* **5**, 2160–2169.

Wiman, B. and Collen, D. (1978a). Molecular mechanism of physiological fibrinolysis. *Nature* **272**, 549–550.

Wiman, B. and Collen, D. (1978b). On the kinetics of the reaction between human antiplasmin and plasmin. *Eur. J. Biochem.* **84**, 573–578.

Ziskind, A. A., Gold, H. K., Yasuda, T., Kanke, M., Guererro, J. L., Fallon, J. T. and Collen, D. (1987). Coronary thrombolysis in dogs with synergistic combinations of human tissue-type plasminogen activator t-PA and single chain urokinase-type plasminogen activator scu-PA. *Clin. Res.* **35**, 337A.

13

Long-Term Follow-Up After Coronary Thrombolysis: The Edinburgh Experience

D. P. de BONO, D. McAREAVEY, M. BEEN and H. PETERSON

Cardiac Department, Royal Infirmary, Edinburgh, UK

1 Introduction

Coronary thrombolysis was first attempted clinically in 1958 (Fletcher *et al.*, 1958) and was the subject of numerous small-scale trials over the next twenty years. Since 1979 there has been increasing evidence that early thrombolytic therapy after myocardial infarction reduces mortality (GISSI study group, 1986; ISIS study group, 1987), improves left ventricular function and reduces infarct size (Serruys *et al.*, 1983). The major benefit is obtained in patients with first anterior myocardial infarcts treated as soon as possible, and certainly within six hours after the onset of symptoms. Questions that remain to be answered include the role of supplementary therapy such as heparin, warfarin, antiplatelet agents and thromboxane antagonists, and the need for and optimal timing of interventions such as coronary angioplasty or coronary artery grafting. The definitive answers will only be given by appropriately designed controlled trials, but careful natural history and follow-up studies can give useful clues to the best design for future trials.

Coronary thrombolysis for acute myocardial infarction started in Edinburgh at the beginning of 1982, and the cumulative treatment rate is shown in Fig. 1. This study is based on the follow-up of the cohort of patients treated before 31 December 1985, who have been followed up for a minimum of 23 and a maximum of 59 months.

HYPERLIPIDAEMIA AND ATHEROSCLEROSIS
ISBN 0.12.675645-7

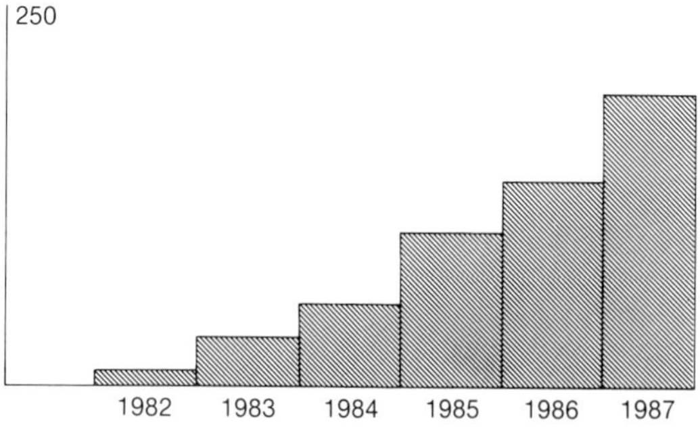

Fig. 1 Thrombolysis in RIE: cumulative total.

2 Patients and methods

One hundred and thirteen patients were treated during the study period. Complete follow-up to 30 November 1987 was available for 100 patients: 91 by clinic attendance, and 9 by postal or telephone enquiry. Follow-up data were incomplete in 13 patients, usually because the patient had moved away from Edinburgh. There were 92 male and 21 female patients; the mean age of male patients was 54.6 years and that of female patients 57.2 years. 100 patients had no previous history of infarction. The distribution of the site of infarction is shown in Fig. 2. Time lag between the onset of symptoms and the start of thrombolytic therapy is shown in Fig. 3—the median delay was 2.6 hours. Fifty-five patients (49%) gave a history of smoking.

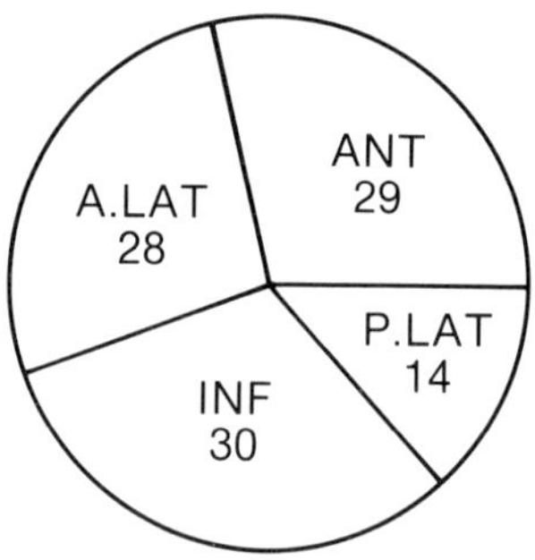

Fig. 2 Site of infarct.

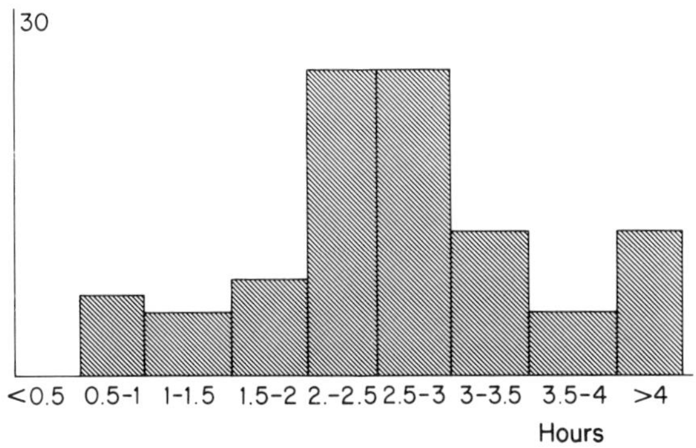

Fig. 3 Length of time to treatment.

2.1 *Treatment*

One hundred of the patients were treated with acylated plasminogen-streptokinase complex (BRL 26921, APSAC, Eminase, Beecham Research Laboratories) (Been *et al.*, 1985, 1986), the remainder with streptokinase (Kabikinase, Kabi-Vitrum). Thrombolytic therapy was given by the intracoronary route in 37 patients and intravenously in 75. The modal dose of APSAC was 30 mg and that of streptokinase 1 500 000 units. Thrombolytic therapy was monitored by measuring fibrinogen concentration, euglobulin lysis time, reptilase time, prothrombin time and thrombin clotting time. Heparin therapy was instituted 6–12 hours after the start of thrombolytic therapy and controlled by the thrombin clotting time. Warfarin was started on day 2 or day 3 and heparin was discontinued when the prothrombin time ratio (corrected INR) was >2. Warfarin was continued for one year (in subsequent cohorts we have discontinued warfarin earlier). In patients for whom warfarin therapy was deemed inadvisable, aspirin 300 mg/day plus dipyridamole (Persantin, Boehringer Ingelheim) 100 mg thrice daily was used instead. Anticoagulant or antiplatelet therapy was not continued if there was evidence *either* that the infarct-related coronary artery was not patent *or* if there had been a definite reinfarction. At the time of discharge, 74 patients were on warfarin, 17 on aspirin + Persantin, and 14 on neither (Fig. 4). Thirty-seven patients had coronary arteriography before treatment, and 82 had subsequent coronary arteriography during the same hospital admission as part of a clinical trial protocol. The results of these angiographic studies have been reported elsewhere (Been *et al.*, 1985, 1986).

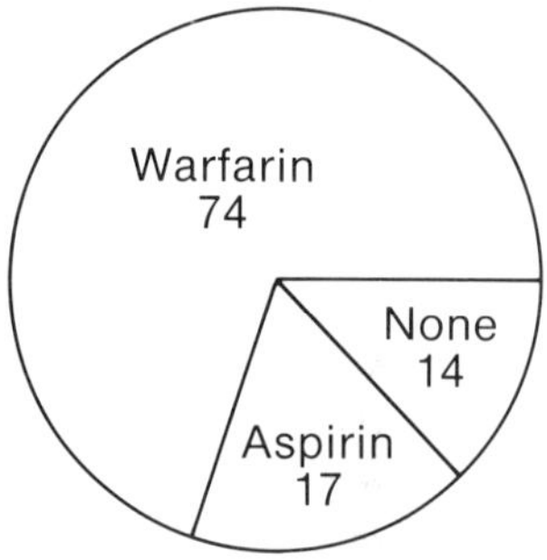

Fig. 4 Anticoagulants at discharge.

3 Results

One hundred and five patients were alive at the time of hospital discharge (in-hospital mortality 7.1%). Ninety-eight patients were alive at 1 year (6 known late deaths and 1 lost to follow-up: a "worst case" one year mortality of 13.3%). Ninety-five patients were known to be alive at 23 months (7 late deaths and 3 lost to follow-up). Of 8 patients who died in hospital, 4 are known to have had angiographic evidence of persisting coronary occlusion, 1 died of papillary muscle rupture and 1 of ventricular rupture with patent coronary arteries, and 2 deaths were possibly related to reinfarction (Table 1).

Table 1 Causes of death after thrombolysis.

Patient	Reperfusion	Reinfarction	Mode of death
In hospital:			
DF	Yes	Possible	Cardiogenic shock
LD	Yes	No	Cardiac rupture
FD	No	No	Cardiogenic shock
ML	No	No	Cardiogenic shock
MMcK	No	No	Cardiogenic shock
HT	No	No	Cardiogenic shock
AG	Yes	No	Pap. muscle rupture
AS	Yes	Possible	Sudden death
Late deaths:			
DF	No	No	Sudden death
AF	Yes	Possible	VF arrest
RF	No	No	Sudden death
GS	No	No	Sudden death
CC	Yes	Possible	Sudden death
JM	Yes	Possible	Sudden death

All of the 7 late deaths were "sudden deaths"; 3 occurred in patients with angiographic evidence of reperfusion failure, the other 4 may or may not have been related to reocclusion.

3.1 Complications

Sixteen patients had bleeding complications, which were "serious" in three patients—two intracerebral bleeds and one major haematemesis. One of the patients with a cerebral bleed had had a head injury at the time of infarction, and the patient with a haematemesis had a stomal ulcer on a gastroenterostomy performed many years before for peptic ulceration. No deaths resulted from bleeding.

Reinfarction (defined as recurrent chest pain, ECG changes and a rise in cardiac enzymes) occurred in 18 patients. Nine cases of reinfarction occurred prior to hospital discharge, the remainder during the first year after treatment. The time distribution of reinfarction is shown in Fig. 5. Two patients had further infarcts after 12 months, but these were in different sites to the original infarct. None of the patients who had definite reinfarction according to this definition died, but reinfarction may have contributed to two of the deaths prior to hospital discharge, and to four of the late deaths. In 7 of the 9 patients who reinfarcted while in hospital, anticoagulation had been deliberately or accidentally discontinued. Four of the nine patients who had out-of-hospital reinfarction in the first year had been prescribed anticoagulants, five had not.

3.2 Intervention

Twenty-six patients (25% of those who were alive at the time of hospital discharge) had an intervention aimed at improving myocardial perfusion. The

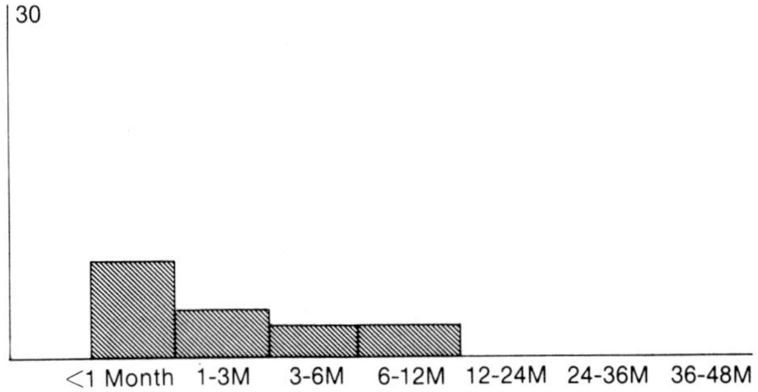

Fig. 5 Time to reinfarction.

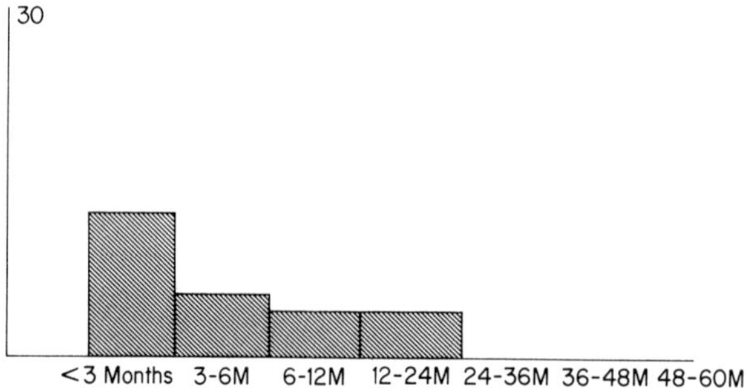

Fig. 6 Time to intervention (PTCA/CAVG).

time distribution of intervention is shown in Fig. 6: half of the interventions were within 3 months of infarction. The most common indication for intervention was persistent post-infarct angina—the prevalence of angina at follow-up clinic attendances is shown in Fig. 7. Intervention took the form of percutaneous coronary angioplasty in 13 patients, coronary bypass grafting in the rest.

4 Discussion

On the basis of our early clinical experiences, we developed a policy for coronary thrombolysis that has in its essentials stood the test of time:

(i) early intravenous thrombolysis;
(ii) follow-up anticoagulation;
(iii) further intervention as indicated for unstable or exercise related angina.

This policy has to be set in the context of other trials and studies.

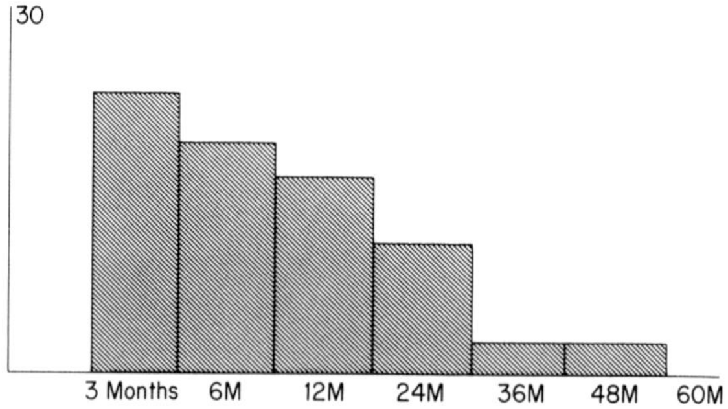

Fig. 7 Post-infarct angina.

4.1 Early intravenous thrombolysis

The GISSI study (1986) conducted in over 10 000 patients has shown a clear-cut reduction in mortality in patients randomized to intravenous thrombolysis with streptokinase compared with controls. The major mortality reduction was seen in patients with first anterior infarcts treated within six hours of the onset of symptoms. The Netherlands Interuniversity Institute Study (Simoons *et al.*, 1986) was too small to show an effect on mortality, but showed a highly significant difference in left ventricular function and infarct size in patients treated with thrombolytic therapy. The ISAM study (1986) showed a trend towards improved survival that did not reach conventional levels of statistical significance; however, in this study the mortality rate in both treated and placebo groups was very low. A preliminary report on the ISIS 2 study comparing intravenous streptokinase with placebo also indicates a significant mortality reduction in the subgroup of patients treated within four hours (ISIS Study Group, 1987). The AIMS study using intravenous APSAC compared with placebo has recently reported a reduction in mortality of over 40% (confidence limits 21–65%) in patients receiving thrombolytic treatment (AIMS Study Group, 1988). It seems that the case for early intravenous thrombolytic therapy has been convincingly established and further placebo-controlled studies are unlikely to be started.

The question of the best drug for thrombolysis is still open. In terms of coronary patency, tissue plasminogen activator (r-TPA) has been shown to be more effective than the "standard" 1 500 000 unit dose of streptokinase (TIMI Study Group, 1985; Verstraete *et al.*, 1985), but attempting to confirm this benefit in terms of improved survival would require a trial of some 10 000 patients. Similarly, although the mortality reduction in the AIMS study using APSAC is impressive, it would be wrong to infer that APSAC was necessarily more effective than streptokinase until the two had been compared directly, and adequate data on this are still lacking.

4.2 Anticoagulation

There is no consensus on the optimal nature of, or indeed the need for, anticoagulation after thrombolysis. Our own experiences and those of Merx and colleagues (1981) would seem to emphasize the need for at least a short period of anticoagulation to reduce the risk of early reocclusion, and in our experience aspirin has been less effective than heparin/warfarin. On the other hand, only 20% of patients in the GISSI study were anticoagulated, and although there was a clear excess of reinfarction in the streptokinase-treated group, it was difficult to correlate this with anticoagulant status. White *et al.*

(1987) have recently described a series of patients treated with intravenous streptokinase followed by heparin for 48 hours with a very low reinfarction rate. Two factors need to be taken into account in interpreting these results, and in designing definitive studies to evaluate the role of anticoagulants. These are that *symptomatic* coronary reocclusion is much more apparent if there is a large area of myocardium at risk, i.e. in patients who have received early and effective thrombolysis, and that late reinfarction (more than two weeks) has in our experience a relatively low mortality, possibly because of myocardial conditioning and/or the establishment of a collateral circulation.

4.3 Intervention

About 70% of patients in whom coronary patency is successfully restored after thrombolysis have a residual coronary stenosis, and in 30% this is severe (Serruys *et al.*, 1983). A severe residual stenosis is one of the risk factors for reocclusion (Harrison *et al.*, 1984), so there has been considerable interest in the possibility of combining thrombolytic therapy with some other intervention, for example, percutaneous coronary angioplasty. The most logical, though not necessarily the most convenient, time to do angioplasty is immediately after restoring coronary patency. Two trials have now compared "immediate" percutaneous coronary angioplasty with "delayed elective" percutaneous coronary angioplasty (the TAMI study) and with a conservative policy of intervention only as required (The European Cooperative Study Group study). In the TAMI study (Topol *et al.*, 1987) there was no benefit of "immediate" over "delayed elective" angioplasty, although a number of patients randomized to elective angioplasty actually had emergency angioplasty because of the recurrence of pain before the elective procedure had been performed. In the European study (Simoons *et al.*, 1988) the trial was discontinued when it became apparent that immediate angioplasty conveyed no benefit in terms of survival, left ventricular function or infarct size, and might even be deleterious.

The question of whether elective delayed angioplasty has advantages over "angioplasty only for symptoms" is being addressed by a number of trials (APSAC-SWIFT in the UK, TIMI II in the United States), but results are not yet available. At present, the pragmatic (and cheaper) policy of angioplasty only as required seems to have many attractions. Despite the conservative attitude we adopted towards "revascularization", the relatively low incidence of clinically significant reinfarction indicates that large-scale trials will be needed to evaluate any potential benefit. Review of the coronary angiograms of the 14 patients who died within the first year indicated that only 3 would have been suited to a revascularization procedure. The patients who would seem to have most to gain from revascularization are probably those with multivessel disease, or with a single severe stenosis in a vessel supplying a substantial area of myocardium. In our experience it is precisely these patients who exhibit post-thrombolysis angina. In considering the cost of thrombolysis, it is appropriate to include the cost of extra procedures such as angioplasty or coronary grafting in up to 25% of patients. However, it should be borne in mind that in our unit 12% of patients in this age group who have infarcts *not* treated with thrombolytic therapy also require a "surgical" procedure within the next 12 months.

References

AIMS Trial Study Group (1988). Effect of intravenous APSAC on mortality after acute myocardial infarction: preliminary report of a placebo controlled trial. *Lancet* **i**, (in press).

Been, M., de Bono, D. P., Muir, A. L., Boulton, F. E., Hillis, W. S. and Hornung, R. (1985). Coronary thrombolysis with intravenous anisoylated plasminogen–streptokinase complex BRL 26921. *Br. Heart J.* **53**, 253–259.

Been, M., de Bono, D. P., Muir, A. L., Boulton, F. E., Fears, R., Standring, R. and Ferres, M. (1986). Clinical and kinetic properties of intravenous APSAC-anisoylated plasminogen streptokinase complex (BRL 26921) in acute myocardial infarction. *Int. J. Cardiol.* **11**, 53–61.

Fletcher, A. P., Alkjaersig, N., Smyrniotis, F. E. and Sherry, S. (1958). The treatment of patients suffering from early myocardial infarction with massive and prolonged streptokinase therapy. *Trans. Assoc. Am. Phys.* **71**, 287–295.

Gruppo Italiano per lo Studio della Streptochinasi nell 'Infarto Miocardico (GISSI). (1986). Effectiveness of intravenous thrombolytic treatment in acute myocardial infarction. *Lancet* **i**, 397–401.

Harrison, D. G., Ferguson, D. W., Collins, S. M., Skorton, D. J., Ericksen, E. E., Kioschos, J. M., Marcus, M. L. and White, C. W. (1984). Rethrombosis after reperfusion with streptokinase: importance of geometry of residual lesions. *Circulation* **69**, 991–999.

The ISAM Study Group. (1986). A prospective trial of intravenous streptokinase in acute myocardial infarction (ISAM). *N. Engl. J. Med* **314**, 1465–1471. ISIS Steering Committee. (1987). Intravenous streptokinase given within 0–4 hours of onset of myocardial infarction reduces mortality in ISIS-2. *Lancet* **i**, 502.

Merx, W., Dorr, R., Rentrop, P., Blanke, H., Karsch, K. R., Mathey, D. G. Kremer, P., Rutsch, W. and Schmutzler, H. (1981). Evaluation of the effectiveness of intracoronary streptokinase infusion in acute myocardial infarction: postprocedure management and hospital course in 204 patients. *Am. Heart J.* **102**, 1181–1187.

Serruys, P. W., Wijns, W., van den Brand, M., Ribeiro, V., Fioretti, P., Simoons, M. L., Kooijman, C. J., Reiber, J. H. and Hugenholtz, P. G. (1983). Is transluminal coronary angioplasty mandatory after successful thrombolysis? *Br. Heart J.* **50**, 257–265.

Simoons, M. L., Serruys, P. W., van den Brand, M., Res, J., Verheugt, F. W., Krauss, X. H., Remme, W. J., Bar, F., de Zwoan, C., van der Laarse, A., *et al.* (1986). Early thrombolysis in acute myocardial infarction: limitation of infarct size and improved survival. *J. Am. Coll. Cardiol.* **7**, 717–728.

Simoons, M. L., Arnold, A. E. R., Betriu, A. *et al.* (1988). Thrombolysis with rt-PA in acute myocardial infarction: no additional benefit of immediate PTCA L. *Lancet* **i**, (in press).

The TIMI Study Group. (1985). The Thrombolysis in Myocardial Infarction (TIMI) study. *N. Engl. J. Med.* **312**, 932–936.

Topol, E. J., Coliff, R. M., George, B. S., Kereiakes, D. J., Abbottsmith, C. W., Candela, R. J., Lee, K. L., Pitt, B., Stack, R. S. and O'Neill, W. W. and the TAMI study group (1987). A randomized trial of immediate versus delayed elective angioplasty after intravenous tissue plasminogen activator in acute myocardial infarction. *N. Engl. J. Med.* **317**, 581–588.

Verstraete, M., Bernard, R., Bory, M., Brower, R. W., Collen, D., de Bono, D. P., Erbel, R., Huhmann, W., Lennane, R. J., Lubsen, J. *et al.* (1985). Randomized trial of intravenous recombinant tissue type plasminogen activator versus intravenous streptokinase in acute myocardial infarction. *Lancet* **i**, 842–847.

White, H. D., Norris, R. M., Brown, M. A., Takayama, M., Marlowski, A., Bass, N. M., Ormiston, J. A. and Whitlock, T. (1987). Effect of intravenous streptokinase on left ventricular function and early survival after myocardial infarction. *N. Engl. J. Med.* **317**, 850–855.

Appendix: Abstracts of Posters

Binding of Apo-Rich HDL Particles by Saturable Sites on Human Blood Platelets Impairs their Responsiveness to Exogenous Agonists.

Kalpna Desai and James S. Owen. *Academic Department of Medicine, Royal Free Hospital School of Medicine, Rowland Hill Street, London NW3 2PF, UK*

Studies in both platelet-rich plasma and in washed platelets have established that physiological concentrations of LDL sensitize platelets[1]. In contrast, conflicting effects of HDL have been found: agonist-induced platelet aggregation is reported to be stimulated, unaffected or inhibited by the presence of isolated HDL (d = 1.063–1.21 g/ml). We have hypothesized that opposing effects of individual HDL subclasses on platelet aggregability may explain these inconsistencies.

Physiological concentrations of HDL_3 (0.8–1.15 mg of protein/ml) had little effect on ADP-induced aggregation of washed platelet suspensions. At 2–3 times above normal levels they sensitized the platelets, increasing aggregation from 45–50% to 60–70%. Normal concentrations of HDL_2 (0.2–0.4 mg of protein/ml) inhibited aggregation by ADP; further subfractionation by heparin–Sepharose affinity chromatography established that the inhibitory effect was largely confined to the particles rich in apoE, termed HDL-E. We conclude that platelet responsiveness in the presence of whole HDL may reflect the relative concentrations of the individual sub-classes in the particular sample[2].

Washed platelets were found to bind radio-iodinated HDL-E. When computer-assisted non-linear curve-fitting analysis was applied to the total binding curve a uniform class of saturable sites was identified; these numbered approximately 2400 per platelet. The binding process was rapid, reaching equilibrium within 15 min at room temperature, and was insensitive to divalent ions. Competition studies showed that modifying HDL-E arginine and lysine residues by cyclohexanedione treatment and by carbamylation respectively abolished the ability of the particles to compete with native HDL-E for binding sites on the platelets. This finding suggests that such positively charged amino acid residues within HDL-E apolipoproteins may be functionally significant for recognition of the lipoprotein particle by the platelet binding site.

Binding of HDL-E by platelets, and its anti-aggregatory action described above, showed a similar rapidity and occurred within the same concentration range. Furthermore, both processes were independent of the presence of calcium ions and were impaired by chemical modification of the apolipoprotein constituents of HDL-E. We therefore conclude that occupation of cell-surface receptors by HDL-E particles impairs platelet responsiveness to exogenous agonists; whether these receptors recognise apoE, or apoA-I or apoA-II, the other major apolipoproteins of HDL-E, remains to be established.

[1] Hassall, D. G., Owen, J. S. and Bruckdorfer, K. R. (1983). *Biochem. J.* **216**, 43–49.
[2] Desai, K., Owen, J. S., Wilson, D. T. and Hutton, R. A. (1986). *Thromb. Haemost.* **55**, 173–177.

Diet-Induced Changes in Rat LDL Binding Sites on Rat Liver Membrane Preparations.

Mukul Rawat and L. M. Srivastava. *Department of Biochemistry, All India Institute of Medical Sciences, New Delhi-110029, India*

Hepatic low density lipoprotein receptor or apoBE receptor is significantly involved in the modulation of lipoprotein metabolism in most animal species studied [1,2]. Epidemiological and experimental studies have established the correlation of dietary factors with lipoprotein metabolism. However, very few studies have been performed to evaluate the effect of dietary factors such as fat, carbohydrate and protein on the receptor[3,4].

We have studied the effect of high carbohydrate (CHO), high protein (PRO) and high fat (FAT) diets on the rat hepatic LDL receptor. Membrane preparations from rat liver were used to study the quantitative and qualitative modulations in the LDL receptor, using radiolabelled rat LDL (rLDL-I^{125}) as ligand and performing receptor-binding assays. The specific binding data were evaluated on a computer program and by graphical method such as Scatchard plot and Rosenthal's plot.

It was observed that high CHO and high FAT diets significantly affected the number of high affinity LDL-I^{125}) binding sites on rat liver plasma membrane preparations (see Table). No qualitative changes were observed. Scatchard analysis of the specific binding data revealed a biphasic curve denoting two affinities.

μg rLDL-I^{125} bound/mg membrane protein
(high affinity binding)

Group	High CHO ($n = 5$)	High FAT ($n = 5$)	High PRO ($n = 5$)	NOR ($n = 5$)
Mean	1.475	0.453	0.954^{NS}	0.804^{NS}
±	±	±	±	±
SD	0.613	0.021	0.641	0.497

High CHO versus High FAT, $p = 0.05$; No other group was significantly different from each other on performing ANOVA.

The results indicate that even unsaturated fat used in the study can affect the receptor in a manner analogous to the saturated fat, though possibly through a slightly different mechanism.

[1] Goldstein, J. L. and Brown, M. S. (1982). *Med. Clin. N. Am.* **66**, 335–362.
[2] Spady, D. K., Stange, E. F., Bilhartz, L. E. and Dietschy, J. M. (1986) *Proc. Natl Acad. Sci. USA* **83**, 1916–1920.

[3] Kovanen, P. T., Bilheimer, D. W. and Goldstein, J. L. *et al.* (1981). *Proc. Natl Acad. Sci. USA* **78**, 1194–1198.
[4] Sirtori, C. R., Galli, G. and Lovati, M. R. *et al.* (1984). *J. Nutr.* **114**, 1493–1500.

A Rapid Screening Assay for Plasma/Serum Cholesterol Ester Transfer/Exchange Protein Activity (CETP).

S. R. Cresswell and D. Ellis. *Smith Kline & French Research Limited, The Frythe, Welwyn, Herts AL6 9AR, UK*

Epidemiological studies have shown that cholesterol carried in LDL is a positive risk factor for atherosclerosis. In man much of this cholesterol is transferred to LDL from HDL via CETP, but there are conflicting views on whether CETP is a positive or negative risk factor for atherosclerosis. In order to study the effects of CETP on plasma lipoprotein profile, a rapid screening assay was needed. The published ultracentrifugational methods were too cumbersome, and so a method based on separation of lipoprotein subfractions by precipitation was developed.

$$\text{HDL. }^{14}\text{C cholesterol oleate} + \text{LDL} \overset{\text{CETP}}{\rightleftharpoons} \text{HDL} + \text{LDL. }^{14}\text{C cholesterol oleate}$$

CETP was added as column fractions or lipoprotein deficient plasma (LPDP), which was prepared by dextran sulphate/$MnCl_2$ precipitation—stored at $-20°C$ for up to 3 months. HDL was radiolabelled in VLDL/LDL-deficient plasma by transfer from a microemulsion of triolein, cholesterol, PC and ^{14}C cholesterol oleate. HDL and LDL were prepared by ultracentrifugation at $\varrho = 1.21$ or 1.063 (Beckman 50.2Ti, 220 000 *g*, 24 or 12 hours respectively) and stored at 4°C, pH 7.4. Lipoprotein fractions and CETP samples were characterized by SDS and native PAGE, cholesterol, cholesterol ester, TG and protein content, as appropriate. Assays contained 50–100 μl LPDP and were carried out at 37°C in 25mM phosphate buffer 2mM DTNB at pH 7.4. Post-incubation separation was achieved by dextran sulphate/$MgCl_2$ precipitation of LDL. Pellets were solubilized in 1 M NaCl and ^{14}C content measured.

Optimization and permissible ranges for the various parameters are described. Assay performance and variability are documented. Time course and applications to column fractions and plasma/serum samples are illustrated.

Human Hepatic Triglyceride Lipase: Molecular Characterization of cDNA and Genomic DNA and mRNA Expression in a Cultured Human Hepatoma Cell Line

Gisela Stahnke[1], Rolf Sprengel[1], Jan Augustin[2] and Hans Will[1]. [1]*Max Planck Institut für Biochemie, 8033 Martinsried/München, FRG;* [2]*Institut für Herzinfarktforschung, Universität Heidelberg, 6900 Heidelberg, FRG*

Human hepatic triglyceride lipase (HTGL) is one of the lipolytic enzymes released into the bloodstream after heparin injection and that is involved in the degradation of triglyceride-rich lipoproteins. However, its precise role in lipid metabolism *in vivo* is not known. *In vitro*, HTGL hydrolyses mono-, di- and triglycerides and phospholipids from artificial substrates and from all plasma lipoproteins. *In vivo*, the enzyme presumably hydrolyses triglycerides of intermediate density lipoproteins (IDL) and phospholipids of high density lipoproteins (HDL), and it may catalyse the conversion of HDL_2 to HDL_3. One familial case of severe HTGL deficiency has been described and appears to lead to lipoprotein abnormalities. As a first step towards a structural and detailed functional analysis of HTGL, we isolated cDNA and genomic DNA of HTGL and studied its expression in a human hepatoma cell line.

By immunoscreening of a human cDNA expression library and by colony hybridization, four cDNA clones of the human triglyceride lipase (HTGL) were isolated which partly overlap and cover the complete coding sequence, including the 3′- and at least part of the 5′-untranslated region. The length of the composite HTGL cDNA (1.7 kb) is consistent in size with that of the mRNA identified in an established human hepatoma cell line. DNA sequence analysis of cDNAs of partially unspliced mRNAs and of cloned genomic DNA indicate that the HTGL coding sequence is split into at least six exons. As predicted from the cDNA, the unprocessed HTGL protein has a molecular weight of 56 kD, three potential glycosylation sites, and a signal peptide of 23 amino acids. Sequence comparison with other lipases including the recently published rat hepatic lipase cDNA (Komaromy and Schotz, *Proc. Natl Acad. Sci. USA* **84**, 1526 (1987)), revealed protein sequence homologies ranging from 30% to 75%. All lipases examined (rat hepatic triglyceride lipase, human lipoprotein lipases, pig pancreatic lipase, rat lingual lipase, human lecithin cholesterol acyltransferase and bovine lipoprotein lipase) share a conserved sequence, which appears to function as the interfacial binding site. From the DNA sequence alone, a region that might represent a lipolytic site common to all lipases could not be deduced. A rather basic sequence at the c-terminus of the predicted HTGL protein sequence is probably involved in heparin binding. The cell culture and sequence data establish that HTGL is a secretory protein with a signal peptide that is produced in the hepatocyte, and that it is synthesized in a permanent cell line of hepatoma origin. Our studies show that HTGL is another member of a lipase gene family that share similar structural and functional domains. The cDNA clones will allow testing for genetic defects in HTGL-deficient patients and for HTGL gene expression in liver diseases, lipoprotein disorders and atherosclerosis.

Transient Hyperlipoproteinemia and Tissue Cholesterol Accumulation in the Developing Chick. A Possible Role of ApoA-I. P. Tarugi, D. Reggiani and S. Calandra. *Istituto di Patologia Generale, Università di Modena, Via Campi 287, 41100 Modena, Italy*

We have previously found that during the embryonic life of the chick, apoA-I mRNA is present only in the liver, while its level in the intestine is relevant only after hatching[1]. Developmental control of apoA-I mRNA level is striking in skeletal muscle, where this mRNA is present at a very high level only a few days after hatching. This high content of apoA-I mRNA occurs during the massive transfer of lipids from the yolk sac to the emerging chick. In this study we investigated the relationship between the developmental changes of apoA-I synthesis and the concomitant changes in plasma lipoproteins and tissue lipids. Plasma and tissue specimens were taken 5 days before (−5) and at 0, 1, 2, 7 and 14 days after hatching. Plasma-free and esterified cholesterol increased from −5 to day 1, but decreased afterwards; in contrast, plasma triglycerides showed a continuous decrease. At day −5 the plasma lipoprotein profile was characterized by a high VLDL level; it decreased in the days after hatching, while the HDL peak progressively increased. Although the plasma apoA-I level paralleled the rise of HDL, in embryonic life and the early post-natal period apoA-I was also found in VLDL and LDL. A high content of esterified cholesterol was found in the liver and in skeletal muscle; it progressively decreased after hatching. Immunohistochemical studies indicate that at day −5 apoA-I was clearly present in hepatocytes but not in the skeletal muscle. However, at day 1 apoA-I was detectable around the lipid droplets and the cell membrane of muscle cells. In contrast, very few lipid droplets and no apoA-I were detected in the muscle cells at day 14. The fall in muscle apoA-I found immediately after hatching coincided with the progressive increase of the plasma apoA-I concentration, thus indicating that the skeletal muscle may contribute to the plasma apoA-I pool.

These findings suggest that the lipid overload that occurs in the chick tissues around the time of hatching may, in some way, stimulate the production of apoA-I, which in turn would facilitate the local distribution of lipids and/or their efflux from tissue to the plasma compartment.

[1] Ferrari, St., Tarugi, P., Drusiani, E., Calandra, S. and Fregni, S. (1987). The complete sequence of chick apolipoprotein A-I mRNA and its expression in the developing chick. *Gene* (in press).

Plasma Cholesterol and Lipase Activities of RICO Rats Fed a Standard Diet Enriched with 0.5% or 1% Cholesterol. F. Sultan[1], L. E. Cardona-Sanclemente[2], C. Lagrange[1], C. Lutton[2] and S. Griglio[1]. [1]*INSERM U.177, 15 rue de l'Ecole de Médecine, 75270 Paris Cedex 06, France;* [2]*Laboratoire de Physiologie de la Nutrition, Université de Paris-Sud, 91405 Orsay Cedex, France*

The effect of cholesterol-enriched diets was tested on genetically hypercholesterolaemic rats (RICO = rat with increased cholesterol) compared with their normocholesterolaemic controls (SW). Three-to-four-month old rats of both genotypes were fed the standard diet (SD) or the same diet enriched with 0.5 or 1% cholesterol, during a one-month period. Plasma lipoprotein lipase (LPL) and hepatic lipase (HL) activities were measured after i.v. injection of 20 U/100 g rat of heparin. When fed the SD diet, RICO rats had higher plasma total cholesterol (1.72 ± 0.04 g/ml vs. 1.01 ± 0.05 (12)) and esterified cholesterol (1.26 ± 0.02 g/ml vs. 0.727 ± 0.04 (12), $p < 0.025$). Their LPL activity was decreased (316 ± 43 mU/ml vs. 485 ± 71 (12), $p < 0.025$), whereas HL activity was comparable (1369 ± 59 mU/ml vs. 1306 ± 89 (12)). HL secretion by isolated hepatocytes after 2 h of incubation in the presence of heparin (5U) was the same (5.61 ± 1.02 mU/10^6 cells (5) vs. 6.16 ± 0.63 (5)) and confirmed the identical plasma values. Cholesterol added to the diet did not modify plasma LPL, which remained lower in the RICO, but increased plasma total cholesterol (19% and 12% for the RICO and SW rats respectively) and decreased HL activity: 14.8% (NS) and 15.6% ($p < 0.01$) with 0.5% cholesterol; 23% ($p < 0.01$) and 19% ($p < 0.005$) with 1.1% cholesterol in the diet for the RICO and SW rats. No difference between genotypes was detected.

Thus the increased hepatic synthesis of cholesterol measured in the RICO rats[1] seemed not to be related to a decrease of their HL activity under the standard diet. Dietary cholesterol that further increased their plasma cholesterol, and particularly chylomicron cholesterol[2], decreased their plasma HL activity. In the latter case, a delayed uptake of chylomicrons may be related to a simultaneous decrease of HL and LPL activities in the RICO rats.

[1] Cardona-Sanclemente, L. E., Verneau, C., Mathé, D. and Lutton, C. (1987). *Biochim. Biophys. Acta* **919**, 205–212.
[2] Cardona-Sanclemente, L. E. (1986). Thèse de Doctorat, Université Paris-Sud, Centre d'Orsay.

Role of Human Apolipoprotein A-IV in Promoting the Formation of Very Small Lipoprotein Particles.

Laurent Lagrost, Philippe Gambert, Stan Bastiras, Anne Athias and Christian Lallemant. *Laboratoire de Biochimie Médicale, Faculté de Médecine 21033 Dijon, France*

ApoA-IV, an apolipoprotein of predominantly intestinal origin, has been identified in several mammalian species and in man. In human plasma, apoA-IV, although present in HDL, is mainly unassociated with lipoproteins[1]. Recent studies have established that this apolipoprotein activates LCAT *in vitro* and have suggested that the formation of HDL cholesteryl esters may regulate apoA-IV binding to HDL[2–4]. Weinberg and Spector[4] have speculated that apoA-IV could function as, or in concert with, a lipid transfer factor. However, its precise function remains obscure. The aim of this study was to examine the effect of apoA-IV on HDL alterations, specifically alterations in particle size distribution, induced by a partially purified serum LTP fraction.

A very small size lipoprotein fraction was formed when total serum lipoproteins were incubated with a partially purified lipid transfer protein and apolipoprotein A-IV. Incubation in the absence of apolipoprotein A-IV induced a general displacement of HDL particles towards the large-size range, as shown by gradient gel electrophoresis. When the reaction mixture was supplemented with apolipoprotein A-IV, the same general HDL size enlargement occurred, but, in addition, there appeared an abundant new small-size lipoprotein fraction of mean diameter 7.4 nm. No cholesterol esterification was detected during the incubations. Immunoblotting experiments showed that apolipoprotein A-IV was not a component of a newly formed lipoprotein fraction and remained in an unassociated form after incubation. Data suggest that apolipoprotein A-IV acts as a cofactor in the complex process of HDL conversion.

[1] Green, P. H. R., Glickman, R. M., Riley, J. W. and Quinet, E. (1980). *J. Clin. Invest.* **65**, 911–919.
[2] Delamatre, J. G., Hoffmeier, C. A., Lacko, A. G. and Roheim, P. S. (1983). *J. Lipid Res.* **24**, 1578–1585.
[3] Steinmetz, A. and Utermann, G. (1985). *J. Biol. Chem.* **260**, 2258–2264.
[4] Weinberg, R. B. and Spector, M. S. (1986). *Biochem. Biophys. Res. Commun.* **135**, 756–763.

The Fate of Cholesterol Derived from HDL_2 in Rat Hepatocyte Monolayers.

William J. Sampson[1], Brian Jackson[1], Keith E. Suckling[1] and Kathleen M. Botham[2]. [1]*Smith, Kline & French Research Ltd, The Frythe, Welwyn, Herts AL6 9AR, UK;* [2]*Royal Veterinary College, Royal College Street, London NW1 0TU, UK*

The synthesis of bile acids by rat hepatocyte monolayers is thought to be limited by the supply of substrate cholesterol. It can be stimulated by a number of sources of additional cholesterol. These include exogenous lipoproteins and mevalonic acid. A number of years ago we showed that rat HDL_2 can stimulate the production of bile acids by rat hepatocyte monolayers. In principle, the cholesterol derived from this lipoprotein could, after release from the lysosomal compartment, be transported directly to the site of bile acid synthesis. Alternatively it could be re-esterified by the action of acyl-CoA : cholesterol acyltransferase (ACAT), stored as cholesteryl ester, which could then be hydrolysed to make the cholesterol available for synthesis of bile acids. We have investigated these possibilities using the ACAT inhibitor, Sandoz compound 58–035. Rat hepatocyte monolayers (2×10^6 cells per dish) were incubated with rat HDL_2 (500 μg) in the presence and absence of 58–035[1]. In all cases mevinolin (5 μM) was added to eliminate the effect of endogenous synthesis of cholesterol. Measurements were made after an incubation period of 5 h in four independent preparations of cells from rats maintained on a diet containing 2% cholestyramine by weight.

HDL_2 caused a stimulation of cholesteryl ester synthesis by 32% and this formation of cholesteryl ester could be inhibited by 58–035. In the same experiments the synthesis and secretion of bile acids was increased by 0.32 ± 0.10 nmol per 2×10^6 cells in 5 h over a basal level of secretion of 2.47 ± 0.46 nmol. Inhibition of cholesteryl ester formation by the additions of 58–035 caused a reduction in bile acid synthesis of 0.37 ± 0.16 nmol below the basal level.

These observations show that the stimulation of bile acid synthesis that is caused by the addition of HDL_2 can be blocked by the inhibition of cholesterol esterification. The implication of this is that cholesterol entering the cell by this route must initially be esterified before it can be made available for other cellular functions. This provides additional evidence for the concept that cholesterol flux in many cell types is highly controlled in a way that is relevant to the metabolic role of the cell and that free diffusion of cholesterol between cell membranes does not occur.

[1] Sampson, W. J., Suffolk, R. A., Bowers, P., Houghton, J. D., Botham, K. M. and Suckling, K. E. (1987). *Biochim. Biophys. Acta* **920**, 1–8.

Specific Removal of Lipoprotein Lp(a) in LDL-Apheresis.

W. Knisel, I. Besenthal, M. Müller, T. Risler and M. Eggstein. *Medizinische Klinik, University of Tübingen, D-7400 Tübingen, FRG*

LDL-apheresis is a new procedure for specific extracorporeal removal of low-density lipoproteins by selective adsorption on Sepharose-bound anti-LDL-antibodies. These monospecific polyclonal antibodies of sheep origin have an anti-apo B-affinity. Therefore we studied the influence of LDL-apheresis on Lp(a), which is an important apolipoprotein-B-containing lipoprotein suggested as an independent risk factor for atherosclerosis.

Serum concentrations of Lp(a) were measured by a commercially available radial immunodiffusion method (Immuno) in addition to other lipid values and various clinical chemical and haematological parameters in a 54-year-old male with familial hypercholesterolaemia type IIa before and after LDL-apheresis within the first ten treatments of one-week intervals.

LDL-apheresis on the average reduced Lp(a) by 65%, total cholesterol by 57%, LDL-cholesterol by 64%, apoB by 65% and total protein by 19%, the latter owing to a dilution within the extracorporeal system (see Table).

Effects of LDL-apheresis on serum levels of Lp(a), other lipid parameters and total protein

	Baseline[a] (mg/dl)	Before[b] (mg/dl)	After[b] (mg/dl)	Reduction
LP(a)	39	34 ± 2.2	12 ± 2.0	65%
Total cholesterol	356	313 ± 24	135 ± 23	57%
LDL cholesterol	147	257 ± 28	93 ± 23	64%
ApoB	147	130 ± 6.1	45 ± 3.0	65%
Total protein	7.1 g/dl	6.5 ± 0.3 g/dl	5.3 ± 0.3 g/dl	19%

[a]Values prior to first treatment.
[b]Mean ± SD of measurements just before and immediately after LDL-apheresis.

Our preliminary results suggest that for the first time we know that LDL-apheresis is a very effective method for specific extracorporeal removal of Lp(a) in addition to the elimination of LDL. Thus LDL-apheresis may augment the therapeutic effectiveness of LDL lowering by an associated decrease of Lp(a).

Dahlen, G. H., Guyton, J. R., Attar, M., Farmer, J. A., Kautz, J. A. and Gotto, A. M. (1986). *Circulation* **74**, 758–765.
Kostner, G. M., Avogaro, P., Cazzolato, G., Marth, E., Bittolo-Bon, G. and Quinci, G. B. (1981). *Atherosclerosis* **38**, 51–61.
Stoffel, W., Borberg, H., Greve, V. (1981). *Lancet* **ii**, 1005–1007.

Is Apolipoprotein E Phenotype Related to the Pathogenesis of Type V Hyperlipoproteinaemia? Marja-Riitta Taskinen, Timo Kuusi and Ritva Kauppinen-Mäkelin. *Second and Third Departments of Medicine, University of Helsinki, Helsinki, Finland*

ApoE phenotypes were first associated with the pathogenesis of type III hyperlipoproteinaemia. In addition, there is both positive and negative evidence indicating that apoE4 plays a role in the development of type V hyperlipoproteinaemia. Therefore, we decided to study apoE phenotype distribution in the type V hyperlipoproteinaemia in the Finnish population, where the gene frequency of apoE4 is high. Twenty-one unrelated probands with type V hyperlipoproteinaemia (18 men and 3 women, age 45 ± 1 years) participated in the study. Their relative body weight averaged 127 ± 3%. The type V diagnosis was based on the level of plasma triglycerides above 1000 mg/dl, the presence of chylomicrons and on the exclusion of lipoprotein lipase and apoCII deficiencies. The reference group for lipoprotein values consisted of 24 normolipidaemic women and 50 men from the office staff of two companies. The mean plasma triglyceride concentration of type V patients was 1262 ± 266 mg/dl and that of cholesterol was 330 ± 33 mg/dl. LDL cholesterol in type V patients with apoE4 ($n = 15$) was not significantly different from that in patients without apoE4 ($n = 3$) (mean ± SEM: 92 ± 14 vs. 63 ± 27 mg/dl). The respective numbers for HDL cholesterol averaged 34 ± 3 and 24 ± 7 mg/dl. Post-heparin plasma LPL activities were lower in both male and female type V patients than in normolipidaemic subjects

(19.5 ± 1.5 vs. 24.9 ±1.0, $p < 0.01$ and 15.9 ± 3.5 vs. 27.2 ± 1.5 μmol FFA/ml per h, $p < 0.01$). The hepatic lipase activity was increased in women with type V (31.0 ± 3.6 vs. 18.7 ± 1.1 μmol FFA/ml per h, $p < 0.001$) but not in men (35.2 ± 3.6 vs. 30.6 ± 1.9 μmol FFA/ml per h). Five different apoE phenotypes were observed upon analytical IEF in type V patients. The apoE phenotype distribution was significantly different from that reported in the normal Finnish population ($\chi^2 = 15.75, p < 0.001$). Accordingly, apoE4 gene frequency (±SD) of the type V subjects was 0.595 ± 0.093, compared with 0.227 ± 0.013 ($p < 0.001$). In contrast, the apoE3 gene frequency of 0.310 ± 0.077 was markedly lower than the respective gene frequency of 0.733 ± 0.017 in the normal population ($p < 0.001$). We suggest that apoE4 is more effective than apoE3 in modulating direct chylomicron and VLDL uptake in liver by downregulation of B/E receptor. The combination of apoE4 phenotype and/or enhanced VLDL production together with subnormal or low removal capacity aggravates hypertriglyceridaemia and leads to the manifestation of type V hyperlipoproteinaemia.

Flow Cytometric Analysis of High Density Lipoprotein Uptake by Human Peripheral Blood T Lymphocytes. Increase During Ageing? K. N. Traill[1], G. Jürgens[2], G. Böck[1], L. Huber[1] and G. Wick[1]. [1]*Institute for General and Experimental Pathology, University of Innsbruck, Austria;* [2]*Institute for Medical Biochemistry, University of Graz, Austria*

The age-related decline in mitogen responsiveness of human peripheral blood lymphocytes (PLB) is said to correlate with an increased membrane cholesterol/phospholipid (CHOL/Pl) molar composition and with serum CHOL/Pl levels. Although PBL can synthesize CHOL themselves, they normally acquire it from plasma low density lipoproteins (LDL) via high affinity apoB/E receptors. Both receptor expression and CHOL biosynthesis are very finely tuned to the cell's requirements for CHOL, so if an imbalance in CHOL homeostasis arises during ageing one/both of these regulatory circuits may no longer be functioning efficiently. We have recently shown that receptor-mediated LDL uptake is increased in freshly isolated T lymphocytes from carefully selected (EURAGE/SENIEUR-Protocol) healthy elderly blood donors[1]. Nevertheless, this would only be expected to lead to CHOL overloading if excess CHOL was not efficiently removed by high density lipoproteins (HDL). The present experiments were undertaken to investigate this, but since very little is known about HDL reactions with lymphocytes it was first necessary to investigate for a specific receptor/binding site on human PBL.

Using fluorescence methodology, we were able to show that dioctadecylindocarbocyanine (Dil)-labelled HDL are taken up by freshly isolated T cells during a 2 h incubation at 37°C; cytoplasmic staining was seen in the fluorescence microscope, indicating that bound HDL had been internalized. In binding studies, performed by means of a fluorescence-activated cell sorter (FACS)[2,3], Dil-HDL uptake was shown to be: (a) saturable during a 2 h incubation at 37°C; (b) specific, since it was competed by HDL (and HDL proteins) but not by LDL; and (c) enhanced 3–6-fold by inclusion of EDTA in the incubation medium as well as by trypsinization of the cells before incubation with Dil-HDL. In preliminary studies to investigate age-related differences in Dil-HDL uptake by human PBL, we found increased levels of uptake. The significance of this with respect to (a) increased LDL uptake and cellular CHOL levels and (b) immune regulation by HDL lipids is under investigation.

[1] Traill, K. N., Jürgens, G., Böck, G., Huber, H., Schönitzer, D., Winter, U. and Wick, G. (1987) *Mech. Ageing Dev.*, in press.
[2] Traill, K. N., Böck, G., Winter, U., Hilchenbach, M., Jürgens, G. and Wick, G. (1986) *J. Histochem. Cytochem.* **34**, 1217–1221.
[3] Traill, K. N., Jürgens, G., Böck, G. and Wick, G. (1987) *Immunobiol.*, in press.

This work was supported by the Austrian Research Council (Project S-41/01).

Fluorescence Studies of the Mechanism of Action of the Cholesteryl Ester Transfer Protein (CETP) in Human Plasma. T. A. Berkhout, S. Cresswell and D. Ellis. *Smith Kline & French Research Limited, The Frythe, Welwyn, Herts AL6 9AR, UK*

Cholesteryl ester transfer protein (CETP) was purified using phenyl-Sepharose and CM 52 chromatography, followed by micro-emulsion chromatography on a Sepharose 4B column (Hesler *et al.*, *J. Biol. Chem.* **262**, 2275 (1987)). CETP was titrated with vesicles containing phosphatidylcholine,1-pyrene-3β-(*cis*-9-octadecenoyloxy)-22,23, bisnor-5-cholenate (PMC oleate), and trinitrophenylphosphatidylethanolamine (89 : 1 : 10 mol ratio). These vesicles are non-fluorescent as a result of energy transfer between PMC-oleate and the trinitrophenyl moiety. Upon addition of these vesicles to CETP, the pyrene fluorescence increased, indicating complex formation between PMC oleate and CETP in the aqueous phase. When PMC oleate vesicles were titrated with increasing amounts of CETP an increase of fluorescence towards equilibrium levels could also be monitored. Analysis of both titration curves suggested a low affinity of the PMC oleate substrate for CETP. Furthermore, when CETP was incubated with phosphatidylcholine vesicles containing 1% [^{14}C]cholesteryl oleate, it could be shown using isoelectric focusing that part of the total radioactivity had migrated to PKi = 5.2, a value similar to the PKi of CETP.

These results provide evidence for a shuttle mechanism of action for CETP, under the experimental conditions used.

Hepatic Lipase (HL) and Low Density Lipoprotein (LDL) Physical Characteristics. Johan H. Auwerx and John D. Brunzell. *Division of Metabolism, University of Washington, Seattle, WA 98195, USA*

Because of the abnormal lipoprotein characteristics in a family with HL deficiency, an investigation into the effect of HL on LDL physical characteristics was conducted.

The proband was HL-deficient, had beta VLDL in plasma despite an E_3/E_3 phenotype, and lacked the other stigmata of type III hyperlipoproteinaemia. At the time of investigation, his total cholesterol was 196 mg/100 ml while his triglycerides were 389 mg/100 ml. Two of his half-sisters had very low (39 nmol and 31 nmol FFA/min per ml) and his son had low levels (86 nmol FFA/min per ml) of HL activity. Other family members displayed abnormalities in their lipoprotein pattern varying from type IIa, type IV to hyperalphalipoproteinaemia.

Since HL is thought to process VLDL remnants to LDL, these apoB-containing lipoproteins were examined by density-gradient ultracentrifugation and gradient gel electrophoresis. In the proband "LDL" was present in a sharp peak (d = 1.023 g/ml) distributed between classical IDL and LDL, was increased in size (26.4 nm versus 25.3 ± 0.3 nm in control males), was TG-enriched, and contained, like control LDL, very little apoE by PAGGE. His half-sisters had LDL intermediate in size (27.0 nm and 26.5 nm respectively vs. 25.4 ± 0.4 nm in control females), density, and composition between normal subjects and the proband.

	HL (nmol FFA/ min per ml)	LDL Density (g/ml)	LDL composition (mass%)			
			CE	TG	FC	PL
Control M	147 ± 53	1.044 ± .006	58 ± 13	7 ± 3	11 ± 2	24 ± 6
Control F	85 ± 51	1.042 ± .002	58 ± 11	6 ± 3	12 ± 2	24 ± 5
Proband	0	1.023	20	41	7	32
Sister 1	39	1.031	37	15	19	29
Sister 2	31	1.027	—	—	—	—

Incubation of LDL of the proband with HL resulted in a density shift of the LDL from 1.024 to 1.033 g/ml. HL deficiency appears to account for the more buoyant and larger LDL seen in these patients.

We therefore conclude that HL is responsible for part of the processing of VLDL remnants to LDL particles by its effects on lipid composition.

Molecular Cloning of Guinea Pig Lipoprotein Lipase and Some Aspects of its Tissue-specific Regulation.

Sven Enerbäck[1], Henrik Semb[2], Gunilla Bengtsson-Olivecrona[2], Gunnar Bjursell[1] and Thomas Olivecrona[2]. [1]*Department of Medical Biochemistry, University of Göteborg, S-400 33 Göteborg, Sweden;* [2]*Department of Physiological Chemistry, University of Umeå, S-901 87 Umeå, Sweden*

We have isolated and sequenced cDNA clones covering the coding sequence of guinea pig lipoprotein lipase. The expression cDNA library used was constructed in lambda gt 11 with mRNA derived from adipocytes. The deduced amino acid sequence starts with a stretch of 17 amino acids interpreted as a leader peptide. The open reading frame continues with 448 amino acid residues and ends with a TGA. This information, combined with previous established data, allows the assignment of domain borders in the molecule. Clear homologies to pancreatic lipase and bovine lipoprotein lipase are noted.

Northern blot reveals:

(i) a high expression in adipocytes, heart muscle and mammary gland;

(ii) three major transcripts with sizes 3.8 kb, 3.3 kb and 2.1 kb respectively.

Analysis of genomic DNA indicates a single gene locus coding for lipoprotein lipase.

Dot blot analysis indicates a decrease by 20% ($p < 0.001$) of LPL-specific messenger pool after TNF (tumour necrosis factor) and a *decrease* by 82% ($p < 0.0001$) when subjected to starvation, in adipose tissue (these experiments were carried out *in vivo*). In heart muscle *no changes* could be accounted for. In liver we noted an *increase* of LPL-specific message after TNF administration; thus this substance seems to regulate the LPL-message pool in a tissue-specific pattern.

Cell-Specific Regulation of Transcription by the Apolipoprotein B Gene Promoter. Peter Carlsson and Gunnar Bjursell. *Department of Medical Biochemistry, University of Göteborg, Sweden*

A DNA segment containing the promoter of the human apolipoprotein B gene has been positioned in front of the coding sequence of the bacterial chloramphenicol acetyl transferase (CAT) gene. The CAT enzyme activity produced, following transfection of human cell lines and transient expression, is taken as a measure of the transcriptional activity of the apoB promoter. In this assay the apoB promoter is active in the hepatoma-derived cell line HepG2 and inactive in Hela cells. Deletion analysis has defined the minimum amount of 5′-flanking sequences needed to obtain full transcriptional activity in HepG2 cells. It has also made it possible to localize an upstream region necessary to *prevent* activity in Hela cells.

Magnetic Resonance Studies of Acylation-Induced Structural Changes in LDL. David G. Reid[1], David S. Leake[2], Sarah M. Rankin[2] and Duro Oduwole[3]. [1]*Smith Kline & French Research Ltd, The Frythe, Welwyn, Herts AL6 9AR, UK;* [2]*Department of Pharmacology, Kings College, London, UK;* [3]*Chemistry Department, Queen Mary College, London, UK*

Incubation of low density lipoprotein (LDL) with endothelial cells enhances its rate of uptake by macrophages. A similar enhancement can be induced by chemical acetylation of LDL, presumably on the ε-amino positions of lysine residues on apoliprotein B (apoB), by acetic anhydride. The ^{13}C nuclear magnetic resonance (NMR) spectra of native, mouse peritoneal macrophage modified, and acetylated LDL are essentially identical, although only signals from the highly mobile lipid components are discernible. We have labelled LDL with ^{13}C-enriched acetic anhydride, allowing an NMR signal to be observed from acetylated apoB. This signal, unlike signals from lipids such as phosphatidylcholine on the surface of the LDL particle, is practically unaffected by hydrophilic relaxation (i.e. broadening) reagents, such as Mn^{2+}. This implies that the bulk of the ^{13}C label is internally located, probably as the result of a conformational or orientational change on the part of apoB.

We have also used an organic paramagnetic analogue of acetic anhydride to prepare "spin-labelled" LDL, which can be studied by electron spin resonance (ESR). The ESR spectrum of lightly spin-labelled LDL, which has been only briefly incubated with the spin-labelled acylating agent, shows broad resonance lines typical of a slowly but isotropically reorientating species. Prolonged incubation with either more spin-label, or acetic anhydride, sharpens these signals. These findings imply that prolonged acylation increases the reorientation rate of the spin-label. This could be associated with a relocation of the label into the fluid core of the particle.

Post-Receptor Signal Transduction of Specific and Scavenger Low Density Lipoprotein (LDL) Receptors on Human Mononuclear Cells (MNLs).

É. Kovács, Zs. Varga, G. Fóris and Gy. Paragh. *First Department of Medicine, University Medical School, Debrecen, Hungary*

One of the most important biological effects of specific LDL receptors is the inhibition of HMG-CoA reductase, which is responsible for the endogenous cholesterol synthesis. However, its post-receptor signal transduction is unknown.

Our experiments were carried out on MNLs separated of the sera of healthy subjects. It was found that 50–150 μg/ml LDL induced an early cAMP level elevation, which was followed by a later cGMP level increase. The cytosolic free Ca^{2+} level was also increased measured by the Quin 2 fluorescence technique.

The LDL-induced arachidonic acid (AA) cascade could be blocked by the phospholipase C (PLC) inhibitor neomycin.

Finally, the SH-sensitive HMG-CoA reductase activity measured by the incorporation of [^{14}C]acetate is inhibited by O_2^- generation through NADPH oxidase activation by G_i protein–PLC–DAG–AA cascade (DAG diacylglycerol).

The post-receptor signal transduction of scavenger receptors was investigated on monocyte-derived macrophages (MDMs). 50–150 μg/ml acetylated LDL (ac-LDL) induced the apoE secretion of MDMs through the activation of phospholipase A_2 (PLA_2), which could be prevented by pertussis toxin (PT). Therefore the ac-LDL induced PGE_2 secretion through the G_i protein–PLA_2–AA cascade is responsible for the apoE secretion as it is acting extracellularly on the adenylate cyclase itself.

Enhanced Liver Uptake of LDL and HDL Tris-Galactoside-Terminated Cholesterol.

Th. J. C. van Berkel, F. Kuipers, R. J. Vonk and H. J. M. Kempen. *Centre for Bio-Pharmaceutical Sciences, Leiden University, The Netherlands.*

A tris-galactosylated cholesterol derivative (tris-gal-chol), easily soluble in water, is quantitatively incorporated into LDL or HDL upon simple mixing. Tris-gal-chol incorporation into human LDL leads to a rapid galactose-receptor mediated uptake by liver Kupffer cells (*J. Biol. Chem.* **260**, 2694–2699 (1985)), while incorporation into human HDL (apoE-free) induces rapid uptake by liver hepatocytes (*J. Biol. Chem.* **260**, 12203–12207 (1985)). In the present experiments tris-gal-chol was mixed with cholesteryl-ester-labelled rat LDL and HDL and the fate of cholesteryl esters was followed. After intravenous injection into rats a 4–10-fold increase in liver uptake was noticed whereby rat LDL was both cleared by Kupffer cells and hepatocytes while rat HDL was mainly taken up by hepatocytes. After hepatocyte uptake, rapid hydrolysis of the cholesteryl esters occurred (within 20–30 min) and the free cholesterol was directly used for bile acid synthesis. After Kupffer cell uptake, the cholesteryl esters from rat LDL or HDL were first hydrolysed in these cells and then transferred to hepatocytes. The maximum increase of appearance of radioactivity in the bile with rat LDL occurred at a later time after injection than with rat HDL. For both LDL and HDL, upon tris-gal-chol incorporation at 24 h after injection, a two-fold higher percentage of the injected cholesteryl ester radioactivity had appeared in the bile.

Infusion of 10 or 20 mg tris-gal-chol during 4 h caused a dose-dependent decrease of the serum cholesterol concentration (60% with 20 mg of tris-gal-chol), which persists for a further 20 h after stopping the infusion. This effect is specific for tris-gal-chol because tris-glc-chol is ineffective. It can be concluded that tris-gal-chol incorporation into lipoproteins both *in vitro* and *in vivo* leads to a markedly increased catabolism by the liver whereby the cholesterol concentration in the blood can be lowered as a consequence of increased transport of cholesterol (derivatives) to the bile.

Alterations of Human Low Density Lipoprotein under Peroxidative Conditions. G. Jürgens[1], O. Quehenberger[2], S. Zadravec[2], H. Esterbauer[2]. [1]*Institute of Medical Biochemistry and* [2]*Institute of Biochemistry, Karl-Franzens Universität Graz, Graz, Austria*

Human low density lipoprotein (LDL), a carrier of free and esterified cholesterol, phospholipids, triglycerides, lipid-soluble vitamins and certain drugs in the blood, can undergo free-radical-induced peroxidation either in the presence of cells such as endothelial cells or in cell-free systems containing divalent cations like copper or iron[1,2]. The oxidative degradation of polyunsaturated fatty acids only occurs after an almost complete depletion of α- and γ-tocopherol as well as β-carotene[3]. Thereafter, several aldehydic lipid peroxidation products including malondialdehyde, hexanal, propanal, 4-hydroxynonenal (HNE), butanal, 2,4-heptadienal, pentanal, hydroxyhexenal and hydroxyoctenal appeared or increased in concentration[3]. In order to study the role of divalent cations more closely, several copper(II) chloride concentrations were compared with regard to their effect on the concentrations of the tocopherols, β-carotene, peroxides and HNE. All incubations were performed for three hours at room temperature on 0.01 M sodium phosphate buffer, pH 7.4.

Copper (II) chloride (μM)	Tocopherol α- (ng/mg LDL)	Tocopherol γ- (ng/mg LDL)	β-Carotene (ng/mg LDL)	HNE (nmol/mg LDL)	Peroxides (nmol/mg LDL)
0.0	695	76	81	0.04	0.4
0.5	0	30	50	0.04	1.2
1.0	0	2	18	0.06	3.6
2.0	0	0	7	0.06	—
5.0	0	0	0	0.23	5.8
10.0	0	0	0	1.9	7.9

At a concentration of 0.5 μM, LDL was only depleted of α-tocopherol. No lipid degradation products such as HNE and no new fluorophores were formed. Copper(II) chloride concentrations of 2–10 μM led to an increase in the fluorescence intensities at an excitation of 360 nm and an emission of 430 nm of the apolipoprotein solubilized in 5% SDS as well as of the lipids extracted in $CHCl_3 : MeOH = 2 : 1$. For 10 μM copper(II) chloride the increases were 7- and 3.5-fold respectively (compared with native LDL).

Other divalent cations tested in their free or complexed forms showed that free iron(II) as well as its EDTA-chelate or ADP-complex were very weak initiators of lipid peroxidation in LDL, but iron-containing proteins had a high capacity for oxidizing LDL. However, copper(II) ions were the strongest indicators of lipid peroxidation in LDL.

[1] Steinbrecher, U. P., Witztum, J. L., Parthasarathy, S. and Steinberg, D. (1987). *Arteriosclerosis* **7**, 135.
[2] Heinecke, J. W. (1987). *Free Radical Biology and Medicine* **3**, 65.
[3] Esterbauer, H., Jürgens, G., Quehenberger, O. and Koller, E. (1987). *J. Lipid Res.* **28**, 495.

This work was supported by the Östereichischen Fonds zur Förderung der Wissenschaftlichen Forschung (P6176).

Increased Hepatic Clearance of Low Density Lipoprotein Modified by Acetaldehyde. Kari Kervinen, Y. Antero Kesäniemi, Tatu A. Miettinen, Hanna-Kaisa Hyvärinen and Kristian Liewendahl. *Department of Internal Medicine, University of Oulu and Second Department of Medicine, University of Helsinki, Finland*

Plasma low density lipoprotein (LDL) levels are negatively correlated with alcohol consumption. The first metabolite in ethanol oxidation, acetaldehyde (AcA), could be responsible for the low LDL levels in alcohol users. We have studied the metabolism of acetaldehyde-modified LDL (AcA-LDL) in man. LDL was isolated from human volunteers, radiolabelled with either ^{125}I or ^{131}I, incubated in various AcA concentrations (AcA-LDL) and injected back into the donors simultaneously with LDL incubated in identical conditions but omitting AcA (C-LDL). After incubation, the percentage of free amino groups in AcA-LDL (98–54%) showed a negative correlation ($r = -0.99, p < 0.001$) with the final concentration of AcA (0.2–8.0 mM). AcA modification accelerated the *in vivo* catabolism of LDL in such a way that the fractional catabolic rate of LDL was negatively correlated with the percentage of free amino groups in AcA-LDL ($r = -0.87, p < 0.01$). The clearance of AcA-LDL modified in 0.2, 2.0 and 4.0 mM AcA was 1.0, 1.4 and 2.5 times faster than the clearance of C-LDL respectively.

In order to study the tissue distribution and sites of degradation of AcA-LDL we used an external imaging technique utilizing 99m-technetium (Tc) labelled AcA-LDL and C-LDL in healthy volunteers. The uptake of Tc-AcA-LDL in the liver and gallbladder was 1.2 and 2.0 times faster than the uptake of Tc-C-LDL respectively. The uptake of Tc-AcA-LDL and Tc-C-LDL in kidney, spleen and left ventricle did not differ significantly.

These studies show that AcA, at least after *in vitro* treatment, accelerates the catabolism of LDL in man. This accelerated catabolism seems to be mediated by the enhancement in the hepatic uptake of AcA-LDL. The present findings may be one explanation for the low LDL levels in chronic alcoholics, in individuals with high AcA concentrations in the blood and particularly in the liver.

Effects of Thyroid Hormone and a Thyromimetic, SK&F L-94901, on Key Enzymes of Cholesterol Metabolism in Cholesterol-Fed and Hypothyroid Rats. Susan C. Black, David Ellis, Brian Jackson and Keith E. Suckling. *Smith Kline and French Research Ltd, The Frythe, Welwyn, Herts AL6 9AR, UK*

The effects of 3,3′,5-triiodo-L-thyronine (T3) and a thyromimetic (SK&F L-94901) on hepatic and intestinal cholesterol metabolism were investigated on hypothyroid (MTI), cholesterol-fed (HCD) and hypothyroid cholesterol-fed (HCD/MTI) rats. SK&F L-94901 is as effective as T3 at reducing plasma cholesterol levels and stimulating liver function, but has 0.1% of the activity of T3 on cardiac function[1].

T3 and SK&F L-94901 reduced plasma cholesterol in HCD animals from 1.5 ± 0.11 to 1.13 ± 0.14 and 0.9 ± 0.1 mg/ml respectively (control animals = 0.33 ± 0.04 mg/ml). Hypothyroid animals had elevated plasma cholesterol levels of 0.68 ± 0.09 mg/ml, which decreased to 0.41 ± 0.02 and 0.46 ± 0.04 mg/ml by T3 and SK&F L-94901 treatment respectively. The combined effects of cholesterol-feeding and hypothyroidism induced plasma cholesterol levels of 6.28 ± 0.75 mg/ml, which were reduced to 0.59 ± 0.06 and 0.77 ± 0.04 mg/ml with T3 and SK&F L-94901 respectively.

Liver acyl-CoA : cholesterol *O*-acyltransferase (ACAT, EC 2.3.1.26) was reduced in the HCD group by T3 and SK&F L-94901 from 590 ± 150 to 496 ± 154 and 440 ± 108 pmol/min per mg respectively (control = 49.5 ± 17 pmol/min per mg). A similar effect was seen in the MTI group with a reduction from 100 ± 22 to 16 ± 11 and 63 ± 36 pmol/min per mg with T3 and SK&F L-94901 respectively. In the HCDM,TI group ACAT activity (601 ± 76 pmol/min per mg) was not affected by thyroid hormone or analogue.

Liver HMG-CoA reductase (mevalonate : NADP oxidoreductase, EC 1.1.1.34), which was reduced by cholesterol-feeding (2.0 ± 0.9 pmol/min per mg compared with 13.3 ± 8.1 pmol/min per mg in the control group), increased on treatment with T3 and SK&F L-94901 to 5.8 ± 0.9 and 3.8 ± 1.9 pmol/min per mg. This effect was much greater in the MTI group, increasing from 7.6 ± 2.6 to 167 ± 70.2 and 68.4 ± 33.3 pmol/min per mg with T3 and SK&F L-94901 respectively. In the HCD/MTI group the increase was from 0.8 ± 0.6 to 3.6 ± 1.4 and 2.2 ± 1.3 pmol/min per mg respectively.

Intestinal ACAT and HMG-CoA reductase activities were also measured in the three groups of animals; however, no consistent effects of T3 and SK&F L-94901 were observed.

These data indicate that cholesterol feeding has a primary effect on enzyme activities and can mask the effect of thyroid hormones, which are very marked in hypothyroid animals in the absence of cholesterol-feeding.

[1] Underwood, A. H., Emmett, J. C., Ellis, D., Flynn, S. B., Leeson, P. D., Benson, G. M., Novelli, R., Pearce, N. J. and Shah, V. P. (1986). *Nature* **324**, 425–429.

Apolipoprotein Heterogeneity of High Density Lipoproteins Isolated by Immunoaffinity Chromatography. R. W. James, D. Hochstrasser, J.-D. Tissot, A.-F. Muller and D. Pometta. *University Hospital, Geneva, Switzerland*

We have examined the apolipoprotein (apo) heterogeneity of lipoprotein particles (high density lipoproteins, HDL) isolated by successive immunoaffinity chromatography on anti-apo A-II then anti-apoA-I columns. Isolated fractions were analysed by high-resolution two-dimensional gel electrophoresis (2DGE) and compared by computer-assisted gel scanning. Immunoaffinity chromatography was performed on plasma and total HDL ($d = 1.063$–1.21 kg/l) samples from three normolipaemic subjects. Particles containing as the major apolipoproteins apoA-I plus A-II (Lp(AI,AII)) and only apoA-I (Lp(AI)) were isolated from both plasma and HDL and gave qualitatively similar 2DGE profiles. Particles that were isolated directly from plasma were enriched in both the established apos (A-I, A-II, A-IV, C, D and E) and six additional protein bands (termed NA). The latter were identified by their Mr and pI, which were: NA-1, 36–37000, 5.0–5.3; NA-2, 35-39 000, 4.9–5.3; NA-3, 36–37 000, 5.7–6.3; NA-4, 59–62 000, 4.8–5.0; NA-5, 58–66 000, 4.8–5.2; NA-6, 75 000, 5.4–5.5. They were asymmetrically distributed between the two types of particles (plasma-Lp(AI) and plasma-Lp(AI, AII)), as were certain of the established apolipoproteins. The six additional proteins were visible in particles isolated by immunoaffinity chromatography of total HDL, but in trace quantities, suggesting that they were lost during ultracentrifugation. Two of the proteins cover Mr and pI ranges attributed to lipid transfer proteins. The results indicate a more complex protein heterogeneity of HDL particles when they are isolated by immunoaffinity chromatography directly from plasma, with corresponding implications for the metabolic heterogeneity of HDL.

The Effect of Drugs and Physiological Stimuli on Plasma High Density Lipoprotein (HDL) Subfractions in Relation to Coronary Heart Disease. E. R. Skinner, B. A. Griffin, C. Watt, R. J. Maughan, I. C. Reid and G. W. Ashcroft. *Departments of Biochemistry, Environmental and Occupational Medicine and Mental Health, University of Aberdeen, UK*

The value of plasma HDL concentration as an index of coronary risk has recently been challenged[1]. HDL, however, is highly heterogeneous, and we have therefore compared the distribution of its subfractions in subjects of high and low coronary risk and examined the effect of drugs and exercise on the distribution in normal subjects.

Of 272 subjects screened, two groups of male subjects, matched for age and physical fitness (VO_{2max}), were selected on the basis of total plasma cholesterol/HDL-cholesterol as coronary index (CI): Group I, CI > 4.0; Group II, CI < 4.0. All subjects were healthy non-smokers, non-hypertensive and free from medication and previous medical history. Group II subjects contained a higher proportion ($p < 0.01$) of HDL_{2b} (particle diameter 10.57 nm) and lower proportions of HDL_{3b+3c} (7.97 and 7.62 nm) than Group I subjects, as determined by integration of peak areas from gradient gel electrophoresis scans[2]. The mean concentration of an apoE-rich fraction of HDL isolated by heparin–Sepharose affinity chromatography[3] was 24% higher in Group II than in Group I.

When six healthy male volunteers underwent a programme consisting of a 23 mile walk on each of four successive days, the mean percentage of HDL_{2b} increased ($p < 0.01$), while HDL_{2a+3a} (9.16 at 8.44 nm) decreased ($p < 0.01$) when the subjects were maintained on a high-fat diet, but no significant changes were observed with a high-carbohydrate diet. There was no change in the concentration of E-rich HDL with either diet.

The effect of clomipramine on the HDL subfractions of five normal healthy subjects was also investigated. The concentration of HDL_2-cholesterol increased ($p < 0.01$) after two weeks of drug treatment, owing to an increase ($p < 0.01$) in the proportion of HDL_{2a}, with a small and variable increase in HDL_{2b}. There was no change in the level of HDL_3 subfractions.

These studies demonstrate that markedly different profiles of HDL subfractions are observed in subjects with different coronary risk indices and that the distribution is significantly altered in response to physical exercise and drug treatment[4].

[1] Pocock, S. J., Shaper, A. G., Phillips, A. N., Walker, M. and Whitehead, T. P. (1986). *Br. Med. J.* **292**, 515–519.

[2] Blanche, P. J., Gong, E. L., Forte, T. M. and Nichols, A. V. (1981). *Biochim. Biophys. Acta* **665**, 408–419.

[3] Weisgraber, K. M. and Mahley, R. W. (1980). *J. Lipid Res.* **21**, 316–325.

[4] Skinner, E. R., Watt, C. and Maughan, R. J. (1987). *Eur. J. Appl. Physiol.* **56**, 451–456.

Antibody Inhibition of Cholesterol 7α Hydroxylase. Emelyn R. Eldredge[1,2], Brian Jackson[1], C. Roland Wolf[2], and Keith E. Suckling[1]. [1]*Department of Cellular Pharmacology, Smith Kline & French Research Ltd, The Frythe, Welwyn, Herts AL6 9AR, UK;* [2]*Imperial Cancer Research Fund, Department of Biochemistry, University of Edinburgh Medical School, Hugh Robson Building, George Square, Edinburgh EH8 9XD, UK*

The rate-limiting step for bile acid synthesis has long been accepted to be that catalysed by cholesterol 7α hydroxylase. This minor species of cytochrome P-450 has been shown to be unique through substrate specificity studies and is not readily inducible by phenobarbital or 3-methylcholanthrene. We screened nine antibodies as inhibitors of cholesterol 7α hydroxylase, including those raised against cytochromes P-450 from the gene families I, IIA, IIC, and III. Of three antibodies to proteins within family IIC (PB1a, PB1b, and PB2a), an antibody raised against PB2a, a male-specific cytochrome P-450 expressed at adolescence, readily phosphorylated, and also not inducible by phenobarbital, could completely inhibit the microsomal 7α hydroxylation reaction. This finding, together with the fact that cytochromes P-450 are a large multigene family, suggests that cholesterol 7α hydroxylase, being a unique P-450, may share some structural homology with other P-450s in the P-450 IIC gene family.

Failure of the Regulation Function of Specific and Scavenger Low Density Lipoprotein (LDL) Receptors with Unaltered Receptor Density in Acute Myocardial Infarction (AMI). Gy. Paragh, É. Kovács, Zs. Varga, J. T. Nagy and G. Fóris. *First Department of Medicine, University Medical School, Debrecen, Hungary*

In spite of the manifest clinical signs of arteriosclerosis in different diseases, we have not been able to find significant alterations in specific and scavenger LDL receptor activities.

Our investigations were carried out on monocyte-derived macrophages cultured for 72 h (MDM_{72}) of 56 patients with AMI. The binding and degradation of [^{125}I]LDL and [^{125}I]acLDL in the AMI group did not differ significantly from the control values. In contrast, there was a great decrease in the 100 μg/ml LDL-induced inhibition of cholesterol synthesis in 39 patients as well as in the 100 μg/ml acLDL-triggered apoE secretion in 41 patients.

Either the decreased PGE_2 synthesis or the reduced PGE_2 activity with normal cyclo-oxygenase activity of MDM_{72} can be the explanation for the decreased apoE secretion in this latter group of patients.

Hepatic and Intestinal Cholesterol-Metabolizing Enzymes in Two Hyper-cholesterolaemic Animal Models. R. A. M. Devery, P. B. Collins, A. H. Johnson, N. M. G. O'Meara, L. O'Donnell and G. H. Tomkin. *Department of Biochemistry, Royal College of Surgeons in Ireland, Dublin 2, and Department of Metabolic Medicine, The Adelaide Hospital, Dublin 8, Ireland*

This study compares the activities of the key enzymes regulating cholesterol synthesis (3-hydroxy-3-methylglutaryl coenzyme A [HMGCoA] reductase), esterification (acyl coenzyme A : cholesterol-*O*-acyl-transferase [ACAT]) and catabolism (cholesterol 7α-hydroxylase) in the liver and intestine of two hypercholesterolaemic rabbit models, namely the cholesterol-fed and the hypercholesterolaemic diabetic animal. Serum cholesterol levels were similar in the cholesterol-fed (2.35 $\pm$ 0.44 mmol/l, $n = 6$) and diabetic groups (2.5 $\pm$ 0.45 mmol/l, $n = 8$) and were significantly higher ($p < 0.01$) than in the control animals (1.02 $\pm$ 0.20 mmol/l, $n = 5$). The activities of HMGCoA reductase, ACAT and cholesterol 7α-hydroxylase are demonstrated in the table.

HMGCoA reductase activities are significantly reduced in the livers of both groups of hypercholesterolaemic animals relative to control values. In the intestine, while the activity of HMGCoA reductase is reduced in cholesterol-fed animals, it is 2.3-fold higher in diabetic animals. ACAT activities are markedly enhanced in the liver and intestine of cholesterol-fed animals, but are greatly reduced in both tissues from diabetic animals. Hepatic 7α-hydroxylase is twice as active in cholesterol-fed animals as controls but is significantly lowered in diabetic animals. These data highlight the contrasting intracellular situations associated with both hypercholesterolaemic models. The cholesterol-fed model appears to respond by suppression of endogenous cholesterol synthesis, with enhancement of esterification and catabolism. Diabetic

	Control animals	Cholesterol-fed animals	Diabetic animals
HMGCoA reductase			
Liver	0.039 ± 0.005	0.005 ± 0.001***	0.019 ± 0.004*
Intestine	0.026 ± 0.003	0.012 ± 0.004**	0.060 ± 0.022**
ACAT			
Liver	2.15 ± 0.23	14.89 ± 1.47***	0.60 ± 0.07***
Intestine	1.60 ± 0.32	11.69 ± 1.52***	0.39 ± 0.05**
Cholesterol 7α-hydroxylase			
Liver	0.014 ± 0.002	0.028 ± 0.002***	0.006 ± 0.001**

Results (nmol product min^{-1} mg $protein^{-1}$) expressed as mean ± SEM.
*$p < 0.05$, **$p < 0.01$, ***$p < 0.001$—all significantly different from control animals.

hypercholesterolaemia, on the other hand, is characterized by apparent enhancement of intestinal synthesis with partially depressed hepatic synthesis. Cholesterol utilization in this model appears markedly impaired. These differences in cholesterol metabolism between diabetic and dietary-induced hypercholesterolaemic states may underlie the reduced susceptibility of diabetic animals to develop atherosclerosis.

The Role of the Sympathetic Nervous System in the Regulation of Cholesterol Metabolism. N. M. G. O'Meara, R. A. M. Devery, D. Owens, P. B. Collins, A. H. Johnson and G. H. Tomkin. *Department of Biochemistry, Royal College of Surgeons in Ireland, Dublin 2, and Department of Metabolic Medicine, The Adelaide Hospital, Dublin 8, Ireland*

The hypercholesterolaemia associated with acute[1] and chronic[2] stress has not been clearly explained. Although adrenergic mechanisms have been implicated, the exact mechanism by which the sympathetic nervous system regulates cholesterol metabolism is not apparent. This study investigates the effect of chemical sympathectomy on (i) serum lipoprotein cholesterol levels and (ii) the activity of 3-hydroxy-3-methylglutaryl coenzyme A reductase (HMGCoA reductase), the rate-limiting enzyme of cholesterol synthesis, in male New Zealand White rabbits. Sympathectomy was performed by the intraperitoneal administration of 6-hydroxydopamine, lipoproteins were fractionated by ultracentrifugation and the cholesterol content of the lipoprotein fractions was estimated using enzymatic colorimetric methods. Intestinal and hepatic HMGCoA reductase activities were measured by radioenzymatic procedures.

Total serum cholesterol was significantly reduced in the sympathectomized animals ($n = 6$) compared with the non-sympathectomized group ($n = 9$) (0.54 ± 0.04 vs. 0.91 ± 0.12 mmol/l, $p < 0.01$). This was reflected in the VLDL (0.02 ± 0.002 vs. 0.11 ± 0.02 mmol/l, $p < 0.01$), LDL (0.09 ± 0.01 vs. 0.27 ± 0.06 mmol/l, $p < 0.01$) and HDL_3 (0.27 ± 0.02 vs. 0.36 ± 0.03 mmol/l, $p < 0.05$) fractions. This reduced lipoprotein cholesterol concentration in the sympathectomized animals reflected a reduced cholesterol concentration in the lipoprotein particles of these animals. The specific activities of intestinal (0.007 ± 0.002 vs. 0.026 ± 0.003 nmol/min per mg,

$p < 0.001$) and hepatic (0.016 ± 0.005 vs. 0.039 ± 0.005 nmol/min per mg, $p < 0.01$) HMGCoA reductase were significantly reduced in the sympathectomized animals.

The reduced cholesterol concentration in the lipoprotein fractions suggests that the lower VLDL, LDL and HDL_3 cholesterol concentrations in the sympathectomized animals results from a reduced availability of cholesterol for lipoprotein formation in these animals. This may reflect the reduced rate of endogenous cholesterol synthesis in the liver and intestine of the sympathectomized model. It is therefore possible that catecholamines may be involved in the regulation of cholesterol metabolism by influencing cholesterol synthesis. While the molecular basis of such a control feature is currently unclear, it may explain the increased levels of cholesterol in the serum of humans following periods of stress.

[1] Friedman, M., Rosenman, R. H. and Carroll, V. (1958). *Circulation* **27**, 852–861.
[2] O'Donnell, L., O'Meara, N., Owens, D., Johnson, A., Collins, P. and Tomkin, G. (1987). *J. R. Soc. Med.* **80**, 339–342.

An Investigation into the Release of Cholesterol from the Isolated Perfused Rat Spleen.

P. A. Mayes[1], M. A. Mindham[2] and N. E. Miller[2]. [1]*Division of Biochemistry, Department of Veterinary Basic Sciences, Royal Veterinary College, London NW1 0TU, UK;* [2]*Department of Chemical Pathology and Metabolic Disorders, St Thomas' Hospital Medical School, London, UK*

A method was developed that enabled the rat spleen to be loaded with ^{3}H-cholesterol *in vivo*. [^{3}H]Cholesterol in acetone was added dropwise to stirred rat serum at 37°C. The acetone was blown off and blood was reconstituted by mixing the serum with erythrocytes. After incubations for 15 h at 37°C, over 80% of the radioactivity was associated with the erythrocytes, which were washed and suspended in 0.9% NaCl. 1 ml, containing approximately 20 μCi of [^{3}H]cholesterol was injected into a tail vein of a male Wistar rat (350 g). The erythrocytes were taken up rapidly by the spleen, which accumulated a maximum of 21% of the injected dose in 5 h, and then decreased.

In a series of four experiments, the spleens were isolated at 3-4 h following injection and perfused with rat blood at 30% haematocrit for 3 h[1]. Lipoprotein fractions were separated by ultracentrifugation, and extracted in chloroform/methanol (2 : 1). Erythrocytes were washed in 0.9% NaCl and extracted in chloroform/isopropanol (7 : 11).

A mean value of 27.5% of the [^{3}H]cholesterol in the spleen was released into the perfusate over 3 h, $13.4 \pm 1.6\%$ (SEM) was in lipoproteins and $14.1 \pm 1.7\%$ (SEM) was in erythrocytes. The rate of release of radioactivity was constant throughout the perfusion. Although similar amounts of radioactivity were detected in both erythrocytes and serum, the specific activity of cholesterol in the serum was four times as great owing to its lower free cholesterol content. The distribution of radioactivity in the lipoproteins indicated that 78% was in the higher density fractions $d = 1.063$–1.21. [^{3}H]Cholesterol ester represented 22% of the radioactivity released to the lipoprotein fraction $d = 1.075$–1.175 density and 4% of the $d = 1.175$–1.21 fraction. The absence of [^{3}H]cholesterol ester in other lipoprotein fractions is consistent with the absence of a cholesteryl ester transfer protein in rat blood. In addition, the specific activity of the cholesterol released to the HDL, in particular the $d = 1.175$–1.21 fraction, was much higher than other lipoproteins. These results support the view that HDL is the major lipoprotein involved in reverse cholesterol transport. The large amount of radioactivity associated with the erythrocytes, but at low specific activity, suggests a rapid exchange of cholesterol between them and the spleen. When a higher chemical potential of cholesterol is present in spleen cell membranes than in erythrocyte membranes, significant quantities of cholesterol would be expected to be transported from the spleen by this route. This conclusion is in keeping with the demonstration of a role for erythrocytes in cholesterol transport to the liver and the formation of bile acids[2].

[1] Mindham, M. A., Mayes, P. A. and Miller, N. E. *Biochem. Soc. Trans.* (in press).
[2] Laker, M. E. and Mayes, P. A. (1985). *Biochem. Soc. Trans.* **13**, 142–143.

The Role of Insulin, Glucocorticoids and Thyroid Hormones in Controlling Hepatic LDL Catabolism. A. M. Salter[1], N. F. Brown[1], S. C. Fisher[1], R. Fears[2] and D. N. Brindley[1]. [1]*Department of Biochemistry, University of Nottingham Medical School, Queen's Medical Centre, Nottingham NG7 2UH, UK;* [2]*Beechams Pharmaceuticals, Biosciences Research Centre, Epsom, UK*

Rat hepatocytes were incubated in monolayer culture for 20 h in 10% newborn calf serum and then for 16 h in serum-free medium containing 2 g of albumin/l and 10 nM of hormones indicated. Specific, dextran-sulphate-releasable, binding of LDL was determined at 4°C. Results (mean ± SEM) are summarized below.

Addition	n	Relative binding (%)
None	9	100
T_3	9	131 ± 11 (p <0.02)
Insulin	8	128 ± 7 (p < 0.01)
Dexamethasone	9	62 ± 7 (p < 0.001)

Whereas the effects of insulin and dexamethasone were mutually antagonistic, T_3 was unable to reverse the decrease in binding brought about by dexamethasone. The increases in binding brought about by insulin and T_3 were additive. Insulin was found to have a relatively rapid effect with increases in binding being found after 1 h of incubation. In contrast, the effects of T_3 and dexamethasone were longer-term, with maximum responses occurring between 6 and 24 h of incubation. Preliminary results suggest that these changes in binding are accompanied by parallel changes in LDL degradation.

Poorly controlled diabetes and metabolic stress are often associated with elevated plasma cholesterol concentrations and increased prevalence of atherosclerosis. In these conditions the actions of glucocorticoids may prevail over those of insulin. Our results suggest that this would result in a down-regulation in hepatic LDL receptors, which may explain the high plasma cholesterol concentrations. Hypothyroidism is also associated with hypercholesterolaemia. Again this may be explained by a reduced effect of thyroid hormones on the expression of LDL receptors in the liver.

Corneal Arcus and Clinical Ischaemic Heart Disease: Lessons from Familial Hypercholesterolaemia.

A. E. Winder. *Department of Chemical Pathology, Royal Infirmary and Medical School, Leicester LE1 5WW, UK*

Associations between corneal arcus, dyslipoproteinaemia and clinical IHD are generally too soft for individual risk prediction, perhaps because duration and consistency of any lipid abnormality recorded at the time of assessment of arcus and cardiac status is uncertain. Any relationship may be clarified by observations in FH, where the extent of dyslipoproteinaemia is broadly constant from early life to diagnosis and treatment, allowing calculation of integrated exposure to dyslipoproteinaemia. Various clinical and biochemical observations were recorded for 51 male and 55 female FH heterozygotes at presentation, including corneal arcus graded on a scale of 0–4. Arcus progression correlated with age, and correlation was not strengthened by incorporating integrated terms such as cholesterol × age or HDL/TC ratio, suggesting a saturation, time- rather than dose-dependent process. Similar findings arose for seven homozygotes. Having established an association between corneal arcus and age, the relationship with clinical IHD was noted for the 106 new patients, and 84 further FH heterozygotes assessed during treatment. In both series, total age range 8–73 years, patients with clinical IHD showed a below-average expression of corneal arcus with age, and this did not obviously reflect an ascertainment bias in referrals to the lipid clinic.

Corneal arcus is a useful qualitative marker of dyslipoproteinaemia, and in FH may lead to presentation and diagnosis, but progression is not valuable in identifying the patient at high risk of clinical ischaemic heart disease. As this result is quite clear cut, any relationship in less specific lipid disorders is likely to be even less predictive.

Plasma Chylomicron (Remnant) Removal in Patients with Documented Coronary Artery Disease.

P. H. E. Groot, X. H. Krauss, E. van Ramshorst, W. A. van Stiphout, H. Jansen, S. Chin-On and L. Havekes. *Departments of Biochemistry 1 and Epidemiology, Erasmus University Rotterdam; Department of Cardiology, Zuiderziekenhuis Rotterdam; and Gaubius Institute TNO, Leiden, The Netherlands*

To investigate the possible role of chylomicron remnants in atherogenesis, we performed a study on the postprandial handling of a standardized oral fat load in normolipidaemic patients who had recently undergone coronary bypass surgery (CAD patients) and non-atherosclerotic normolipidaemic patients who had undergone coronary angiography for complaints of angina pectoris (P). Exclusion criteria were: LDL-cholesterol >200 mg%, triglycerides >200 mg%, hypertension or diabetes. All patients (20 CAD and 20 P) were males of ages between 35 and 65 years. To obtain comparable populations, CAD and P entering the study were matched for age (52 ± 1 and 51 ± 1 years), Quetelet index (25 ± 0.6 and 25 ± 0.4) and fasting levels of cholesterol (220 ± 8 and 215 ± 6 mg%). Fasting plasma levels of LDL-cholesterol (158 ± 6 vs. 152 ± 6 mg%), VLDL-cholesterol (26 ± 3 vs. 23 ± 4 mg%) and triglycerides (145 ± 8 vs. 126 ± 8 mg%) were not different in CAD and P, but HDL-cholesterol (33 ± 2 vs. 43 ± 2 mg%) and HDL-3-cholesterol (24 ± 1 vs. 31 ± 2 mg%) were statistically significantly lower ($p < 0.003$, unpaired two-tailed t-test). The oral fat load, consisting of cream (77.5 g fat/m^2) supplemented with cholesterol in egg yolks (0.5 g/m^2) and retinyl palmitate (27 000 IU/m^2) was given to patients after an overnight fast. No drugs that could affect lipoprotein metabolism were used in the period before and during the study. Blood samples were obtained every 2 h for 14 h, and a final sample was obtained 24 h after the fat load. During this period no other nutrients were taken. Plasma samples were analysed for total and $d < 1.019$ g/ml and $d > 1.019$ g/ml cholesterol, triglycerides and retinyl palmitate concentrations. Total plasma cholesterol hardly changed (peak values 225 ± 8 vs. 221 ± 6 mg% for CAD and P respectively). Plasma values for plasma triglycerides (TG) and retinylpalmitate (RP) increased in CAD and P in parallel and peaked at $t = 6$ h (456 ± 46 vs. 386 ± 54 mg% and 2102 ± 245 vs. 1917 ± 256 μg/ml. In the descending phase of the post-prandial response, significant differences were found between CAD and P: 10 h TG, 184 ± 18 vs. 124 ± 19 mg%*; 10 h RP, 1204 ± 195 vs. 649 ± 124 μg/ml*; 12 h TG, 136 ± 11 vs. 92 ± 7**; 12 h RP, 696 ± 118 vs. 350 ± 53 μg/ml**; 14 h TG, 114 ± 8 vs. 90 ± 6 mg%*; 14 h RP, 470 ± 74 vs. 251 ± 28 μg/ml**; 24 h TG, 138 ± 8 vs. 119 ± 7 mg%; 24 h RP, 211 ± 25 vs. 136 ± 12 μg/ml** (*$p < 0.03$; **$p < 0.01$ unpaired two tailed t-test). Similar differences were found in the $d < 1.019$ g/ml fractions. These data indicate that chylomicron remnant removal is delayed in normolipidaemic CAD patients compared with P, while HDL cholesterol levels are lower.

Abnormalities of Receptor- and Non-Receptor-Mediated Catabolism of Low-Density Lipoprotein (LDL) in Hypertriglyceridaemia.

Markku J. Savolainen and Y. Antero Kesäniemi. *Department of Internal Medicine, University of Oulu, Kajaanintie 50, SF-90220 Oulu, Finland*

Several abnormalities of LDL metabolism have been reported in hypertriglyceridaemic patients. Low LDL levels in these subjects have been suggested as being due to the increased catabolism of LDL as a result of the enhanced receptor-induced LDL degradation. On the other hand, altered LDL composition in hypertriglyceridaemia with small, dense and triglyceride-rich, cholesteryl-ester-poor particles has been shown to poorly suppress the LDL receptor activity in cell culture studies, suggesting increased receptor-mediated mechanism for LDL removal. We therefore undertook this study to specifically investigate the role of receptor and non-receptor pathways for LDL catabolism in hypertriglyceridaemia.

Nine subjects with various plasma triglyceride levels were recruited for the study. The quantitation of the receptor- and non-receptor-mediated catabolism of LDL apoprotein B was performed by using autologous native and glucosylated LDL, radio-labelled with either iodine 131 or 125. The fractional catabolic rate (FCR) of native LDL (total LDL catabolism) ranged from 0.299 (pools/day) to 1.078, that of the glucosylated LDL (non-receptor pathway) from 0.038 to 0.258, and that of the receptor-mediated LDL clearance (the difference between the total catabolism and the catabolism for glucosylated LDL) from 0.245 to 0.819. Plasma triglyceride values among the subjects were between 1.28 and 6.79 mmol/l.

A significant correlation was observed between the plasma triglyceride values and the FCRs for total LDL catabolism ($r = 0.819$). This was due to the close correlation between the triglyceride levels and the FCR values for the receptor-mediated removal of LDL ($r = 0.889$). However, the non-receptor-mediated catabolism of LDL was also increased in parallel with the elevation of the plasma triglycerides ($r = 0.841$). Overall, the relative proportion of the receptor pathway for LDL catabolism remained quite constant (72.6% ± 6.1, SD) regardless of the plasma triglyceride concentration ($r = -0.063$). These data indicate multiple abnormalities of LDL metabolism in hypertriglyceridaemic subjects. The enhanced LDL receptor activity is seemingly mainly responsible for the remarkably fast clearance of LDL in hypertriglyceridaemia, but the accelerated receptor-independent pathway is also a contributing factor. The latter may well be related to the development of premature atherosclerosis observed in some hypertriglyceridaemic patients.

"Fit statt Fett" (Fit instead of Fat)—An Austrian Interventional Programme against Atherosclerosis. J. Kaliman, P. Fitscha, E. Rasinger, G. Pakesch, H. Sinzinger, K. Widhalm and M.-T. Trauttmansdorff. *Atherosclerosis Research Group (ASF) Vienna, Atherosclerosis and Thrombosis Research Group of the Austrian Academy of Sciences (ATK) Vienna, and Austrian Assoc. Res. Atherosclerosis (AMFA), Vienna, Austria*

In Austria the death rate from cardiovascular disease approached 54% in 1986. Whereas in other Western countries there has been a decline in coronary artery disease, in Austria it is still increasing. Major reasons for this are a total fat intake of nearly 50% of total energy, an annual increase of 1% in energy consumption and a high rate of animal fat intake. Therefore in 1987 we started a campaign consisting of a variety of information activities and screening of the population with regard to cholesterol and triglyceride levels. The aim of these activities is to reduce the cardiovascular death rate by 1% a year as of 1988. Our programme has included the following.

1. General information about atherosclerosis and everyday new dietary recommendations are given over a Viennese telephone line (15 72).
2. In cooperation with the Viennese physicians' organization, a banking institute and the Austrian television and broadcasting company, a one-month promotion programme has been carried out in order to inform the population about the risk factors for atherosclerosis and, in particular, about hypercholesterolaemia.
3. A representative population inquiry has been launched to evaluate the knowledge of the population and physicians and their readiness to cooperate.
4. Regular information in newspapers is supporting this campaign.
5. Screening of the population for risk factors takes place in factories and companies to discover people at high risk. The first data on the response of the population and preliminary screening results are presented.
6. An Austrian consensus has been edited giving new "normal values" for cholesterol and proposing screening strategies.

Screening for Cardiovascular Risk—The Role of the General Practitioner.

Shirley R. McEwan. *2 Russell Place, Dundee DD3 7RU; Department of Clinical Pharmacology, Ninewells Medical School, Dundee*

Serum lipid levels in the population need to be reduced to favourably affect the incidence of cardiovascular disease in Britain[1]. Population and high-risk approaches are complementary—not mutually exclusive[2]. General practitioners have unique access to their patients for identifying individuals particularly at risk and securing their compliance with treatment strategies[3].

This study aims to characterize the cardiovascular risk profile by systematic screening of the full cohort of 400 apparently healthy men in the 35-55 age group in one Scottish east coast urban practice and to identify which of these risk factors respond to appropriate counselling by the family doctor.

Patients are initially contacted directly by telephone—89% response as compared with 50% response to letter invitation. Patients are then screened by the practice nurse, using a single-page proforma that facilitates recording, patient assessment and computerization for data analysis.

A pilot study of 100 patients, randomly selected from the target group and re-assessed at six months, showed a much higher than suspected incidence of cardiovascular risk factors, particularly cigarette smoking 55%, hypertension (>150/90) 43%, hypercholesterolaemia (>6.5 mmol/l) 55%, excess alcohol consumption (>21 units/week) 31%, and obesity (BMI >27.6) 18%[4].

Smoking and hypertension respond favourably to counselling, but measures to reduce hypercholesterolaemia, obesity and alcohol abuse are less readily accepted.

	Initial	6/12 Follow-up	
Cigarette smoking	55%	44%	$p < 0.001$
Hypertension (>150/90)	43%	16%	$p < 0.001$
Cholesterol (mean mmol/l)	6.67	6.39	NS
Alcohol excess	31%	26%	NS
Obesity	18%	17%	NS

Conclusion: Cigarette smoking and hypertension can both be ameliorated by effective CP screening and counselling. Successful measures to modulate hypercholesterolaemia, obesity and excess ethanol intake still need to be devised.

[1] *Br. Cardiac Soc. Working Group Report on C.D. Prevention* (1987), p. 4.
[2] *Study Group of European Atherosclerosis Society (1987) Eur. Heart J.* **8**, 78–80.
[3] *RCGP Report* No. 19 (1981), pp. 1–6.
[4] McEwan, S. R. (1987) *The Practitioner* (in press).

Modulation of LDL Binding by Cyclic AMP in Human Vascular Smooth Cells and Skin Fibroblasts.

Aliya Middleton, Nicola Bonser and Bruce Middleton. *Department of Biochemistry, University of Nottingham Medical School, Queen's Medical Centre, Nottingham*

The role of cAMP in LDL metabolism in vascular smooth muscle cells (SMC) and fibroblasts is not well understood, and the existing evidence is conflicting. Raising cellular cAMP has been reported to inhibit LDL metabolism by some authors[1,2], whereas others have found no effect[3,4].

In this study cellular cAMP was increased by using the cAMP analogues db-cAMP (1 mM) and CTP-cAMP (1 mM), forskolin (0.1 mM)—an adenylate cyclase activator—and methyl isobutyl xanthine (MIX) (0.25 mM)—a phosphodiesterase inhibitor. Cultures were incubated for 24 h in a medium containing human lipoprotein-deficient serum (LPDS) with or without these agents. LDL binding, measured at 4° for 2 h, was stimulated in fibroblasts by db-cAMP (140% of control values), CTP-cAMP (222%) and forskolin (160%); MIX, however, caused an inhibition (57%). In SMC (obtained from the veins of human umbilical cords) db-cAMP increased binding at 4° (192%) and binding (154%), internalization (136%), and degradation (150%) measured at 37°.

In another series of experiments, fibroblasts or SMC were incubated with LPDS medium for 24 h to up-regulate the number of LDL receptors, followed by short (3 h) or long (24 h) exposure to cAMP elevating agents. The results are presented in the Table.

LDL binding at 4° (percentage of binding with LPDS alone)

Addition time (h)	Fibroblasts			SMC	
	db-cAMP	Forskolin	MIX	Forskolin	MIX
3	80 ± 12	63 ± 3**	75 ± 4**	73 ± 4**	78 ± 5**
24	118 ± 3**	201 ± 4***	85 ± 2*	146 ± 1**	56 ± 5**

*$p < 0.02$; **$p < 0.01$; ***$p < 0.001$.

The magnitude and direction of the effects are clearly time-dependent. A short incubation with all three agents reduced LDL binding. Continuing the incubation for 24 h reversed the effect exerted by forskolin to cause an increase in LDL binding, whereas the inhibition caused by MIX was maintained. The time dependence of the effect could explain the conflicting results reported in the literature[1–4]. The reason for the difference between the action of forskolin and MIX after 24 h is as yet unclear.

These results suggest that changes in cellular cAMP levels could play an important role in regulating LDL metabolism in fibroblasts and SMC.

[1] Maziere, J. C. *et al.* (1983), *Biochem. Biophys. Res. Commun.* **112**, 795.
[2] Stout, R. W. and Bierman, E. L. (1983). *Atherosclerosis* **46**, 13.
[3] Schonfeld, G. *et al.* (1980). *J. Clin. Endocrinol Metabol.* **51**, 662.
[4] Brown, M. S. and Goldstein, J. L. (1975). *Cell* **6**, 307.

Is Atherosclerosis a Disease of the Outside of the Artery? Robert F. G. Booth, Andrew C. Honey, David G. Hassall, Julian Beesly, Salvador Moncada and John F. Martin. *The Wellcome Research Laboratories, Beckenham, Kent, U.K.*

Accumulation of macrophages in the intima, migration into and proliferation of smooth muscle cells within the intima, foam-cell formation and accumulation of cholesteryl esters are the earliest changes observed to occur during the development of atherosclerosis. Many studies have suggested that these changes occur subsequent to endothelial cell damage and platelet deposition. We now present evidence that atherosclerotic lesions can occur rapidly in the presence of a morphologically intact endothelium as a result of manipulation of the outer layer of the vessel wall. Twenty-four rabbits were separated into two dietary groups, one fed normal laboratory chow, the other the same diet supplemented with 1 g/day cholesterol. At day 0 of the diet a hollow silastic collar was positioned around the outside of the left carotid artery (LCA) and filled with sterile saline (0.9% w/v). The right carotid artery (RCA) was sham-operated and no collar positioned. At day 14, in half of the animals from each group, the carotid arteries were removed, washed, freeze-clamped and the lipids extracted. The arterial content of cholesterol (C) and cholesteryl ester (CE) was measured. In the remaining animals the arteries were perfuse-fixed *in situ*. The LCAs were subdivided into three regions: a mid-region from within the collar (MR), a regional proximal to the collar (PR) and a distal region (DR). These regions were subdivided for histology and scanning EM. Medial/intimal ratios (M/I) of transverse sections of each region were evaluated by image analysis.

	Normal diet		High-cholesterol diet	
	M/I	CE (pmol/mg)	M/I	CE (pmol/mg)
LCA-PR	19.6	1.01	16.6	2.00
LCA-MR	6.5	1.72	5.0	3.83
CLA-DR	17.0	0.92	12.6	2.22
RCA	21.7	0.66	19.7	0.72

Histology revealed intimal monocyte infiltration and SMC proliferation. Scanning EM revealed no observable endothelial damage. There was foam-cell formation in the high-cholesterol group. The lesion was highly focal. We conclude that early atherosclerotic lesions may result from damage to the outer layers of blood vessels.

Monocyte Adherence and Chemotaxis are Inhibited by Carbacyclin. David G. Hassall, Judi Ward, Salvador Moncada, John F. Martin and Robert F. G. Booth. *The Wellcome Research Laboratories, Beckenham, Kent, U.K.*

The adherence of blood monocytes to the arterial endothelium and subsequent migration into the arterial intima are early events in the development of atherosclerotic lesions. After migration to the intima, it is believed that the monocytes/macrophages may release growth factors that stimulate smooth muscle cell proliferation. The precise factors that stimulate monocyte adherence and chemotaxis are undefined. However, it is known that exposure of endothelial cells to either low density lipoproteins (LDL), very low density lipoproteins (VLDL) or Interleukin I increased the adherence of monocytes; moreover, oxidized LDL and certain factors secreted by both smooth muscle cell and endothelial cell cultures are chemotactic for monocytes. The factors that oppose these pro-adherent and pro-chemotactic factors are unknown. In the present series of experiments it is confirmed that exposure of endothelial cell monolayers to LDL (100 μg/ml) causes a two-fold increase in human peripheral blood monocyte adherence and it has been demonstrated that carbacyclin (1×10^{-7} M), a stable prostacyclin analogue, inhibits the LDL potentiation of monocyte adherence. In the presence of the monocyte chemotactic agent f-Met-Leu-Phe (FMLP, 5×10^{-8} M) the migration of monocytes is stimulated five-fold. Exposure of monocytes to carbacyclin (1×10^{-6} M) reduces monocyte chemotaxis to FMLP (20% inhibition), and in the additional presence of the cAMP phosphodiesterase inhibitor HL725 (1 μm) the inhibition of monocyte chemotaxis is potentiated (50%), suggesting a cAMP-dependent inhibition of chemotaxis. Direct measurements of intracellular cAMP levels in monocytes have confirmed that an elevation in cAMP correlates with an inhibition of monocyte chemotaxis. Prostacyclin (1×10^{-7} M) also inhibits monocyte chemotaxis in response to FMLP (36% inhibition). These results suggest that the production of prostacyclin by the vessel wall may be important in the regulation of monocyte behaviour. Moreover, the impairment of vessel wall prostacyclin production that is observed in hyperlipidaemia may directly contribute to increased monocyte adherence and migration.

Binding of LDL to Heparin-Sepharose and Arterial Proteoglycans: Inhibition by Serum High-Molecular-Weight Components. H. J. Kempen and R. Buytenhek. *Gaubius Institute TNO, Herenstraat 5d, 2313 AD Leiden, The Netherlands*

In the first part of this study the interaction of human LDL with heparin immobilized on Sepharose was reinvestigated. Binding of isolated LDL (stabilized with human serum albumin) was compared with that of LDL in full serum.

(1) Binding of isolated LDL was decreased by 10 or 30 mM $CaCl_2$ but was not affected by $MgCl_2$. In contrast, with full serum LDL binding was increased by divalent cations.

(2) In both situations binding of LDL was saturable, but the maximum degree of binding that could be reached was much higher with isolated LDL than with LDL in full serum. This could be ascribed to an inhibitory action of factor(s) found in the lipoprotein-free fraction (LPF) of serum. The effect of this factor(s) was diminished in the presence of $CaCl_2$, or $MgCl_2$, which suggests that the stimulation of LDL-binding by these cations in full serum is due to suppression of the inhibitory activity of this factor(s).

(3) The inhibitory factor(s) in the LPF fraction can be partially purified by absorption to heparin-Sepharose, followed by elution with 6 M guanidine choloride. The resulting preparation had an about 50-fold higher specific activity.

(4) Upon gel filtration, the inhibitory activity has an apparent molecular weight of

greater than 900 kD. It seems to be a protein since it is trypsin-sensitive, with free amino groups and S—S bridges being essential for its activity, since activity loss occurs upon acetylation and reduction with dithiothreitol.

In subsequent experiments the interaction of LDL with bovine arterial proteoglycans was studied. The above-described inhibitory effects of LPS could essentially be reproduced.

Investigation of the Control of Gene Expression in Cholesterol-loaded Macrophages. Lesley Graham, John Davison, Joost Jobsis and Steve Humphries. *Charing Cross Sunley Research Centre, Lurgan Avenue, London W6 8LW, UK*

Cholesterol-loaded macrophages or "foam cells" form a significant proportion of atherosclerotic tissue, and are believed to be derived from circulating blood monocytes. Since foam cells have been identified in fatty streaks, it seems possible that they may play a major role in lesion formation. Although a great deal is now known about cholesterol homeostasis in macrophages, the exact mechanism of *in vivo* foam cell formation remains unknown. We have used standard methodology to induce *in vitro* foam-cell formation in order to investigate whether levels of mRNA for certain specific "candidate" genes are altered in cholesterol-loaded macrophages.

Peripheral blood monocytes were isolated and cultured according to standard procedures. RNA was extracted from control and acetyl-LDL (AcLDL) treated macrophages and analysed by slot blot analysis using cDNA probes for ApoE, actin and the LDL-receptor. Preliminary studies demonstrated that ApoE mRNA levels were increased in cholesterol-loaded macrophages, whereas LDL-receptor and actin mRNA levels were unchanged relative to controls. Further studies are in progress to establish whether the human cell lines U937, HL-60 or THP-1 yield similar results and could therefore be used as model systems for studying mechanisms of foam-cell formation.

Macrophage Protease Activity towards Native and Modified Low Density Lipoproteins. Sara M. Rankin, Marion E. Knowles and David S. Leake. *Department of Pharmacology, King's College London, Strand, London WC2R 2LS, UK*

Macrophage-derived foam cells are a prominent feature of atherosclerosis. It has been shown that LDL is oxidized by arterial cells or macrophages and then internalized rapidly by acetyl-LDL receptors on macrophages and degraded in lysosomes[1,2]. We have shown previously that sonicates of mouse resident peritoneal macrophages contain both acidic (probably lysosomal) and neutral protease activities toward LDL[3].

The identity of the neutral proteases is unknown, but they are inhibited substantially by preincubation at 70°C for 10 min and by incubation with foetal calf serum (1%) but not with bovine serum albumin (50 mg/ml), α_1-antitrypsin (100 μg/ml), α_2-macroglobulin (50 μg/ml), aprotinin (2 μg/ml), PMSF (806 μM) or TLCK (135 μM).

A comparison was made of the activities of macrophage proteases toward native and modified LDL. ^{125}I-Labelled LDL (125 μg protein/ml) in F10 medium with added $FeSO_4$ (3 μM) was incubated for 24 h with cultured macrophages (macrophage-modified LDL) or cell-free dishes (control LDL). LDL was also incubated for 24 h in F10 with added $CuSO_4$ (100 μM). The LDLs were then reisolated by ultracentrifugation. These LDLs, and also native and acetylated LDL, were incubated at pH 4.5 for 24 h at 25 μg protein/ml with a macrophage sonicate (25 μg protein/ml) containing 1 mM EDTA and 5 mM dithiothreitol. The non-iodide, trichloroacetic-acid-soluble degradation products were measured.

Type of LDL	Proteolysis of LDL by a macrophage sonicate at pH 4.5 (μg protein in 24 h; mean $\pm$ SEM, $n = 4$)
Native	1.53 $\pm$ 0.01
Acetyl	2.00 $\pm$ 0.04
Control	1.36 $\pm$ 0.02
Macrophage-modified	0.369 $\pm$ 0.017
Cu^{2+}-oxidized	0.148 $\pm$ 0.004

The acidic proteases were much less active towards macrophage-modified and Cu^{2+}-oxidized LDL than towards native or control LDL. This may be due to alterations in the structure of apolipoprotein B100 or to protease inactivation by LDL oxidation products.

Neutral protease activity at pH 8.5 was also much less active toward Cu^{2+}-oxidized than native LDL, but, in contrast with the acidic proteases, was less active toward acetyl-LDL.

Macrophages in culture degraded macrophage-modified and Cu^{2+}-oxidized LDL much faster than native LDL. This suggests that lysosomal degradation is not the rate-limiting step in the handling of modified LDL by macrophages. The relatively small amounts of radioactivity that did accumulate in the cells, however, were considerably greater for macrophage-modified and Cu^{2+}-oxidized LDL than for native or acetylated LDL. It has yet to be determined if this is of any significance as regards atherogenesis.

[1] Henriksen, T., Mahoney, E. M. and Steinberg, D. (1981). *Proc Natl Acad Sci USA* **78**, 6499.
[2] Rankin, S. M. and Leake, D. S. (1986). *Biochem. Soc. Trans.* **14**, 1084.
[3] Rankin, S. M. and Leake, D. S. (1987). *Biochem. Soc. Trans.* **15**, 485.

Hypocholesterolaemic Action of 1-Ethoxysilatrane. Prashant P. Mehta, T. Ramasarma and C. K. R. Kurup. *Department of Biochemistry, Indian Institute of Science, Bangalore-560 012, India*

Silatranes are a class of organo-silicon compounds that are heterocyclic derivatives of pentacoordinate silicon. They have been shown to possess a variety of biological activities, including antitumour, insecticidal, antimicrobial and wound-healing effects as well as promotion of the growth of connective tissue and hair[1]. The concentration of silicon in aortic walls has been reported to decrease in atherosclerosis, and it has been suggested that silicon possesses antiatheromatous and antisclerotic action[2]. The hypocholesterolaemic action of 1-ethoxysilatrane has been investigated. When administered intraperitoneally to the rat (5–50 mg/day per animal) for 3 weeks, the levels of cholesterol in the circulation decreased. The concentration of triacylglycerols in serum was unaffected, while phospholipids showed a significant decrease. Mitochondria isolated from the livers of silatrane-administered animals showed no significant change in oxidative or phosphorylating activity. The population of mitochondria in liver showed no significant increase. To gain insight into the mechanism of action of the compound, the specific activity of HMGCoA reductase in liver microsomes was assayed and was found to decrease by 43% in the silatrane-administered animals. Thus the action of 1-ethoxysilatrane appears to be confined to cholesterol biosynthesis, unlike other hypocholesterolaemic agents such as clofibrate[3] and diethyl hexyl phthalate[4], which show additional effects. The compound therefore offers a good model for the study of the regulation of HMGCoA reductase and an answer for the renewed efforts to find more specific and less toxic agents for use in the control of hypercholesterolaemia.

Effect of administration of 1-ethoxysilatrane on the concentration of serum cholesterol in the rat

Silatrane (mg/rat per day)	Serum cholesterol (mg/dl)		Decrease (%)
	Control	Silatrane-treated	
1	74 ± 4	62 ± 0.1	16 ± 3
5	73 ± 4	55 ± 4	24 ± 3
10	70 ± 7	53 ± 7	24 ± 3
25	70 ± 15	53 ± 7	21 ± 9
50	70 ± 3	53 ± 2	25 ± 1

Effect of administration of 1-ethoxysilatrane on serum and liver components

Component	Control	Silatrane-treated
Serum		
Cholesterol (mg/dl)	73 ± 4	55 ± 4
Triacylglycerols (mg glycerol/dl)	27.3 ± 1.0	22.8 ± 3.0
Phospholipids (mg phosphorus/dl)	6.1 ± 0.7	3.2 ± 0.7
Liver		
HMGCoA Reductase (pmol mevalonate formed/min per mg microsomal protein)	651 ± 120	371 ± 135

[1] Voronkov, M. G. (1979). *Top. Curr. Chem.* **84**, 78–135.

[2] Loeper, J., Loeper, J. and Fragny, M. (1978). In *Biochemistry of Silicon and Related Problems* (ed. G. Bendz and I. Lindquist, pp. 281–296. Plenum Press, New York.

[3] Kurup, C. K. R., Aithal, H. N. and Ramasarma, T. (1970). *Biochem. J.* **116**, 773–779.

[4] Nair, N. and Kurup, C. K. R. (1986). *Biochem. Pharmacol.* **35**, 3441–3445.

Immunological Investigation of the Changes in the Antigenic Structure of Human Aortic Elastin in Ageing and Atherosclerosis. St. Baydanoff, G. Nicoloff and Ch. Alexiev. *University School of Medicine, Department of Biology, 5800 Pleven, Karl Marx Street 1, Bulgaria*

It is well known that the antigenic determinants on elastin can be classified functionally into two categories: major determinants, related to the cross-linking domain, which show cross-reactivity between species; and limited, species-specific, determinants in non-cross-linked regions of the molecule[1]. This work describes an investigation for determination of the antigenic changes of human aortic elastin from healthy subjects of different age, killed by accident, grouped into seven age groups within the age range between human foetus and 75 years. All the preparations (up to group VI) were taken from regions without any visible changes along the intima. Group VII (60–75 years old) was divided into two sub-groups: VII A—including preparations from the macro- and microscopically normal areas between atherosclerotic plaques; and VII B—including preparations from the very atherosclerotic plaques from the same aortas. Anti-elastin immune serum was produced by subcutaneous immunization of young male sheep with aortic alpha-elastin from group VII A. The anti-elastin antibodies, showing cross-reactivity, were consumed by incubation with insoluble chick aortic elastin. Then the serum was tested by an enzyme-linked immunosorbent assay (ELISA) with the alpha-elastins from the different age groups, and some age-related changes in their antigenic structure were established. The highest extinction values were found with the VII A group and the lowest with group VII B, the difference being statistically significant ($p_t = 0.001$). Probably, the atherosclerotic process may first involve the phylogenetically younger, species-specific part of the elastin macromolecule, while the cross-reacting cross-linked regions seem to be more stable.

[1] Mecham, R. P. and Lange, G. (1982). *Biochemistry* **21**, 669–673.

Blood Serum Atherogenicity Associated with Coronary Atherosclerosis (Non-Hyperlipidaemic): Evidence for Non-Lipid Factor Providing Atherogenicity of Low Density Lipoproteins. A. N. Orekhov. *Institute of Experimental Cardiology, USSR Cardiology Research Centre, 121552 Moscow, USSR*

To reveal the presence of atherogenic potential in the blood serum obtained from patients with angiographically assessed coronary atherosclerosis (non-hyperlipidaemic), we used primary cultures of subendothelial cells isolated by collagenase from unaffected human aortic intima. We have already demonstrated that such cultures are made up mostly of typical and modified smooth muscle cells[1]. Within 24 h of cultivation with a 40% sera of patients suffering from coronary atherosclerosis, the total intracellular cholesterol level increased two- to five-fold[2]. Cultivation with the sera of healthy subjects had no effect on the intracellular cholesterol level. The sera of patients were separated by ultracentrifugation into two fractions: total lipoprotein fraction containing the main classes of lipoproteins; and a lipoprotein-deficient fraction. The former, but not the lipoprotein-deficient fraction, was characterized by atherogenicity, i.e. the ability to induce the accumulation of intracellular cholesterol. Lipoproteins of the patients' serum were separated into main classes: low density lipoproteins

(LDL), very low density lipoproteins (VLDL) and high density lipoproteins (HDL_2 and HDL_3). An atherogenic component of the serum capable of stimulating the deposition of intracellular cholesterol was represented by LDL and, in one case, VLDL, but not by other classes of lipoproteins. LDL and other lipoproteins isolated from the blood serum of healthy subjects failed to raise the cholesterol content in cultured cells, i.e. they were non-atherogenic. Stimultaneous addition to the culture of a lipoprotein-deficient fraction from the patients' blood serum and the total lipoprotein fraction or LDL isolated from the serum of healthy subjects brought about the accumulation of intracellular cholesterol, which suggests that the patients' serum contains a non-lipoprotein component capable of imparting atherogenic properties to the initially non-atherogenic LDL. Atherogenicity of the patients' serum can be sharply reduced or even completely eliminated by passing it through a sorbent containing LDL immobilized on agarose. After this procedure, regeneration of the column by glycine buffer, pH 2.5, was performed. We failed to detect measurable amounts of cholesterol or apoB in the eluate, although pooling of the pH 2.5 eluate with the serum that lost atherogenicity after passing through the LDL-sorbent partially restored its atherogenic potential. Simultaneous addition to the culture of the eluate derived from atherogenic serum of a patient and LDL obtained from the serum of a healthy donor caused a substantial accumulation of intracellular cholesterol, whereas LDL taken separately failed to alter the cholesterol level.

[1] Orekhov, A. N., Tertov, V. V., Novikov, I. D. *et al.* (1985). *Exp. Mol. Pathol.* **42**, 117–137.
[2] Chazov, E. I., Tertov, V. V., Orekhov, A. N. *et al.* (1986). *Lancet* **ii**, 595–598.

Homogeneity of Thromboxane Receptors in the Dog.

G. T. G., Swayne, J. Maguire and D. A. A. Owen. *Department of Pharmacology, Smith Kline & French Research Ltd, The Frythe, Welwyn, Herts AL6 9AR, UK*

Evidence for the existence of multiple receptor sites has classically been derived from differential potencies of antagonists when assayed in different tissues. The availability of structurally different thromboxane receptor antagonists has allowed investigation of receptor homogeneity. The possibility that the thromboxane receptor is different from platelets and vascular tissue is largely based on experimental findings in the dog[1,2]. We have assayed the potency of a variety of structurally different antagonists (ICI 185282, SQ 29548, Sulotroban (BM 13177), Daltroban (BM 13505), L-636499 and L-640035) on human/dog platelet binding and aggregation as well as dog saphenous vein contraction.

The binding assay used was that of Mais *et al.*[3], which measured the specific displacement of [^{125}I]PTA-OH binding on human/dog washed platelets. Platelet aggregation induced by the thromboxane-mimetic U46619 was performed on human/dog washed cells based on that of Born[4]. Isolated strips of dog saphenous vein were mounted in organ baths containing Krebs solution. Changes in isometric tension were recorded to cumulative increases in concentration of U46619 to just maximum, whereupon cumulative concentrations of the antagonist were added to the bath from which a concentration that produced a 50% inhibition was derived (IC_{50}). All values are derived from dose response graphs. Linear correlation coefficients were determined by the least squares method.

The results shown in the Table clearly indicate a similar rank order of potency in each of the five assay systems used. ICI 185282 and SQ 29548 were found to be most potent with activities varying from 1.6×10^{-9} to 6.6×10^{-8} M, depending on the assay used. L-640035 was consistently the least potent.

Potency of TXA_2 antagonists: IC_{50}, molar (rank order)

	Human binding	Dog binding	Dog aggregation	Dog saphenous	Human aggregation
ICI 185282	7.0×10^{-9}(1)	3.0×10^{-8}(3)	4.3×10^{-9}(2)	6.6×10^{-8}(2)	3.9×10^{-8}(3)
SQ 29548	1.1×10^{-8}(2)	1.2×10^{-8}(1)	N/A	2.0×10^{-8}(1)	1.6×10^{-9}(1)
BM 13505	2.9×10^{-8}(3)	1.6×10^{-8}(2)	1.4×10^{-9}(1)	2.0×10^{-7}(3)	1.5×10^{-8}(2)
BM 13177	9.3×10^{-7}(4)	7.0×10^{-7}(4)	4.3×10^{-7}(4)	2.4×10^{-6}(4)	2.8×10^{-6}(4)
L-636499	1.7×10^{-6}(5)	2.6×10^{-6}(5)	2.0×10^{-7}(3)	1.0×10^{-5}(5)	3.2×10^{-6}(5)
L-640035	6.2×10^{-5}(6)	1.4×10^{-4}(6)	1.6×10^{-5}(5)	3.0×10^{-4}(6)	8.8×10^{-5}(6)

The linear correlation coefficients between each assay were all statistically significant, $p < 0.01$, with the exception of that between dog platelet aggregation and saphenous vein contraction, which was $p < 0.05$ for $n = 5$. This evidence suggests that a similar TXA_2 receptor exists on dog platelets and vascular tissue as well as on human platelets.

[1] Mais, D. E., Saussy, D. L., Chaikhouni, A., Kochel, P. J., Knapp, D. R., Hamanata, N. and Halushka, P. V. (1985). *J. Pharm. Exp. Ther.* **233**, 418–424.
[2] Halushka, P. V., Mais, D. E. and Saussy, D. L. (1987). *Fed. Proc.* **46**, 149–153.
[3] Mais, D. E., Burch, R. M., Saussy, D. L., Kochel, P. J. and Halushka, P. V. (1985). *J. Pharm. Exp. Ther.* **235**, 729–734.
[4] Born, G. V. R. (1962). *Nature* **194**, 927–929.

Genetic Variation at the Fibrinogen Locus is Involved in Determining Plasma Fibrinogen Levels. S. E. Humphries[1], M. Cook[1], F. Green[1], Y. Sterling[2], and T. W. Meade[2]. [1]*Charing Cross Sunley Research Centre, Lurgan Avenue, London W6 8LW, UK;* [2]*MRC Epidemiology and Medical Care Unit, Northwick Park Hospital, Watford, Harrow HA1 3UJ, UK*

High plasma fibrinogen concentrations are strongly associated with an increased risk of ischaemic heart disease. We have used three restriction fragment length polymorphism (RFLPs) of the fibrinogen genes to study the role of genetic variation at this locus, in the determination of plasma fibrinogen levels. In a sample of 91 individuals, significant differences in mean fibrinogen levels were found in those with different RFLP genotypes. The strongest association was observed with a polymorphism detected with the β-fibrinogen probe and the enzyme BclI. The probe detects two alleles that we designate B1 and B2. The group of individuals with the genotype B1B1 have a mean fibrinogen level of 2.74 g/l, those with the genotype B2B2 have a mean fibrinogen level of 3.69 g/l, while the group of individuals heterozygous for the two alleles, with the genotype B1B2, have an intermediate mean level of 2.98 g/l. In this study, genetic variation at the fibrinogen gene locus detected with these RFLPs accounts for 15% of the total phenotypic variance in fibrinogen levels. We have also used these polymorphisms to study the contribution of variation at this locus to determine fibrinogen levels in families, and in a panel of individuals on whom repeat measurements of fibrinogen have been carried out. Our results suggest that study at the DNA level of the fibrinogen genes, and in particular the β-fibrinogen gene, will be useful in elucidating at least part of the underlying mechanism of the genetic control of plasma fibrinogen levels.

Prevention of *In Vitro* Effects of rt-PA on the Haemostatic System by the Use of Fibrinolytic Inhibitors. E. Seifried[1,3], P. Tanswell[2], D. C. Rijken[3] and C. Kluft[3]. [1]*Abt. Innere Medizin III, Universität Ulm, FRG;* [2]*Fa. Dr Karl Thomae GmbH, Biberach, FRG;* [3]*Gaubius Institute TNO, Leiden, The Netherlands*

Laboratory monitoring of haemostatic parameters in patients undergoing thrombolytic therapy with rt-PA showed a decrease of fibrinogen, plasminogen and α_2-antiplasmin. The rapid increase of these proteins after termination of the rt-PA infusion suggested *in vitro* plasminogen activation during freezing and thawing before assaying the samples. Therefore, simulating blood collection procedures during therapy, *in vitro* effects of rt-PA on fibrinolytic and coagulation assays were investigated.

In the absence of a fibrinolytic inhibitor, 45 min incubation at 0°C with 2 μg rt-PA/ml blood (3.4 μg/ml plasma) caused prolongation of clotting-time assays and decreases of plasminogen (to 44% of the control value), fibrinogen (to 27%), α_2-antiplasmin (to <5%), F VIII (to 41%) and F XIII (to 16%). In other experiments rt-PA effects were found to be correlated with the incubation time, but not with the incubation temperature. Remarkably, decrease of the storage temperature from +25 to 0°C did not reduce depletion of haemostatic parameters. To prevent *in vitro* plasminogen activation, three inhibitors were tested. A specific polyclonal anti-rt-PA antibody prevented interferences in all fibrinolytic and most clotting assays. D-Phe-Pro-Arg-CH_2Cl (PPACK) enabled correct assays of fibrinogen and fibrinolytic parameters but interfered with coagulometric assays dependent on endogenous thrombin generation. Aprotinin was suitable only for a restricted range of both assay types. Most *in vitro* effects were observed only with rt-PA plasma concentrations in excess of therapeutic values. Nevertheless, it is concluded that, for clinical application, collection of blood samples on either specific antibody or PPACK is essential for a correct assessment of *in vivo* effects of rt-PA on the haemostatic system in patients undergoing fibrinolytic therapy.

Pharmacological Comparison of Lys_{77}-Plasminogen and Glu_1-Plasminogen Forms of APSAC. R. Fears, H. Ferres, H. Greenwood and R. Standring. *Beecham Pharmaceuticals Research Division, Great Burgh, Epsom, Surrey, KT18 5XQ, UK*

The pro-enzyme APSAC (anisoylated plasminogen-streptokinase activator complex, Eminase) is a novel thrombolytic agent, liberating free activator at a defined rate, that achieves high reperfusion and low reocclusion rates when administered as a single injection to patients with acute myocardial infarction. There is, however, relatively little comparative data on APSAC, which is the lys_{77}-plasminogen form, and the corresponding glu_1-plasminogen form of the activator, although it has been suggested that lys-plasminogen itself is bound to fibrin to a greater extent than is glu-plasminogen.

It was the purpose of the present studies to compare the pharmacological characteristics of the two prodrugs. Uptakes into preformed clots prepared from platelet-poor volunteer plasma at 37°C in non-lysing conditions (aprotinin present), were measured using acylated activator complexes radiolabelled with ^{125}I in glu- or lys-plasminogen. The progressive uptake of the glu-plasminogen complex was consistently and significantly lower than the uptake of the lys-plasminogen homologue. An equivalent difference in uptake between the two complexes was also obtained using clots that had been aged for 6 h. The relative uptakes of the glu- and lys-plasminogen substrates were much lower than the uptakes of the activators, and lys-plasminogen was bound to a greater extent than glu-plasminogen. Further evidence for differences in binding was obtained by measuring accumulation during clot formation from human plasma, when the order of binding was again lys-APSAC > glu-form of the activator complex > lys-plasminogen > glu-plasminogen. Lys-APSAC was also bound to a greater extent than SK-glu-plasmin(ogen), the form of the activator that is produced when SK is administered.

In enzyme kinetic studies it was found that the free activator form of the glu-plasminogen-streptokinase complex showed slightly higher basal activity with respect to the activation of lys-plasminogen substrate than the lys-plasminogen-streptokinase activator complex, but there was a similar enhancement of enzyme activity (mediated by an effect on Km) for both complexes in response to a fibrin mimic (CNBr-digested fibrinogen). This maintenance of high enzymic activity together with the increased uptake by human plasma clots explains the greater fibrinolytic activity for lys-APSAC compared to the glu-form of the complex demonstrated in other studies using a human plasma clot lysis system.

Both forms of the acylated complex were cleared slowly from the bloodstream after administration to guinea pigs. Thus, a continuing uptake of the agent into the thrombus *in vivo* is also likely, as a consequence of the long residence time of APSAC in the bloodstream.

The Measurement of Plasma Fibrinogen as a Thrombotic Risk Factor: A New HPLC-Based Micro-Assay Able to Detect Increased Fibrinogen Synthesis.

Christopher Southan. *Haematology Department, Charing Cross and Westminster Medical School, London W6 8RP, UK. (Present address, Department of Medical Chemistry, Smith Kline & French Research Ltd, Welwyn, Herts AL6 9AR, UK*

Several studies have established that high fibrinogen levels constitute a significant predictive risk factor both for stroke and coronary heart disease (Meade, T. W. *et al. Lancet,* **ii**, 533–537 (1986); Wilhelmsen, L. *et al. N. Engl. J. Med.* **311**, 501–505 (1984)). Although a number of different fibrinogen assays are available, those with good accuracy are time-consuming and require carefully collected venepuncture samples. This work describes a new method of fibrinogen quantitation using high-pressure liquid chromatography (HPLC) to measure the fibrinopeptides that are cleaved from fibrinogen during the conversion to fibrin by thrombin (Southan, C. *et al. Thromb. Res.* **43**, 195–204 (1986)). Although the test was initially developed to screen for fibrinopeptide defects in congenital dysfibrinogenaemia, it has a number of features that make it particularly suitable for the type of study referred to above. The method basically consists of adding an excess of thrombin to the plasma for quantitative fibrinopeptide cleavage, followed by dilution, heating and filtration. When analysed by HPLC, the height of the released fibrinopeptide peaks, when compared with a standard, allows direct measurement of fibrinogen concentration. The assay is potentially automatable and requires only 50 μl of plasma, obtainable by finger-prick sample. By the use of microbore columns, this could be reduced to 10 μl. Results can be obtained retrospectively on samples stored with different anticoagulants and even from reconstituted freeze-dried plasma. Another advantage of this method is the ability to measure the extent to which fibrinopeptide A (FpA) is present in its phosphorylated form (FpAP). This parameter has recently been shown to be related to the rate of fibrinogen synthesis *in vivo* (Southan, C. *et al. Thromb. Haemost.* **56**, 193–197 (1986)). This effect was most clearly demonstrated in the acute-phase response to surgery, where rising fibrinogen concentrations were preceded by raised FpAP levels. There was also some evidence of an association between constitutive high fibrinogen levels and increased amounts of FpAP. Because of the features described above, this new fibrinogen assay has two potential applications to the investigation of thrombotic risk. In the chronic hyperfibrinogenaemic risk group it is important to establish if they are also characterized by high FpAP levels indicative of increased rates of synthesis. For acute hyperfibrinogenaemia following surgery, FpAP levels might be used to identify those with increased risk of post-operative thrombosis.

Index